PATHOLOGY and MICROBIOLOGY for MORTUARY SCIENCE

David F. Mullins, PhD

Licensed Funeral Director and Embalmer

Former Instructor of Funeral Service Technology
and Current Vice President of Institutional Research,
Advancement, Technology, and Accreditation

East Mississippi Community College
Scooba, Mississippi

THOMSON
DELMAR LEARNING

Australia Canada Mexico Singapore Spain United Kingdom United States

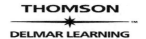

Pathology and Microbiology for Mortuary Science
by David F. Mullins, PhD

Vice President,
Health Care Business Unit:
William Brottmiller

Editorial Director:
Cathy L. Esperti

Acquisitions Editor:
Marah Bellegarde

Developmental Editor:
Debra Flis

Editorial Assistant:
Jadin Babin-Kavanaugh

Marketing Director:
Jennifer McAvey

Health Care Channel Manager—
Education:
Tamara Caruso

Marketing Coordinator:
Kimberly Duffy

Senior Production Editor:
James Zayicek

Art and Design Coordinator:
Alexandros Vasilakos

Library of Congress Cataloging-in-Publication Data:
Mullins, David F.
    Pathology and microbiology for mortuary science / David F. Mullins.
        p. cm.
    Includes index.
    ISBN: 1-4018-2519-2
    1. Pathology. 2. Medical microbiology.
3. Undertakers and undertaking. I. Title.

RB112.M856 2006
616.9'041—dc22

2005041351

NOTICE TO THE READER

Publisher does not warrant or guarantee any of the products described herein or perform any independent analysis in connection with any of the product information contained herein. Publisher does not assume, and expressly disclaims, any obligation to obtain and include information other than that provided to it by the manufacturer.

The reader is expressly warned to consider and adopt all safety precautions that might be indicated by the activities described herein and to avoid all potential hazards. By following the instructions contained herein, the reader willingly assumes all risks in connection with such instructions.

The publisher makes no representations or warranties of any kind, including but not limited to, the warranties of fitness for particular purpose or merchantability, nor are any such representations implied with respect to the material set forth herein, and the publisher takes no responsibility with respect to such material. The publisher shall not be liable for any special, consequential, or exemplary damages resulting, in whole or part, from the readers' use of, or reliance upon, this material.

This book is dedicated to the challenge!

The challenge to those who teach:
The lecturer should give the audience full reason to believe that all his powers
have been exerted for their pleasure and instruction.

—Michael Faraday (1791–1867), apprentice to a bookbinder at 14,
chemist who isolated benzene at 34, and a lecturer at 70.

The challenge to those who learn:
If you study to remember, you will forget; but, if you study to understand,
you will remember.

—Author unknown

Contents

Preface

Finally, there is a comprehensive textbook for the study of both pathology and microbiology written specifically with funeral service professionals in mind. *Pathology and Microbiology for Mortuary Science* is written as a textbook for mortuary science students, as a resource for educators, and as a reference for funeral directors and embalmers. Never before has it been so important for funeral service personnel to be familiar with the study of diseases and death. Advances in modern transportation make it possible for people to be halfway around the world in only hours, and every traveler carries microorganisms along for the ride. The increasing number of multidrug-resistant diseases, the risk of bioterrorism, and the high rate of immunosuppressing diseases worldwide makes the study of the effects of microorganisms and pathological conditions on human remains an essential component of lifelong learning for every funeral director and embalmer.

THE DEVELOPMENT OF THE BOOK

Many learners appear to be intimidated by the study of both pathology and microbiology. Introductory textbooks for college-level survey courses offer far too much material for the needs of the beginning embalmer, and they do not contain pertinent materials that funeral service practitioners will use throughout their careers. Mostly, they are not integrated into the overall scheme of instruction in mortuary colleges. This book, however, resolves those limitations by following a pedagogy specific to funeral service instruction.

Throughout its pages, this book provides both ease of reading for learners and a sound pedagogical approach for instructors. Advanced scientific concepts and complex language are presented in a straightforward and nonintimidating manner through the inclusion of numerous tables, illustrations, and real-life examples. And, although the principles of pathology and microbiology are conveyed in their simplest forms, there is no loss of scientific integrity or accuracy. *Pathology and*

Microbiology for Mortuary Science provides the reader with the knowledge necessary to distinguish between infectious and noninfectious disease characteristics and the knowledge necessary to protect both the practitioner and the public from the spread of pathogenic microorganisms.

PREREQUISITES AND ASSUMPTIONS

The only prerequisite this book has is that the reader is already somewhat familiar with the basics of embalming and has a rudimentary knowledge of human anatomy. Since much of the study of pathology and microbiology is based on an understanding of anatomy and physiology, brief reviews of anatomical structures are included as appendices for quick reference. The book offers suggestions concerning embalming techniques and refers at times to various embalming chemicals.

Most important, this book is not an embalming textbook, and it is not designed to replace the experiences of either an instructor or a practitioner. The embalming suggestions provided herein are only applicable given the set of circumstances implied in the corresponding section of the text, and they may not apply in all situations. One of the first steps in preparing to embalm human remains is to complete a thorough case analysis, which requires the practitioner to prioritize and balance the advantages and disadvantages of specific embalming techniques in an attempt to obtain an appropriate level of disinfection, preservation, and restoration of the deceased. The embalming suggestions in this textbook are only offered as potential contributors to the completion of such a balanced case analysis. Their purpose is to highlight the potential effects of disease conditions on the postmortem preparation of the deceased.

ORGANIZATION

The entire book is designed around the current American Board of Funeral Service Education's Curriculum Outlines for pathology and microbiology. These outlines are developed and approved by instructors from accredited mortuary science programs and other funeral service professionals across the United States. The glossary definitions are taken directly from these outlines and from *Taber's Cyclopedic Medical Dictionary*, which is referenced in all of the science portions of the ABFSE Curriculum Outlines. In addition, the author has attempted to include in this book each element within the outlines. However, the book is not limited to the content of these outlines, as it includes some diseases and conditions not specifically mentioned in the outlines. These diseases and conditions are presented because of their current importance or because they add to a fuller scope and understanding of the material presented. This book takes a global approach to the study of diseases, and although some diseases mentioned are rare in the United States, they may be significant in other countries.

UNIQUE FEATURES OF THE BOOK

The chapters in this book begin with comprehensive learning objectives for the reader. A list of key terms follows the learning objectives, and each key term is highlighted in the book where it is defined. Each of the key terms is also included in the glossary at the end of the book. Prior to reading each chapter, the reader is directed to an appendix for a brief review of pertinent anatomy and physiology. Each chapter ends with review questions that contain both multiple choice and matching styles. Chapters in which specific diseases are discussed also contain case analyses at the end of the chapters. The answers to the review questions and the case analyses are located at the end of the book.

INSTRUCTOR'S MANUAL

The *Instructor's Manual to Accompany Pathology and Microbiology for Mortuary Science* provides additional instructor support with quizzes, tests, midterm and final exams, and crossword puzzles.

ACKNOWLEDGMENTS

The author and Thomson Delmar Learning would like to acknowledge the following individuals for their review of the manuscript and helpful suggestions:

James M. Dorn, BS, MS
    Chairman, Department of Embalming Sciences
    Cincinnati College of Mortuary Science
    Cincinnati, Ohio
Estelle Hagedorn, MS, RNC, RD
    Pittsburgh Institute of Mortuary Science
    Pittsburgh, Pennsylvania
Keven E. Patterson
    Funeral Director/Embalmer
    St. Petersburg College
    Funeral Services Faculty
    St. Petersurg, Florida
Thomas Shaw, MBA
    Associate Professor
    Mortuary Science and Funeral Service
    Southern Illinois University Carbondale

    I would like to thank Dr. Thomas L. Davis, Jr. (President Emeritus, East Mississippi Community College) for his advice, support, and friendship. I would also like to thank Dr. Rick Young (President, East Mississippi Community College) for his encouragement toward my completing my doctorate and for his friendship and trust. I would also like to thank my friends, colleagues, and students, without their support, this book would not be possible.

I would also like to thank Deb Flis, developmental editor, for her understanding attitude and for patiently nudging me toward completion. Several times I would have abandoned this project, were it not for her support. I would also like to thank Beehive Production Services, for painstakingly copyediting the manuscript and preparing it for production.

ABOUT THE AUTHOR

David F. Mullins began his undergraduate education at Purdue University and received his BMS from the Cincinnati College of Mortuary Science. He also holds both an MS in higher education administration and a PhD in sociology from Mississippi State University.

Dr. Mullins began his career as a firefighter and EMT in aircraft crash rescue, where he also trained in hazardous materials management and mass fatality response. He has also sold cemetery property and served the community as a licensed funeral director and embalmer in both small and large funeral homes. In 1996, Dr. Mullins started teaching funeral service technology. He helped write the Mississippi Model Curriculum in Funeral Service Technology, and served on both an ICFSEB National Board Exam item writing team and an ABFSE Curriculum Subcommittee.

In 2002, Dr. Mullins was honored by the lieutenant governor by being named faculty honoree for the Mississippi HEADWAE award. Dr. Mullins received the ABFSE Graduate Scholarship several times, and was named Outstanding Doctoral student by the Alpha Kappa Delta international sociology honor society. Currently, he is vice president of Institutional Research, Advancement, Technology, and Accreditation at East Mississippi Community College, where he also authored *The Illustrated Guide to Anatomy and Physiology: An Introductory Text for the Study of Embalming and Disease.*

Introduction

THE ABFSE AND THE ICFSEB

One of the steps required to become a licensed funeral service professional in most places in the United States is to complete a degree at an accredited program of funeral service education. The agency that currently accredits programs of funeral service education in the United States and Canada is known as the American Board of Funeral Service Education (ABFSE). The ABFSE comprises various funeral service organizations and representative educators from the more than 50 currently accredited programs of funeral service education.

As of January 2004, one of the requirements to graduate from an ABFSE accredited program of funeral service education is to take the National Board Exam. The International Conference of Funeral Service Examining Boards (ICFSEB) consists of members who represent licensing agencies, and it is the agency responsible for the National Board Exam. The questions on the National Board Exam are based on the curricula used in all ABFSE accredited programs of funeral service education.

GOALS OF THIS BOOK

All of the anonymous reviewers of the draft manuscript of this book suggested that the book should strictly follow the format of the ABFSE Curriculum Outlines in Pathology and Microbiology. This book, therefore, is based on the same national outlines used by all accredited programs of funeral service. It is designed to help learners prepare for portions of the National Board Exam. In addition, exams in the classroom will likely cover the majority of the material in this book. This book is also intended to serve as a reference for apprentices/interns and for licensed funeral directors and embalmers. To that end, the book has many of the same goals and objectives as those emphasized by the ABFSE.

The Preamble to the Accreditation Standards of the ABFSE states the following:

> Funeral service is a profession practiced by men and women who are required to meet certain educational, societal, and governmental standards. Some are administrative and logistical, while others concern health and sanitation. The primary focus of funeral service lies in competent, ethical service to the public. Accreditation of Funeral Service Education Programs is intended to help ensure that those academic ingredients necessary to the successful practice of funeral service are offered each student in a consistent and universal manner. (*Manual on Accreditation*, 2002:9-1)

The ABFSE requires each program to have the following aims and purposes:

> Each program in funeral service education shall have as its central aim recognition of the importance of funeral service education personnel as (1) members of a human services profession, (2) members of the community in which they serve, (3) participants in the relationship between bereaved families and those engaged in the funeral service profession, (4) professionals knowledgeable of and compliant with federal, state and provincial/territorial, and local regulatory guidelines, as well as (5) professionals sensitive to the responsibility for public health, safety and welfare in caring for human remains (*Manual on Accreditation*, 2002:9-3).

Each program must have at least the following objectives:

- To enlarge the background and knowledge of students about the funeral service profession.
- To educate students in every phase of funeral service, and to help enable them to develop the proficiency and skills necessary of the profession, as defined in the preceding excerpt from the Preamble.
- To educate students concerning the responsibilities of the funeral service profession to the community at large.
- To emphasize high standards of ethical conduct.
- To provide a curriculum at the postsecondary level of instruction.
- To encourage research in the field of funeral service.

This textbook is written in a manner consistent with these stated goals and objectives of the ABFSE. This book has three overreaching goals:

1. To inform the reader of the most common educational, societal, and governmental standards related to pathology and microbiology as they apply to the practice of funeral service.
2. To help prepare learners to engage bereaved families, members of the healthcare industry, and the public in a competent, ethical, and professional manner.
3. To help readers learn the proper application of sanitation methodologies designed to protect the funeral service practitioner and the public from biohazardous risks associated with the funeralization of human remains.

ORGANIZATION OF THIS BOOK

The book is divided into two parts. Part One covers the study of pathology and pathological disorders of the human body. It focuses upon inflammatory disorders, degenerative disorders, and traumas to the body. Part Two covers the study of microbiology. It focuses primarily on disease-causing microorganisms, their classification, anatomy, requirements for growth, and methods of control. Part Two concludes with a description of human diseases caused by significant microorganisms. The appendices at the end of the book offer helpful information that compliment material within the book but that is not directly part of the study of pathology or microbiology.

The Glossary is based on definitions found in the ABFSE Curriculum Outlines.

The color insert provides a reference for practitioners to compare with specific lesions on the deceased. The insert also helps learners visualize information in the text.

PART ONE

PATHOLOGY

ABFSE Subject Description for Pathology

The study of pathological disease conditions and how they affect various parts of the body, with particular emphasis on those conditions that relate to or affect the embalming or restorative art process.

ABFSE Objectives for Pathology:

Upon satisfactory completion of a course in pathology, the learner should be able to:

- Identify the pathological conditions and etiological factors that require special procedures in the removal, handling, preparation, and disposition of human remains.
- Demonstrate a knowledge of diseases and related terminology that will enable competent communication with members of the medical community, allied health professionals, and surviving family members.
- Describe the benefits derived from the postmortem examination of human remains.

CHAPTER 1

Introduction to Pathology

Learning Objectives

Upon completion of the chapter, review questions, and case analysis, the reader should be able to:

- Compare and contrast the cellular theory of disease with the germ theory of disease.
- Define pathology.
- Describe the various divisions of pathology.
- Explain the benefits of the autopsy.
- Distinguish between a burn wound, a gunshot wound, and a stab wound.

Key Terms

autopsy
cause of death
etiology
general pathology
hypothermia
lesion

manner of death
mechanism of death
pathogenesis
pathology
special pathology

 ## HUMORS AND DISEASE

Hippocrates was born on the Greek island of Cos around 450 BC, and between that time and about 380 BC, he and other writers developed what has become known as the Hippocratic approach to the study of disease (Boyland 2002). At the time, religious beliefs guided common knowledge about disease and its causes. For example, Hippocrates rejected the notion that epilepsy was the result of a "divine visitation" and could be cured only through an appeal to the gods or magic. He argued for a naturalistic approach to the study of disease. Hippocrates and his colleagues of the time formed the basis of both modern ethics of medicine and the treatment of disease.

Humors

Hippocrates and his colleagues argued that disease was the result of imbalances in the natural fluids in the body. The basic fluids in the body were known as *humors*. The four humors are blood, phlegm, black bile, and yellow bile (serum). Healthy people were believed to have the proper balance, concentration, and mixture of these humors. Disease was thought to be the result of either bile or phlegm becoming too dry, too moist, too cold, or too hot. The imbalance of the humors was believed to result from wounds, smells, sounds, sights, or the pursuit of or indulgence in sexual pleasures.

Cellular Theory of Disease

Rudolph Virchow believed that disease was due to one diseased cell creating another diseased cell. In 1858, Virchow argued that all living cells were the products of other living cells with the Latin phrase, *omnis cellula a cellula*, which means "all cells arise from cells." Since the human body is actually a collection of individual cells, Virchow contended that disease was not an affliction of the body at-large or the body's humors. He argued, instead, that if healthy cells derived from healthy cells, diseased cells must likewise result from already diseased cells. Virchow's cellular theory of disease is premised on the concept that changes to cells, whether originating from within the cell or outside the cell, are the cause of disease. Virchow died as a result of trauma in 1902, when he fell while boarding a streetcar.

All deaths can be classified into one of the following three categories by cause: (1) deaths due to diseases-causing microorganisms like those that cause AIDS, tuberculosis, or the flu; (2) deaths due to degenerative pathological disorders like heart disease or strokes; or (3) deaths due to by-products of the social environment as in the cases of suicide, murder, or vehicular accidents (Weeks 1999). Part One of this textbook focuses on pathological diseases that are due to inflammation, degeneration, congenital defects, or social environment.

DIVISIONS OF PATHOLOGY

Literally translated, **pathology** is the study (*logos*) of suffering (*pathos*). Pathology incorporates aspects of clinical practice as well as basic science. Pathologists study both the **etiology**, or underlying causes, of diseases and the **pathogenesis** of disease, which is the mechanism that results in the manifestations of signs and symptoms in the body. Embalmers are interested in both the etiology and pathogenesis of disease because the changes in the body associated with pathological disorders often inhibit proper distribution and diffusion of embalming chemicals. These changes may also alert embalmers to the need for alternative embalming techniques, calling for a thorough case analysis prior to beginning each embalming procedure. For example, cancer of the liver is marked by changes in blood composition that alter its characteristics. The potential presence of bilirubin in such cases calls for the use of embalming fluids specifically designed to limit the potential of bilirubin-biliverdin conversion, which may cause a visible green discoloration in the deceased. Embalmers, therefore, must be familiar with aspects of several divisions of pathology. Table 1-1 lists the different divisions of pathology and defines them.

PLAN OF STUDY IN PATHOLOGY

Structure and function are closely related in the body. For example, the ureters are the tubes that transport urine from the kidneys to the urinary bladder. The ureter attaches toward the lower portion of the urinary bladder. As the bladder fills with urine, it exerts pressure on the ureter, helping prevent the urine from traveling back into the ureter and kidneys. The structures in the urinary system are directly related to their functions.

The study of pathology focuses largely on changes in structures and functions of the body. Pathologists use contemporary molecular, microbiological, and immunological techniques to study the changes that occur in cells, tissues, and organs. Much of what pathologists do in their diagnosis of disease and management of therapies is to identify changes in the gross or microscopic appearance of cells and tissues.

The field of pathology has traditionally been divided into general pathology and special pathology. **General pathology** focuses on the cellular and tissue responses to pathologic stimuli. Basically, general pathology deals with the study of the widespread processes of disease such as inflammation, degeneration, necrosis or cellular death, and repair, without reference to particular organs or

Table 1-1 Divisions of Pathology

Pathological anatomy	Also known as morbid anatomy, this is the study of structural changes in the body caused by disease. It includes both gross pathology and histopathology.
Gross pathology	The study of changes in the structure of the body that are readily seen with the unaided eye as a result of disease.
Histopathology	Also known as microscopic pathology, this is the study of microscopic changes that cells, tissues, and organs undergo as a result of disease.
Surgical pathology	The study of tissue specimens excised surgically during operations.
Clinical pathology	The study of disease by means of body secretions, excretions, and other body fluids in the diagnosis of disease.
Physiological pathology	The study of changes in body function due to disease.
Medicolegal pathology	Also known as forensic pathology, this is the study of disease to ascertain the cause and manner of death.

organ systems. In contrast, **special pathology** deals with the specific features of disease in relation to particular organs or organ systems, which is why special pathology is also referred to as systemic pathology (Kumar et al. 2003).

THE IMPORTANCE OF LESIONS

The study of lesions is extremely important to pathologists, and it is of primary concern to the funeral service practitioner as well. A **lesion** is a circumscribed area of pathologically altered tissue. In addition to being caused by disease, it may also be the result of an injury or a wound. A single patch in a skin disease is also referred to as a lesion. Lesions include everything from boils to tumors to moles; or they may include scars, scales, ulcers, or hives. Generally speaking, lesions are the pathological changes in structure that an embalmer or funeral director can see on the body. One of the reasons that funeral service professionals study pathology and microbiology is to be able to distinguish one lesion from another. For example, if a lesion is present on the deceased's lip, it is important for the embalmer to know if it is a mark left on the lip due to an intubation tube, which is used in hospitals to help maintain a patient's airway, or a chancre due to syphilis, which is the result of a sexually transmitted disease. In this example, the embalmer cannot be injured by a lesion left by an intubation tube; however, it is possible to become ill from a syphilis infection in the deceased.

Throughout this book, lesions are described in relation to the diseases that cause them. The color insert in this book depicts many lesions so that the reader may become familiar with those that signal potentially infectious conditions.

AUTOPSIES

One of the ABFSE's objectives associated with the study of pathology is for learners to be able to describe the benefits derived from the postmortem examination of human remains. When people die, it is often in the best interest of the community to determine the cause of death. Although an **autopsy** is frequently an investigation into the circumstances of a person's death for the purposes of legal issues, there are many other reasons why a postmortem investigation may be necessary. An autopsy, which is also known as a necropsy, provides the community with three important pieces of information.

First, autopsies confirm or alter the clinical diagnosis and treatment of the disease. For example, if the autopsy reveals that the deceased died of heart failure due to high blood pressure, then it will be important for the deceased's children to more closely monitor their own blood pressures throughout their lifetimes. Second, autopsies advance medical knowledge and research. Suppose a child has a rare form of cancer and lives to be 23 while participating in experimental drug therapies. An autopsy would reveal the effects the drugs had on the anatomical structures of the deceased. Third, autopsies are routinely used to assist in medicolegal cases to determine the identification of the deceased and the specific cause and manner of death.

There is a difference in the cause, manner, and mechanism of death. The **cause of death** is any injury or disease that produces a physiological derangement in the body that results in the death of the individual. A gunshot wound to the head, a stab wound to the chest, lung cancer, or a blood clot in an artery of the heart are examples of a cause of death. The **mechanism of death** is the physiological derangement produced by the cause of death that results in death. Examples of mechanisms of death include bleeding, blood poisoning, or a faulty heart beat. Finally, the **manner of death** explains how the cause of death came about. The manner of death is generally classified on death certificates as either natural, homicide, suicide, accident, or undetermined/unclassified.

Appendix A describes some of the most common procedures conducted during an autopsy.

TRAUMA-RELATED DEATHS

Humans die from disease-causing microorganisms, degenerative pathological conditions, and social manners of death such as murder, suicide, or motor vehicle accidents. Social manners of death, so called because they generally stem from social behaviors, are largely due to human behavior, human interaction, and the environment in which humans live. For example, a case of alcohol poisoning that leads to death at a college fraternity party results from social interaction. In general, social causes of injury and death are traumas. **Trauma** is the process or event leading to an injury or wound. The remainder of this chapter focuses on some of the most common forms of trauma-induced deaths.

Drug Abuse

Drug abuse can be defined as the use of mind-altering substances in a way that differs from generally approved medical usage. There are several classes of drugs including sedatives, stimulants, opiods, cannabinols, psychedelics, and inhalants.

Cocaine. Cocaine is a stimulant with many derivatives extracted from the leaves of the coca plant. Typically, it is prepared as a water-soluble powder diluted with talcum powder. When it is formed into a crystal, it is referred to as "crack," which gets its name from the crackling sound it makes when heated. Although the body's response to cocaine in its powder form and in the form of crack is the same, crack is a much more potent drug. Cocaine can be snorted, smoked by mixing it with tobacco, swallowed, or injected.

Cocaine produces an intense, euphoric high, which is a feeling of well-being and joy. Cocaine's physical effect on the body is to cause the accumulation of dopamine and adrenaline in the nervous system, which results in excess stimulation of the nervous system. Cocaine also starves the heart for blood by constricting the coronary artery and accelerating blood clot formation by facilitating platelet aggregation (see Appendices C and D for a review of related anatomy). Cocaine also causes the heart to beat improperly by disturbing the balance of normal levels of potassium, calcium, and sodium ions. The effects of cocaine on the nervous system and cardiovascular system are not dependent on the dose, and cocaine has caused sudden death in first-time users.

Heroin. Heroin is an opiate derived from the poppy plant, and it is closely related to morphine. It is usually diluted by the seller with talcum powder or quinine, making the strength of the dose unknown to the buyer. Heroin is usually injected, and its effects may include euphoria, hallucination, or sedation. Sudden death results from respiratory failure or heart failure. Long-term use of heroin causes lung edema, lung abscess, infections, kidney failure, and clumping of talcum powder in the blood and lungs. Heroin use also leaves lesions on the body at the sites of injection, which may be anywhere, including the arms, between the fingers, between the toes, or in the male scrotum. These lesions are known as needle tracks (Figure 1-1).

Gunshot Wounds

In the United States in 1998, there were 30,708 deaths from gunshot wounds, including 17,424 suicides, 12,102 homicides, 866 accidents, and 316 gunshot deaths by undetermined causes (Surveillance 2001). The type of weapon, the type of bullet, and distance from the weapon all affect the extent of tissue injury (Belkin 1987; Chapman & McClain 1984).

Color Plate 1 and Color Plate 2 picture an entrance wound and an exit wound, respectively. Notice that an exit wound is typically much larger than an entrance wound, depending on the ballistics of the weapon and tissue characteristics. There is also a marked difference between gunshot wounds and stab wounds, which are pictured in Color Plate 6.

Ballistics. The term *ballistics* refers to the science of the travel of bullets in flight. A short, high-velocity bullet begins tumbling more rapidly in tissue, displacing more tissue and imparting more energy into the tissues. Figure 1-2 illustrates the

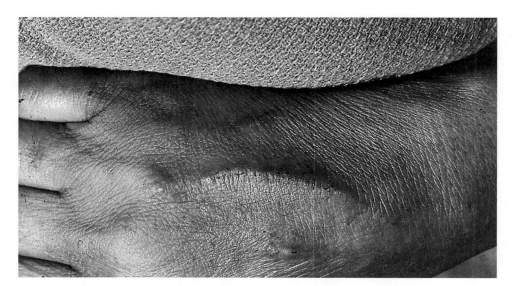

Figure 1-1 Needle track. (Reprinted with permission from Vincent J. DiMaio and Dominick DiMaio, 2001, *Forensic pathology*, 2nd ed. Copyright CRC Press, Boca Raton, FL.)

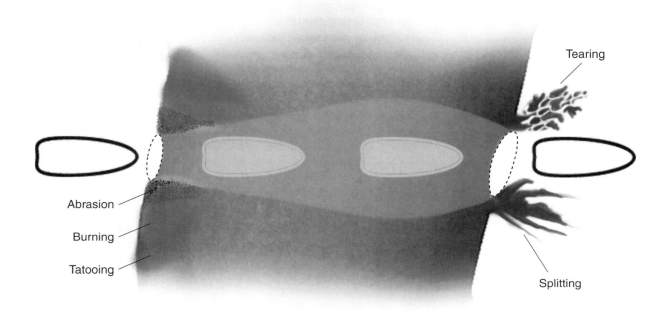

Tearing

Abrasion

Burning

Tatooing

Splitting

Figure 1-2 Comparison of entrance and exit wounds.

types of damage bullets can cause in the tissues. The level of tissue damage is largely determined by the speed (velocity) and size (mass) of bullets. For example, an M-16 (.223 caliber) rifle produces large surface wounds from its high-velocity, low-mass bullets that tumble, cavitate, and release energy quickly. In comparison, a hunting rifle (.308 caliber or greater) has a larger-mass bullet that penetrates deeper to kill large animals at a distance.

Bullets produce tissue damage in three ways, as described in Table 1-2 (Adams 1982; Fackler 1996).

Table 1-2 Injuries Inflicted by Bullets

Laceration and crushing	Handguns cause primarily crushing injuries because they use low-velocity bullets that travel less than 1,000 feet per second.
Cavitation	A cavity is caused by the path of the bullet itself combined with the continued forward acceleration of the tissue in the wake of the bullet, which stretches out the wound. Cavitation occurs with projectiles traveling in excess of 1,000 feet per second.
Shock waves	Tissues are compressed by shock waves that travel ahead and to the sides of the bullet. Shock waves last only a few microseconds causing little tissue damage at low velocity.

Bullet design is also important in determining the level of tissue injury due to gunshots. Some bullets have full metal jackets around their lead core, which limits their ability to expand within the tissues. Low-velocity handgun cartridges may fire bullets with a soft lead point or a "hollow point" designed specifically to explode in tissues on impact.

The distance of the target from the weapon also plays a large role in the level of tissue damage sustained in a gunshot wound. Most bullets fired from handguns lose their energy at 100 yards, while high-velocity military .308 rounds still have considerable energy at 500 yards. Bullets fired from military and hunting rifles have more wounding potential at a greater distance than do handguns and shotguns.

Density and Elasticity of Tissues. The density and elasticity of tissues also affects the extent of damage associated with gunshot wounds. More damage occurs in dense tissues with low elasticity. For example, lung tissue is dense and elastic, so it suffers less damage than muscle tissues, which is higher in density but much less elastic. The liver, spleen, and brain have almost no elasticity, so they are injured easily in shootings. It is also possible for fluid-filled organs such as the bladder, heart, intestines, and large blood vessels to burst when impacted by a bullet, generating waves of pressure within body cavities. Bone tends to fragment, sending numerous bone projectiles throughout the tissues. A bullet must travel at least 163 feet per second to penetrate skin and 213 feet per second to break bone (Adams 1982).

Contact wounds characteristically have soot, a muzzle imprint, and laceration of the skin (Zeichner et al. 1992). Intermediate-, or close-range wounds have a wide zone of powder stippling, but lack a muzzle imprint and laceration. Distant-range wounds lack powder stippling and leave a hole approximately the size of the bullet. The entrance wound will have more gunshot residue than the exit wound, if the exit wound has any gunshot residue at all. Often there is no exit wound because bullets are designed to cause the greatest damage by expanding and expending all their energy in the tissues. When present, exit wounds are larger than entrance wounds, due to the expansion and tumbling of the bullet on its axis as illustrated in Figure 1-3.

Guns and Suicide. Suicide is a significant cause of death, and the presence of multiple gunshot wounds in a suicide victim is possible. There is an association between the type of weapon used and the area of the body in which the fatal gunshot occurs. The three most common sites of injury for suicides involving a handgun are the right temple, the mouth, and the chest. The three most common sites of injury for suicides involving a rifle are the right temple, the forehead, and the chest. The three most common sites of injury for suicides involving a shotgun are the mouth, the chest, and under the chin. The differences in shooting sites among weapons are largely due to the requirements of physically firing the weapon (Kohlmeier, McMahan, & DiMaio 2001).

Contrary to movie and television stereotypes, the force from a handgun shooting typically does not throw the victim backwards to the ground. The majority of persons shot with handguns report no noticeable effect on impact. In

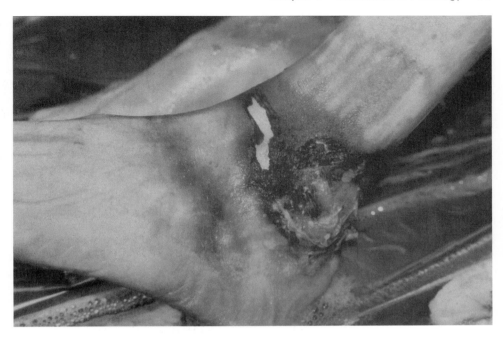

Figure 1-3 An exit wound near the ankle.

most cases, it is only when systemic changes occur after being shot with a handgun that victims realize the severity of their injury (Fackler 1998).

Electrical Injuries

Death and injury due to electricity are due to electrons flowing through the body depolarizing muscle and nerves, disrupting heart and brain function, and producing electrical burns of body tissues (Wright 2001). Electrical burns occur as a result of heating the tissues by the physical property of friction as electrons pass through the body and by the destruction of cell membranes. Electrical injuries are commonly associated with severe damage at the site where the electricity entered and exited the body. There are three broad categories of electrical injuries including lightning, low-voltage injuries, and high-voltage injuries.

Lightning. The survival rate from lightning is over 50 percent; however, survival may be in a vegetative state due to severe brain damage. There are a wide variety of possible effects on the body associated with lightning strikes. Burns are not always present, but they may occur in males under the scrotum and on the penis. There is also a high likelihood of bleeding behind the eardrum and rupture of the eardrum.

High Voltage. High-voltage injuries occur when objects such as poles, sailboat masts, antennas, or cranes make contact with an overhead high-voltage power line. Occasionally, mostly through occupational exposures, individuals come in contact with switching equipment, and they directly touch energized components of high-voltage electrical systems.

Low Voltage. Low-voltage injuries most frequently occur when children bite into electrical cords. The resulting injuries include severe burns of the lip, face, and tongue. The other common cause of low-voltage electrical injuries occurs when adults become grounded while touching appliances or other energized objects.

Burns

A burn involves the destruction of skin cells and sometimes the underlying structures of muscle, subcutaneous tissues, or bone. The young, the elderly, the physically challenged, and the mentally challenged are all at increased risk of burn injuries. Such increased risk may be due to an inability to care for themselves, curiosity, sensory changes associated with aging, or an inability to fully comprehend cause-and-effect relationships. The severity of a burn is a function of the tissues' ability to withstand the duration of contact and the characteristics of the causative energy source. Possible sources of energy that may cause burns include heat sources, cold sources, and chemicals.

According to the National Safety Council (2003), there were approximately 3,309 deaths in the United States due to smoke, fire, and flames. Most of these accidental deaths occur in the home and are caused by smoking, defective electrical wiring, defective or misused heaters, children playing with matches, or clothing catching fire, which occurs with greater frequency among the elderly.

Deaths associated with burns are largely a result of the extent of the burned area, the severity of the burn, the age of the victim, and the presence of inhalation injuries. The level of burn largely depends on the thickness of the person's skin. Both the young and the elderly have thin skin. One attribute of those who survive burns for even short durations before death is the presence of extreme swelling of the tissues as illustrated in Color Plate 3.

Rule of Nines. In living individuals, the extent of a burn is expressed as a percentage of the body surface area as determined by the "rule of nines" (Figure 1-4). Assuming that the body surface area is 100 percent, then the head is 9 percent, the upper extremities are each 9 percent, the front of the torso is 18 percent, the back is 18 percent, each of the lower extremities is 18 percent, and the genitals are 1 percent.

Severity of Burns. There are four degrees of burn severity, and Figure 1-5 illustrates the first three degrees. In first-degree burns, which are also referred to as superficial burns, the skin is red without blisters. Microscopically, this tissue contains dilated congestion in the dermal layer of the skin, and the epidermis becomes necrotic and peels. A minor sunburn that peels is an example of a first-degree burn.

In a second-degree burn, or partial-thickness burn, the skin is moist, red, and blistered. The extent of the damage has reached the dermal layer of the skin. The hair and sweat glands are generally not involved, and they act as the source

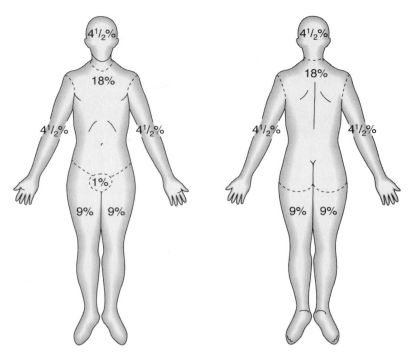

Figure 1-4 Rule of nines—used to calculate percentage of the body surface burned.

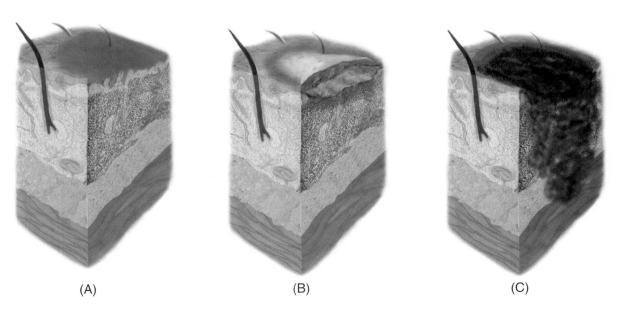

(A)   (B)   (C)

Figure 1-5 Depth of burn wounds: (A) first degree, (B) second degree, and (C) third degree.

of regeneration of the epidermis. Second-degree burns eventually heal without scarring.

Third-degree burns, which are also known as full-thickness burns, are characterized by necrosis of the epidermis and the dermis. On the surface, the skin usually has a dry, white, leathery appearance. There are no blisters, and the lesions may also appear charred, with a brown or black discoloration. Third-degree burns heal with a scar. Color Plate 4 provides a visual comparison of the first three degrees of burns.

In fourth-degree burns, there are incineration injuries extending deep into the tissues. Deaths due to flames may include large areas of fourth-degree burns in which entire tissues are evacuated, which means that they were entirely consumed by the fire. Cremation is an example of total soft-tissue evacuation and would be classified as a fourth-degree burn.

Frostbite. Color Plate 5 illustrates burns of the hands and feet resulting from frostbite, which is a cold-related injury characterized by freezing of tissue. Most cases are encountered in soldiers, in those who work outdoors in the cold, and among winter outdoor enthusiasts (Mechem 2001). Tissue changes include ice crystal formation, cellular dehydration, protein denaturation, inhibition of DNA synthesis, abnormal cell wall permeability, damage to capillaries, and pH changes. Rewarming causes blood clots, edema, loss of blood flow to tissues, and tissue death. Typically, frostbite does not lead to death unless the wound becomes infected and the infection spreads, but when the body's core temperature drops too low in a condition known as hypothermia, it may be fatal. Normal body temperature is 98°F (37°C), and severe **hypothermia** is defined as a body temperature below 80°F (27°C). Funeral service practitioners may encounter deaths due to hypothermia among newborns, the elderly, and homeless populations during the winter months due to overexposure to cold.

Stabbing

Stab wounds are produced by pointed instruments, and most such wounds causing death are the result of homicides. The edges of the wound in the skin are typically sharp, as indicated in Color Plate 6. Stab wounds are usually referred to as incisions because of the clean cut through the skin, as opposed to lacerations, which have jagged edges and result from a tear in the skin due to blunt force. The most commonly used weapon in stabbings is a knife; however, other devices capable of causing incised wounds include ice picks, scissors, screwdrivers, broken glass, and pens or pencils.

The sharpness of the point of the knife determines its ability to pass through the skin. The sharper the tip, the easier the knife will penetrate the skin. Once the tip perforates the skin, it will pass through the organs with little force. Unless the tip strikes bone, the depth of penetration does not indicate the degree of force required to inflict the stab wound. The depth of the stab wound and the degree to which different parts of the knife are in contact with the skin influences the appearance of the stab wound. If great force is used, and the entire length of the blade enters the wound, the skin may be bruised by the handle of the knife.

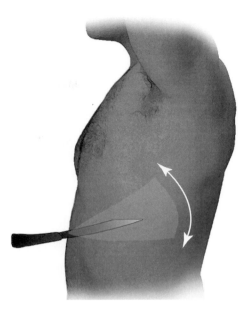

Figure 1-6 Twisting of the blade during stabbing creates a cone-shaped zone of damage.

The shape of the wound is determined both by the shape of the blade and the properties of the skin. If the skin is stretched during the stabbing, the wound will have a short, broad appearance when the skin relaxes. Much like the grain of wood, skin has a unique pattern of growth known as Langer's lines that are similar between individuals. Surgeons take advantage of Langer's lines to reduce scarring. If a stab wound crosses Langer's lines, the skin will pull apart at the edges of the wound creating a gaping wound. Figure 1-6 illustrates the degree of internal damage that can occur if the knife is twisted or if the victim moves during the stabbing. Stab wounds associated with twisting of the weapon or movement of the victim typically produce a Y- or L-shaped wound on the skin.

Motor Vehicle Accidents

Motor vehicle accidents are often due to impairment of drivers by alcohol, drugs, or a combination of the two. The drugs need not be drugs of abuse, but can be prescription medications. Another potential cause of fatal motor vehicle accidents is human error, which includes such events as reckless driving and falling asleep, eating, caring for children, reading, or talking on the phone while driving. Anything that distracts the driver from the road can result in a fatal accident. Another common cause of motor vehicle accidents is environmental hazards, such as bad weather, slick or icy roads, poorly marked roads, and poorly constructed roads. Finally, motor vehicle accidents may result from defective vehicles or natural diseases such as an individual suffering heart failure while driving.

Figure 1-7 illustrates what happens to the driver's body in front impact collisions. If the driver is unrestrained by a seatbelt or airbag, the individual will continue in a forward movement, even after the vehicle has stopped. Injuries will generally occur in the following order: The driver's knees will impact the instrument panel, the chest will impact the steering wheel, and the head will strike the windshield or sun visor region of the vehicle. Objects protruding from the instrument panel, such as levers or knobs, can produce patterned abrasions on the body. Figure 1-8 shows the imprint of a steering wheel on the chest of a man who died in a motor vehicle accident.

It is important to the embalmer to note that the extent of injury due to motor vehicle accidents often leaves little or no signs on the deceased. However, there may be extensive damage to the blood vasculature and internal organs. Such injury can inhibit the proper distribution of embalming fluid during arterial injection due to the nonintact blood vasculature. It is also possible that injuries to the head may result in multiple fractures of the skull that are not apparent on the surface. As the arterial embalming fluid enters the tissues, the head may swell uncontrollably at normal injection pressures. This swelling does not occur before death in such cases because death is sudden, and the heart stops beating before swelling can occur. The injection of fluids simulates the action of the heart and swelling can then occur.

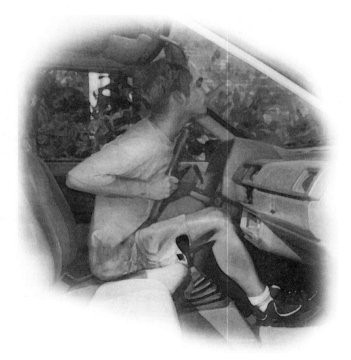

Figure 1-7 Up-and-over sequence of frontal collisions.

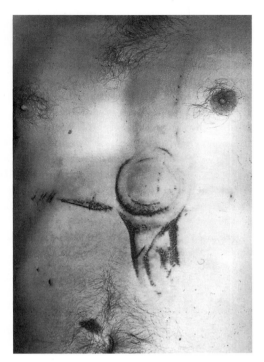

Figure 1-8 Imprint of steering wheel on chest. (Reprinted with permission from Vincent J. DiMaio and Dominick DiMaio, 2001, *Forensic pathology*, 2nd ed. Copyright CRC Press, Boca Raton, FL.)

Following an embalming technique known as a "head freeze" may prevent swelling of the head. A head freeze includes the use of astringent embalming fluids and short bursts of injection directly into the head via the carotid arteries while it is manually held in place by the embalmer or, preferably, by a second embalmer. Each side of the head is injected separately. The theory is that the embalming fluid will fixate the tissues before they have the opportunity to swell. While this technique can be effectively utilized to restore the head without distention, there is debate as to the depth of penetration of the embalming chemicals within the deeper tissues of the head. It could be argued that the use of a head freeze technique is a trade-off between preservation and restoration, which may be necessary in certain situations.

REVIEW QUESTIONS

Matching

1. _____ lesion
2. _____ Virchow
3. _____ autopsy
4. _____ pathology
5. _____ humors

a. necropsy
b. once believed to be the basic fluids in the body
c. literally means the "study of suffering"
d. a circumscribed area of pathologically altered tissue
e. credited with the discovery of the cellular theory of disease

Multiple Choice

1. Of the following weapons, which would be least likely to leave an exit wound?
   a. high-caliber military rifle
   b. high-caliber hunting rifle
   c. shotgun
   d. low-caliber target pistol
2. Which of the following is the study of microscopic changes that cells, tissues, and organs undergo as a result of disease?
   a. surgical pathology
   b. gross pathology
   c. histopathology
   d. clinical pathology
3. Which of the following is not a benefit of an autopsy?
   a. Autopsies describe the progression of the death struggle.
   b. Autopsies confirm or alter clinical diagnosis and treatment.
   c. Autopsies advance medical knowledge and research.
   d. Autopsies assist in medicolegal cases to determine identification of the deceased and the cause and manner of death.
4. In cases of motor vehicle deaths, why is it important to be more cautious than usual concerning the deceased's head during embalming?
   i. The accident may have caused lacerations to the scalp that are not obvious because they may be covered by the hair.
   ii. The accident may have caused bruising to the face.
   iii. Glass shards and other foreign debris that might cause injury to the embalmer may not be obvious because they may be covered by the hair.
   iv. The absence of bruising and other obvious trauma does not preclude the presence of skull fractures that may lead to swelling during arterial injection.
      a. i and iii
      b. ii and iii
      c. i, ii, and iv
      d. i, iii, and iv

5. According to the rule of nines, what percentage of the body is burned if the burn covers the entire chest and abdomen?

   a. 9%
   b. 15%
   c. 18%
   d. 27%

Putting Learning to Work!

The purpose of the following case analysis is to allow you to apply the information you have learned in a real-world situation. Read the case carefully and try to answer the following questions:

What disorder do you suspect the person had at the time of death?

What potential embalming complications do you anticipate?

What precautions should you take as the embalmer to limit the effects of these complications?

Case Analysis

A 65-year-old male died in the emergency room from injuries sustained in a boating accident. The man had received injuries in the Vietnam War that resulted in the amputation of both of his arms. His prosthetic arms were welded together during the incident that led to his death. He has burns on his penis and the underside of his scrotum. Blood is also present in the auditory meatus of his left ear.

Bibliography

Adams, B. (1982). Wound ballistics: A review. *Military Medicine, 147,* 831–835.
Belkin, M. (1987).Wound ballistics. *Program Surgery, 16,* 7–24.
Bird, C., Conrad, P., & Fremont, A. (Eds.). (2000). *Handbook of medical sociology* (5th ed.). Upper Saddle River, NJ: Prentice Hall.
Boyland, M. (2002). Hippocrates (c. 450 BCE to 380 BCE). In *The Internet encyclopedia of philosophy*. Retrieved May 28, 2003, from http://www.utm.edu/research/iep/h/hippocra.htm#The Four Humors.
Brown, P. (2000). *Perspectives in medical sociology* (3rd ed.). Prospect Heights, IL: Waveland Press.
Campbell, W. (2002). *The germ theory calendar*. Retrieved June 26, 2003, from http://germtheorycalendar.com/.

Chapman, A., & McClain, J. (1984). Wandering missiles: Autopsy study. *Journal of Trauma, 24,* 634–637.

DiGiovanni, J. (2002). *Rudolph Virchow: Founder of modern pathology.* Retrieved May 28, 2003, from http://www.suite101.com/article.cfm/14014/95171.

DiMaio, V., & DiMaio, D. (2001). *Forensic pathology* (2nd ed.). Boca Raton: CRC Press LLC.

Fackler, M. L. (1996). Gunshot wound review. *Annals of Emergency Medicine, 28,* 194–203.

Fackler, M. L. (1998). Civilian gunshot wounds and ballistics: Dispelling the myths. *Emergency Medicine Clinics of North America, 16,* 17–28.

Hubble, M., & Hubble, J. (2002). *Principles of advanced trauma care.* Clifton Park, NY: Thomson Delmar Learning.

Kohlmeier, R., McMahan, C., & DiMaio, V. (2001). Suicide by firearms. *American Journal of Forensic Medicine and Pathology, 22,* 337–340.

Kumar, V., Cotran, R., & Robbins, S. (2003). *Robbins basic pathology* (7th ed.). Philadelphia: Saunders.

Levine, R., & Evers, C. (1998). *The slow death of spontaneous generation (1668–1859).* Retrieved June 26, 2003, from Access Excellence, The National Health Museum at http://www.accessexcellence.org/AB/BC/Spontaneous_Generation.html.

Mayer, R. (2000). *Embalming: History, theory, & practice* (3rd ed.). New York: McGraw-Hill.

Mechem, C. (2001). *Frostbite.* Retrieved July 27, 2003, from eMedicine at http://www.emedicine.com/emerg/topic209.htm.

Myers, J., Neighbors, M., & Tannehille-Jones, R. (2002). *Principles of pathophysiology and emergency medical care.* Clifton Park, NY: Thomson Delmar Learning.

Neighbors, M., & Tannehill-Jones, R. (2000). *Human diseases.* Clifton Park, NY: Thomson Delmar Learning.

Pathology for funeral service. (1999). Dallas, TX: Professional Training Schools.

Rudolph Virchow (1821–1902). (2003). Retrieved July 25, 2003, from the Department of Diagnostic Medicine/Pathobiology at Kansas State University at http://www.vet.ksu.edu/depts/dmp/personnel/faculty/virchowbioe.htm.

Shelton, H. (1992). *Boyd's introduction to the study of disease* (11th ed.). Philadelphia: Lea & Febiger.

Surveillance for fatal and nonfatal firearm-related injuries—United States, 1993–1998. (2001). *Morbidity and Mortality Weekly Review, 50,* 1–34.

Thagard, P. (1997). *The concept of disease: Structure and change.* Retrieved May 28, 2003, from the Philosophy Department, University of Waterloo at http://cogsci.uwaterloo.ca/Articles/Pages/Concept.html.

The World Health Report 2002: Reducing risks, promoting healthy life. (2002). Geneva, Switzerland: World Health Organization.

Venes, D. (Ed.). (2001). *Taber's cyclopedic medical dictionary* (19th ed.). Philadelphia: F. A. Davis.

Weeks, John R. 1999. *Population: An introduction to concepts and issues* (7th ed.). Belmont, CA: Wadsworth Publishing.

What are the odds of dying? (2003). Retrieved July 27, 2003, from the National Safety Council at http://www.nsc.org/lrs/statinfo/odds.htm.

Wright, R. (2001). *Electrical injuries.* Retrieved May 27, 2003, from eMedicine at http://www.emedicine.com/emerg/topic162.htm.

Zeichner, A., Levin, N., & Dvorachek, M. (1992). Gunshot residue particles formed by using ammunitions that have mercury fulminate based primers. *Journal of Forensic Science, 37,* 1567–1573.

CHAPTER 2

Nature of Disease

Learning Objectives

Upon completion of the chapter and review questions, the reader should be able to:

- Define disease.
- Classify complications of disease as either signs or symptoms.
- Begin using the key terms to describe disease.
- Explain why certain conditions predispose people to disease.
- Explain how physical agents, chemical agents, and infectious agents cause disease.
- Discuss the difference between lifespan and longevity.

Key Terms

acquired	infection
acute	infestation
allergies	intoxication
chronic	morbidity rate
communicable	mortality rate
complications	nosocomial
congenital	occupational disease
deficiency	organic
diagnosis	pandemic
endemic	prevalence
epidemic	prognosis
exacerbate	recurrence
febrile	remission
fulminating	signs
functional	sporadic
hereditary	symptoms
iatrogenic	syndrome
idiopathic	

DISEASE, DISORDERS, AND ILLNESS

What is a disease? Most people would agree that disorders caused by microorganisms, such as mumps, AIDS, the common cold, and hepatitis, are diseases. But what about disorders like alcoholism, obesity, and depression? Before discussing the nature of disease, it is important to adopt a uniform understanding of the word *disease*.

A person with a disease typically experiences discomfort, dis-ease, or disharmony with the environment. A healthcare provider recognizes diseases by a set of signs or symptoms. The pathologist, on the other hand, may recognize disease by structural, functional, cellular, or molecular changes in the tissues, which may be observed with the naked eye or with instruments such as microscopes or through the use of advanced tests designed to detect specific types of genetic abnormalities.

Boyd's Introduction to the Study of Disease is a pathology textbook that was first published in 1938, and it states that, "disease is the pattern of response of a living organism to some form of injury" (Shelton 1992). This definition focuses on the significance of alterations in normal function due to the body's response to injuries, infections, and stress.

Taber's Cyclopedic Medical Dictionary (Venes 2001) is used as a reference for many terms in the ABFSE Curriculum Outlines, and most of the definitions in this book are, therefore, taken from *Taber's*. A disorder is defined by *Taber's* as, "A pathological condition of the mind or body. See: Disease." The definition of disease is then given as, "A condition marked by subjective complaints, a specific history, and clinical signs, symptoms, and laboratory or radiographic findings. The concepts of disease and illness differ in that disease is usually tangible or measurable, whereas illness (and associated pain, suffering, or distress) is highly individual and personal."

By combining these definitions, a distinction can be made between disorders, diseases, and illnesses. A *disorder* is typically a measure of specific changes associated with a pathological condition. For example, someone born with a cleft lip is typically recognizable by an altered appearance of the lip, altered speech, and altered function of the mouth and nose. It is the alteration from normal that distinguishes one pathological disorder from another. *Diseases*, however, are recognizable by certain patterns of deviation from health. The common cold is a disease in which a person might experience runny nose, headaches, sinus pressure, watery eyes, and a sore throat. A person can, however, have a disease and not experience any illness. The symptoms and signs of disease are indicated by the term *illness*. For example, high blood pressure is a serious disease that may not cause any illness until the person dies from sudden failure of the heart. Based on these definitions, it is possible for a person to have a disease and experience no illness until the disease progresses to the point of noticeable disorder of the body.

So, although there are differences in the definitions of the words *disorder, disease,* and *illness,* in this textbook they are used interchangeably. The important concept to remember is that, regardless of the choice of words, there are ways to recognize disease by changes in the body; however, not all diseases are accompanied by characteristics lesions. **Organic** diseases are accompanied by specific anatomical changes, such as the red spots associated with measles or the yellow discoloration of the skin that often accompanies hepatitis. In contrast, **functional** diseases, such as schizophrenia, have no recognizable change in anatomy. In other words, organic diseases are those accompanied by changes in anatomical structure, while functional diseases are those accompanied by changes in physiological function. It is also important to note that functional diseases are not devoid of physical changes like chemical imbalances that may be detectable by diagnostic tests.

Some diseases are due to infections. An **infection** is the state or condition in which the body or a part of it is invaded by a disease-causing agent that, under favorable conditions, multiplies and produces injurious effects. Diseases caused by microorganisms are considered infections. Other diseases are not caused by microorganisms at all; instead, they may be due to deficiencies. A **deficiency** is a lack of dietary or metabolic substance that can lead to disease. Still other diseases are the result of genetics. A **hereditary** disease is one based on genetic characteristics transmitted from parent to offspring.

Although there have been tremendous strides made in medicine since the mid-1800s, many scientists believe that humans are on the verge of one of the most potentially significant eras in medical history. Computers are allowing scientists to conduct medical research into the genetic causes of disease that has never before been possible. Between 1990 and 2003, scientists used computers to identify the sequence of human genes through the Human Genome Project (2004). One of the greatest potentials of the human genome database is the ability to understand life. Knowing the sequence of human genes, and the sequence of microbial genes, will allow scientists to create better disinfectants and to create drugs that destroy microorganisms' genetic material with few or no side effects to patients. It is believed that scientists will be able to predict genetic diseases by testing parents' DNA prior to having children, and then they may be able to correct the genetic failure to prevent the disease from being inherited. It is impossible to say exactly what discoveries will be made in the near future, but drastic changes in the treatment of disease are expected. It is certainly not inconceivable that such changes will also affect the funeral service industry. Effective communication between the healthcare community and funeral service practitioners is extremely important.

DESCRIPTIVE TERMINOLOGY

Anyone who wishes to study illness and death must become familiar with the special vocabulary that the healthcare profession uses. Acquiring a working knowledge of the terminology is a prerequisite for understanding the literature of health and medicine. In the study of illness, it makes sense to begin with the diagnosis of disease. Diagnosis is the term denoting the naming of the disease or syndrome. Basically, the **diagnosis** is the recognition of the nature of a particular disease. In lay terms, the diagnosis occurs when the health professional determines from which specific illness a person suffers. If a diagnosis is made, the illness will likely have a prognosis. The **prognosis** is the prediction of the outcome of a particular illness, while the manner in which the disease develops is referred to as its pathogenesis.

The course of an illness is influenced by its complications. Any unfavorable conditions arising during the course of a disease are referred to as **complications**, and they manifest as either signs or symptoms. **Signs** are the objective disturbances produced by a disease that can be observed by other people. Examples of signs of a disease include increased heart rate, a change in the color of the skin, or swelling around the mouth. Each of these disturbances can be witnessed by other people; however, some disturbances are only observed by the person with the illness. **Symptoms** are the subjective disturbances caused by a specific disease that are felt or experienced only by the patient but are not directly measurable. Examples of the symptoms of a disease include pain, nausea, anxiety, numbness, or loss of sensation in the limbs. Any disturbance that others can observe is a sign, while those disturbances that are felt by the patient are symptoms. Those diseases associated with fever are referred to as **febrile** diseases.

The appearance and persistence of different illnesses are not uniform. Diseases that are present at birth are referred to as **congenital**, while diseases present after birth are **acquired**. Some illnesses appear suddenly and last only a short time, while others are only noticeable after a long period and remain for a long time. **Acute** diseases have a rapid onset and a short duration, while **chronic** diseases have a slow onset and a long duration. **Fulminating** diseases are a special type of acute disease characterized by a rapid and severe onset, and they are usually fatal.

Illnesses do not necessarily occur continuously either. **Remission**, which is similar to abatement, is the temporary cessation of the symptoms of a disease, while the reappearance of the symptoms of a disease after a period of remission is referred to as the **recurrence** of a disease. A word that may appear similar to recurrence at first, but is actually quite different in meaning, is exacerbation. The word **exacerbate** means that the severity of a disease has increased. If a person had cancer, and the cancer was not present for a period of time, it would be said that the cancer was in remission. If the signs and symptoms of the cancer appeared again at a later time, it would be referred to as recurrence. If, during the period of recurrence, the cancer began to spread, it would be said to have exacerbated.

A **communicable** disease is one that can be transmitted directly or indirectly from one individual to another. These infectious diseases can spread between populations, or they can remain within a population. The number of cases of disease present in a specific population at a given time is known as the **prevalence** of the disease. A disease that is continuously present in a community is said to be **endemic**. Hansen's disease—a form of leprosy—is an endemic disease with over 70 percent of the 700,000 cases in 2000 having occurred in India, Myanmar, and Nepal, while only 108 cases occurred in the United States during 1999 (*The World Health Report 2002*). This information means that Hansen's disease is endemic to India, Myanmar, and Nepal.

A disease that is currently in higher than normal numbers is referred to as an **epidemic**. An epidemic does not necessarily mean that there are many people who are infected with the disease. In 2000, the Centers for Disease Control and Prevention (CDC) declared that the West Nile virus was a newly emergent epidemic disease in the United States with only seven deaths in New York and only 62 positive cases in the country in 1999.

Sporadic diseases occur occasionally in a random or isolated manner. A new variety of a rare neurological disorder known as Creutzfeldt-Jakob disease, which typically infects people over 65 years of age, has been isolated in the United Kingdom. This new variety of CJD is known as variant Creutzfeldt-Jakob disease (vCJD), and it has affected people at the age of 29. Variant Creutzfeldt-Jakob disease is considered sporadic because it affected 101 people in the United Kingdom between 1996 and 2001, with only three cases in France and one case in Ireland during that same time (New variant CJD 2003).

A disease that is epidemic, widespread, or even a worldwide event is known as a **pandemic** disease. AIDS is an acronym for acquired immune deficiency syndrome. A **syndrome** is a set of signs and symptoms associated with a particular disease, and AIDS is an example of a pandemic disease. The World Health Organization (*The World Health Report 2002*) estimates that over 40 million adults and children were living with HIV/AIDS at the end of 2001. It is also estimated that over 5 million people became infected with AIDS worldwide in the year 2001. Of the 5 million newly infected cases in 2001, more than 800,000 of those cases were children. The vast majority of people with HIV are unaware that they carry the virus that causes AIDS. There were approximately 3 million deaths related to AIDS in 2001 worldwide, with approximately equal numbers of men and women dying from the disease. In sub-Saharan Africa, AIDS is the number one cause of death, while AIDS currently ranks as the fourth leading cause of death in the world.

LIFESPAN VERSUS LONGEVITY

There are over 6 billion people in the world today. The United States Bureau of the Census (2004) projects that the world's population will reach 7 billion in the next 10 years and 8 billion by the year 2028. The primary reason for the world's ever-growing population is not that more people are being born; it is because people are dying at an older age. Instead of dying in their 40s, people routinely live past their 70th birthday in much of the industrialized world.

There is a difference in how long a person can possibly live and the ability to remain alive from one year to the next. The word *lifespan* refers to the oldest age to which human beings can survive, while the word *longevity* refers to a person's life expectancy. A French woman named Jeanne Louise Calment died at the age of 122, which is the oldest authenticated lifespan of any human who ever lived (Weeks 1999). The average life expectancy or longevity for the world is approximately 66 years of age. However, longevity varies among countries due largely to social causes. For example, Japan has the highest longevity of any country at 80 years, the United States has a life expectancy of 76 years, and Zimbabwe has a life expectancy of only 39 years of age.

Demographers are social scientists who study trends in population, including diseases and deaths. The study of the occurrence of disease is known as *morbidity*, while the study of death due to specific causes is termed *mortality*. The relative incidence of a disease in the population, or the number of cases of a disease in a given time in a given population, is referred to as the **morbidity rate** for a disease. The number of deaths in a given time or place, or the proportion of deaths to a population, is referred to as the **mortality rate**. Stated in simpler terms, the morbidity rate describes how many cases of a disease there are at a certain time and place, while the mortality rate describes how many deaths there are at a certain time and place.

As mentioned in Chapter 1, all deaths can be classified into one of the following three categories by cause: (1) deaths due to disease-causing microorganisms, (2) deaths due to degenerative pathological disorders, or (3) deaths due to by-products of the social environment, which are most often trauma-induced deaths. Table 2-1 compares the ten leading causes of death in the United States with the ten leading causes of death in Africa in 2000 (*The World Health Report 2002*).

There are many reasons why some people die sooner than others. Although scientists cannot explain precisely why people in Japan experience a greater longevity than people in Zimbabwe, they realize that the reason is not entirely biological. Although certain deaths occur from biological, degenerative pathologies like cystic fibrosis—which is directly inherited from one's parents—other deaths are strongly correlated with social causes such as low income, lack of education, or race.

PREDISPOSING CONDITIONS AND DISEASE

In the study of the etiology, or cause, of illnesses, it is important to distinguish between those factors that predispose someone to disease and those factors that are the immediate causes of disease. *Predisposing conditions* make someone more likely to develop illness, while *immediate causes of disease* directly result in illness. It is also important to recognize that science has not yet determined the etiology of all illnesses. Those illnesses for which the cause is unknown are re-

Table 2-1 The Ten Leading Causes of Death in the United States and Africa in 2000

United States	Africa
1. Diseases of the heart	1. Parasitic infections
2. Cancer	2. AIDS
3. Cerebrovascular diseases	3. Respiratory infections
4. Respiratory infections	4. Malaria
5. Accidents	5. Diarrheal diseases
6. Diabetes mellitus	6. Cancer
7. Influenza and pneumonia	7. Childhood diseases
8. Alzheimer's disease	8. Perinatal conditions
9. Glomerulonephritis	9. Accidents
10. Septicemia	10. Tuberculosis

ferred to as **idiopathic**. Other illnesses are the result of medical treatment. For example, one treatment for certain types of arthritis is to inject gold directly into the affected joint. Gold injections, as well as some treatments for high blood pressure or heart disease, have been known to result in a purplish-red rash with flat bumps on the skin known as lichen planus. When illnesses like lichen planus result from medical treatment they are called **iatrogenic** illnesses. Infections acquired in a hospital or other healthcare setting are referred to as **nosocomial** infections.

Predisposing conditions are not immediate causes of illness, but, rather, they are those elements of diseases that make one person more likely to suffer injury than another person. Age is one predisposing condition to illness because certain diseases are more likely to occur among certain age groups. For example, childhood diseases like measles generally do not affect the elderly, and babies do not normally develop Alzheimer's disease. There are also illnesses that are sex specific. For example, women do not develop testicular cancer, and men do not develop ovarian cysts.

The sex-based predisposition to illness is more complicated than simple differences in anatomy, however. It is widely known that women tend to outlive men, and that men are more likely to die from accidents, gunshot wounds, and addiction-related causes such as alcoholism, tobacco usage, and drugs. This tendency is believed to be largely the result of men engaging more frequently in risk-taking behaviors. Table 2-2 compares the ten leading causes of death in 2000 by sex (*National Center for Health Statistics* 2003).

Some people are predisposed to certain illnesses due to their race. Table 2-3 compares the ten leading causes of death among African Americans, American Indians, Asian Americans, and Caucasians in 2000 (*National Center for Health Statistics* 2003). It is difficult to separate race from more social predisposing conditions to illness such as occupation, nutritional status, economic status, and environment. Because people of low socioeconomic status are frequently forced

Table 2-2 The Ten Leading Causes of Death in 2000 by Sex

Women	Men
1. Heart disease	1. Heart disease
2. Cancer	2. Cancer
3. Cerebrovascular diseases	3. Cerebrovascular diseases
4. Chronic lower respiratory diseases	4. Accidents
5. Diabetes mellitus	5. Chronic lower respiratory diseases
6. Influenza and pneumonia	6. Diabetes mellitus
7. Alzheimer's disease	7. Influenza and pneumonia
8. Accidents	8. Suicide
9. Nephritis	9. Nephritis
10. Septicemia	10. Liver disease

Table 2-3 The Ten Leading Causes of Death among African Americans, American Indians, Asian Americans, and Caucasians in 2000

African Americans	American Indians	Asian Americans	Caucasians
1. Heart disease	Heart disease	Cancer	Heart disease
2. Cancer	Cancer	Heart disease	Cancer
3. Cerebrovascular diseases	Accidents	Cerebrovascular diseases	Cerebrovascular diseases
4. Accidents	Diabetes mellitus	Accidents	Chronic lower respiratory diseases
5. Diabetes mellitus	Cardiovascular diseases	Chronic lower respiratory infections	Accidents
6. Homicide	Liver disease	Influenza and pneumonia	Influenza and pneumonia
7. AIDS	Chronic lower respiratory diseases	Diabetes mellitus	Diabetes mellitus
8. Chronic lower respiratory diseases	Suicide	Suicide	Alzheimer's disease
9. Nephritis	Influenza and pneumonia	Nephritis	Nephritis
10. Influenza and pneumonia	Nephritis	Perinatal period	Suicide

to work in dangerous occupations in hazardous environments, they are predisposed to contract illnesses that people with high educations and high incomes are less likely to contract. A disease with an abnormally high rate of occurrence in members of a particular workforce is referred to as an **occupational disease**. Coal miners in Appalachia once frequently developed an occupational disease known as black lung, or anthracosis, from inhaling the fine coal dust in the coal mines.

The poor do not have the economic resources to afford healthy lifestyles that include diets rich in fresh fruits and vegetables and frequent trips to the doctor. Even when they are able to acquire medical care, they may not use an entire prescription; instead, they may save it for the next time the illness arises (Bird et al. 2000; Brown 2000). Even though people from any socioeconomic level may not seek health care or follow prescribed treatment, the poor and undereducated are more likely to experience poor health (Brooks-Gunn et al. 1997; Duncan and Brooks-Gunn 1997; Hauser et al. 1997; Thorton 2004). Although age, sex, race, nutritional status, occupation, environment, economic status, and genetics are part of the etiology of illness, none of these factors are the direct cause of illness, though they do predispose certain groups of people to a poorer quality of health.

IMMEDIATE CAUSES OF DISEASE

The immediate causes of illness include trauma, physical agents, chemical agents, infectious agents, deficiencies of essential substances, and allergens. Traumas include such events as gunshot wounds, automobile accidents, and blunt force injuries that might result from being struck with a baseball bat or a similar object. Although traumas are typically caused by mechanical agents, other more common physical agents may also be dangerous. For example, temperature is a physical agent that can cause hyperthermia and sunburns on the beach or hypothermia and frostbite in a snowstorm. There are a variety of chemical agents that are poisonous to the human body. Children are frequently accidentally poisoned by ingesting household cleaners, eating lead-based paint chips; adolescents, by sniffing glues or aerosols such as spray paint for their intoxicating effects. **Intoxication** is a state of being poisoned by a drug or toxic substance.

Infectious agents can be spread from one person to another through various means and are a leading cause of death throughout the world. The harboring of animal parasites, especially macroscopic forms, such as ticks or mosquitoes is known as **infestation**, and some diseases related to exposure to animal parasites are isolated within high-risk groups such as rabbit breeders or ranchers who shear sheep for a living. Certain disease-causing microorganisms may infest animal hides, manure, and other animal products, which explains the higher risk for these diseases among ranchers and others who make their living working with animals.

Deficiencies of essential substances can also be the direct cause of disease. Pernicious anemia, for example, results from a lack of intrinsic factor in the stomach of some people. Intrinsic factor is a necessary component in the digestion and absorption of vitamin B_{12} in the body. Although people with pernicious anemia may ingest sufficient quantities of iron, they are unable to use the iron, resulting in a failure of their bodies to transport adequate amounts of oxygen in the blood. Finally, allergens are the immediate cause of illness for many people. People may be allergic to anything from bee stings and pollen to animal dander and poison ivy. **Allergies** are defined as having a hypersensitivity to a substance that does not normally cause a reaction.

REVIEW QUESTIONS

Matching

1. _____ organic diseases
2. _____ syndrome
3. _____ pathogenesis
4. _____ congenital
5. _____ exacerbate

a. a set of complications associated with a disease
b. diseases present at birth
c. diseases accompanied by specific anatomic changes
d. to increase the severity of illness
e. the manner in which disease develops

Multiple Choice

1. Which of the following describes a disease characterized by a sudden onset with a relatively short duration?
   a. fulminant disease
   b. recurrent disease
   c. chronic disease
   d. acute disease

2. Which of the following terms is used to describe a disease continuously present in a community?
   a. epidemic
   b. pandemic
   c. endemic
   d. sporadic

3. Which of the following terms best describes this statement: "In 1997, 61.8 people per 100,000 died of stroke in the United States?"
   a. mortality rate
   b. morbidity rate
   c. epidemic
   d. fulminating disease

4. Which of the following is not a predisposing condition of disease?
   a. sex
   b. race
   c. age
   d. deficiencies

5. Which of the following is not a cause of disease?
   a. chemical agents
   b. economic status
   c. deficiencies
   d. infectious agents

Bibliography

Anderson, R. (2002). Deaths: Leading causes for 2000. *National Vital Statistics Reports, 50* (16).
Bird, C., Conrad, P., & Fremont, A. (Eds.). (2000). *Handbook of medical sociology* (5th ed.). Upper Saddle River, NJ: Prentice Hall.
Brooks-Gunn, J., Duncan, G. J., & Aber, J. L. (Eds.). (1997). *Neighborhood poverty*. New York: Russell Sage.
Brown, Phil. 2000. *Perspectives in medical sociology* (3rd ed.). Prospect Heights, IL: Waveland Press.
Duncan, G. J., & Brooks-Gunn, J. (1997). *Consequences of growing up poor*. New York: Russell Sage.
Hauser, R. M., Brown, B. V., & Prosser, W. R. (1997). *Indicators of children's well-being*. New York: Russell Sage.
HIV and its transmission. (2002). Retrieved July 26, 2003, from the National Center for HIV, STDs, and TB Prevention, Division of HIV/AIDS Prevention, Centers for Disease Control and Prevention at http://www.cdc.gov/hiv/pubs/facts/transmission.htm.

HIV infection and AIDS: An overview. (2003). Retrieved July 22, 2003, from the National Institute of Allergy and Infectious Diseases, National Institutes of Health, U.S. Department of Health and Human Services at http://www.niaid.nih.gov/factsheets/hivinf.htm.

Human Genome Project. (2004). Retrieved March 20, 2004, from the Department of Energy and the National Institutes of Health at http://www.ornl.gov/sci/techresources/Human_Genome/home.shtml.

Human immunodeficiency virus type 2. (1998). Retrieved July 22, 2003, from the National Center for HIV, STDs, and TB Prevention, Division of HIV/AIDS Prevention, Centers for Disease Control and Prevention at http://www.cdc.gov/hiv/pubs/facts/hiv2.htm.

Kumar, V., Cotran, R., & Robbins, S. (2003). *Robbins basic pathology* (7th ed.). Philadelphia: Saunders.

Mayer, R. (2000). *Embalming: History, theory, & practice* (3rd ed.). New York: McGraw-Hill.

McNeil, D. (2003, June 16). Tenth of HIV cases in a study in Europe are resistant to drugs. *New York Times*: A-1.

Medical terminology. (2003). Retrieved July 24, 2003, from English Centre at http://ec.hku.hk/mt/.

National Center for Health Statistics. (2000). *National mortality data, 1998*. Hyattsville, MD: Author.

National Center for Health Statistics (NCHS) Vital Statistics System. (2003). Retrieved July 24, 2003, from the Office of Statistics and Programming, National Center for Injury Prevention and Control, Centers for Disease Control and Prevention at http://wonder.cdc.gov/.

Neighbors, M., & Tannehill-Jones, R. (2000). *Human diseases*. Clifton Park, NY: Thomson Delmar Learning.

New variant CJD. (2005). Retrieved January 8, 2005, at http://www.cdc.gov/ncidod/diseases/cid/cjd_fact_sheet.htm.

Pathology for funeral service. (1999). Dallas, TX: Professional Training Schools.

Shelton, H. (1992). *Boyd's introduction to the study of disease* (11th ed.). Philadelphia: Lea & Febiger.

Thagard, P. (1997). *The concept of disease: Structure and change*. Retrieved May 28, 2003, from the Philosophy Department, University of Waterloo at http://cogsci.uwaterloo.ca/Articles/Pages/Concept.html.

Thornton, A. (Ed.). (2004). *The well-being of children and families*. Ann Arbor, MI: The University of Michigan Press.

The World Health Report 2002: Reducing risks, promoting healthy life. (2002). Geneva, Switzerland: World Health Organization.

United States Bureau of the Census. (2004). Retrieved January 8, 2005, at http://www.census.gov/popest/estimates.php.

Venes, D. (Ed.). (2001). *Taber's cyclopedic medical dictionary* (19th ed.). Philadelphia: F. A. Davis.

Weeks, J. (1999). *Population: An introduction to concepts and issues* (7th ed.). New York: Wadsworth.

What are the odds of dying? (2003). Retrieved July 27, 2003, from the National Safety Council at http://www.nsc.org/lrs/statinfo/odds.htm.

CHAPTER 3

Cellular Reaction to Injury

Learning Objectives

Upon completion of the chapter and review questions, the reader should be able to:

- Compare and contrast cellular swelling and cellular infiltration.
- Compare and contrast fatty degeneration and amyloid degeneration.
- Compare and contrast moist gangrene, gas gangrene, and dry gangrene.
- Compare and contrast physiological changes in cells and pathological changes in cells.
- Compare and contrast atrophy, hypertrophy, hyperplasia, metaplasia, and regeneration.

Key Terms

amyloid	gout
atrophy	hypertrophy
calcification	infiltration
caseous	necrosis
degeneration	pigmentation
gangrene	regeneration

CELLS AND THEIR ENVIRONMENTS

All cells exist within an environment, and changes to that environment result in changes within the cell. The attempt by cells to maintain a relatively stable environment is known as *homeostasis*. As the cell adjusts to its internal and external environments through feedback systems, a state of dynamic equilibrium is reached. The cell is constantly interacting with its changing environment to remain stable, but never achieves complete stability because its environment is constantly changing. It is, therefore, fair to say that cells are stable if they are capable of changing in response to changes in their environment. As cells encounter changes in their environments, they respond through a process of adaptation. If the changes exceed their capacity to adapt, the cell experiences regressive degeneration leading to its ultimate death. **Degeneration** is defined as the deterioration of tissues with corresponding functional impairment as a result of disease or injury.

While reading this chapter, review cellular anatomy by referring to Appendix B.

POTENTIAL CAUSES OF CELLULAR INJURY

There are many causes of cellular injury. The loss of oxygen is known as oxygen deprivation or *hypoxia*. One form of oxygen deprivation is carbon monoxide poisoning. Chemical agents such as prescription drugs, illicit drugs, air pollutants, alcohol, asbestos, and pesticides also damage cells by altering their osmotic environment. The infectious agents described in Part Two of this textbook cause injury to cells as well. A cell may also become damaged by the body's own defense system. These autoimmune diseases result in what are known as immunological reactions in which the immune system attacks the body's cells and tissues.

Cells are also injured due to genetic defects, which may be as subtle as the substitution of a single amino acid in the hemoglobin of individuals with sickle cell anemia. Nutritional imbalances can injure cells through both the extremes of starvation and obesity. Trauma, temperature extremes, radiation, and electric shock are all physical agents that can result in cellular injury. Finally, the aging process itself damages cells. A process known as *cellular senescence* leads to alterations in cells' abilities to replicate and repair, resulting in cellular degeneration and the eventual death of the cell.

REGRESSIVE CELLULAR CHANGES

One of the first signs of almost all cellular injury is the presence of cellular swelling, which occurs when cells are unable to maintain the proper balance and concentration between ions and fluid levels, which is the basis of osmotic pressure. The balance between cellular fluids and ions can be explained through the analogy of a tropical aquarium. Tropical fish can only survive in saltwater that has the correct balance of salt and water for the specific species of fish. Additionally, there must be an adequate total amount of saltwater in the tank. If the tank is only half full, it cannot support as many fish. In a similar fashion, cells react to changes in their environment by altering both the total quantity of intracellular fluids and ion concentration within that fluid.

Osmotic pressure is defined as the pressure that develops when two solutions of different concentrations are separated by a semipermeable membrane. Osmotic pressure varies with concentration of the solution and with temperature increase. Human cells have an osmotic pressure approximately equal to that of the fluid in which they circulate (e.g., blood, lymph, cerebrospinal fluid). Solutions exerting the same osmotic pressure as that within the cell are said to be *isotonic*. Solutions with a stronger osmotic pressure than the cell are called *hypertonic* solutions, and solutions with a weaker osmotic pressure than the cell are *hypotonic*. A cell placed in a hypertonic solution will shrink, while a cell placed in a hypotonic solution will swell. The shrinkage of a cell placed in a hypertonic solution is known as *crenation*. Arterial embalming fluid affects cells in a similar manner. *Desiccants* are hypertonic embalming fluid solutions that remove excess moisture from the tissues, while *humectants* are hypotonic embalming fluid solutions that add moisture to dehydrated tissues.

Cellular Swelling

When an entire organ or tissue experiences cellular swelling, there is a loss of color (*pallor*), and the cells become distended (*turgor*). It is important for the embalmer to note that cellular swelling cannot always be removed during the embalming processes. Cellular swelling is usually reversible when the cell recovers from the injury (e.g., mosquito bites). If the person dies, cellular swelling will persist, causing disfiguration.

Fatty Degeneration

Another form of reversible change that cells sometimes undergo is fatty degeneration. Fatty changes occur in cells due to the accumulation of triglycerides, which are the result of three hydroxyl groups of an ester reacting with fatty organic acids. Basically, triglycerides are the result of the digestion of fats. Fatty changes often occur in cells nearby dead cells. Fatty changes may be present in cells of the heart, skeletal muscle, kidney, and other organs. Possible causes of fatty degeneration include toxins, protein malnutrition, diabetes mellitus, obesity, and starvation. The most common cause of fatty change in the liver, however, is alcohol abuse. In severe forms, fatty changes may precede cellular death, although cells may die without undergoing fatty change.

Amyloid Degeneration

In certain diseases, cells undergo amyloid degeneration. **Amyloid** is a waxy, translucent, complex protein that resembles starch. The process of amyloid degeneration is sometimes called waxy degeneration or lardaceous degeneration. Amyloid degeneration may occur in certain cancers, chronic inflammatory diseases, chronic renal failure, Alzheimer disease, and type two diabetes mellitus.

Infiltration

Cells can also be changed through **infiltration**, which is the process of seepage or diffusion of a substance into tissues that should not normally be present in the cells. Infiltration occurs prior to cellular swelling. Cells undergo pigmentation when they become infiltrated with pigments. **Pigmentation** is defined as the coloration caused by either deposit or lack of colored material in the tissues. Exogenous pigments are colored substances that come from outside the body, while endogenous pigments are colored substances that are synthesized within the body.

Exogenous Pigmentation. One example of an exogenous pigment that infiltrates the cells of the body is carbon found in coal dust. A disease known as coal workers' pneumoconiosis, or black lung, affected many coal miners in Appalachia. Miners were exposed to extremely fine coal dust, which they inhaled into their bodies. Phagocytes in the lungs of the miners transported the carbon deposits throughout the lymphatic system of the miners. The lungs of the miners, as well as their lymph nodes, became blackened due to the carbon.

Endogenous Pigmentation. One of the most common forms of endogenous pigment infiltration is the local excess of blood found in a bruise. The red-blue discoloration that occurs in the tissues is the result of the presence of hemoglobin in the blood. The hemoglobin is transformed into biliverdin, which is green, and bilirubin, which is a rust color. The iron ions of hemoglobin break down into a golden-yellow compound.

Calcification. A wide variety of diseases result in a common processes within injured cells known as calcification. In all cases of cellular death due to necrosis, calcium deposits are present. **Calcification** implies the depositing of calcium salts, magnesium, iron, and other minerals within the cells. Calcification of the lymph nodes present in cases of tuberculosis can actually turn the lymph node to stone. The embalmer will most commonly encounter calcification of the arteries. In cases of atherosclerosis, fine, white granules, or clumps that feel like gritty deposits, are present in the arteries. It may be impossible to introduce the arterial tube into the artery for the injection of arterial embalming fluids due to the process of calcification.

Gout. **Gout** is a common form of arthritis that causes swelling and pain in some of the body's joints. In particular, gout typically affects a joint in the big toe, but it also affects other joints of the feet and ankle, as well as other parts of the body. Gout is a disorder caused by the accumulation of excess amounts of uric acid in the tissues. Uric acid is a chemical that is a natural end product of the normal process of purine metabolism. In other words, the body breaks down foods and builds up tissues by utilizing chemicals that naturally form uric acid in the body. When excess levels of uric acid are found in the blood, the condition is referred to as *hyperuricaemia*. Uric acid is normally dissolved in the body; however, the presence of excess levels of uric acid in the blood can lead to the formation of microscopic crystals that infiltrate the tissues of the joints. The presence of these uric acid crystals—which are technically known as monosodium urate crystals—causes the inflammation of the joints and the pain, swelling, and loss of function of the affected joints that accompanies cases of gout-related arthritis.

Gout often appears suddenly, and it may become chronic, in which case joint deformity is not uncommon. In chronic cases of gout, larger crystals known as *tophi* may appear in the joints. Tophi may appear in any affected joint, and they are sometimes present in the ears. Gout may be an inherited condition, but certain foods result in higher levels of uric acid through purine metabolism. These foods include, but are not limited to, beans, red meat, shellfish, organ meats (e.g., liver, kidneys, tongue), peas, and lentils. The two aspects of treatment of gout include drugs and diet designed to lower uric acid levels, as well as anti-inflammatory and pain medications to relieve discomfort.

CELLULAR DEATH

Necrosis is a sequence of structural changes that follow cell death in living tissue. All dead cells are not necrotic. Tissue placed in a specimen bottle and treated with a fixative is dead, but it is not necrotic. The process of necrosis includes cellular swelling, changes in the nature of cellular proteins—which is known as *denaturation*—and the breakdown of cellular organelles. The morphologic changes in necrotic cells are the result of two concurrent processes.

The first necrotic process is the denaturation of cellular proteins. Proteins are denatured when their molecular structure is changed due to heat, radiation, pH changes, or other mechanisms that destroy or diminish their original properties. For example, as heat is added in the process of frying an egg, the proteins in the egg are denatured.

The second necrotic process is the self-digestion of the cell through a process known as *autolysis*. As the lysosomes within the cell begin to break down the cell's internal structures, the cell undergoes morphological changes altering its appearance. Autolytic enzymes alter not only the individual dead cells, but they also change the entire area of necrotic tissue, which manifests as caseation or gangrene.

Caseous necrosis is a distinct form of necrosis present in cases of tuberculosis. The term *caseous* means cheeselike, and the center of caseous necrotic tissue has a cottage-cheese appearance. Caseous necrosis is characterized by pink areas of necrosis surrounded by inflammatory granules.

Gangrene is a term commonly used to refer to several types of necrosis. Wet, or moist gangrene, is a form of liquefactive necrosis that results from bacterial or fungal infections that develop in areas of dead, necrotic tissue. The tissues become swollen, discolored, and blistered. When accompanied by gas gangrene, wet gangrene may exhibit a crackling sound known as *crepitation* when it is touched due to the presence of gas in the tissues.

Clostridium perfringens, which is described in greater detail in Part Two of this book, is a gram-positive, endospore-forming bacterium that causes gas gangrene (see Color Plate 7). It causes the fermentation of carbohydrates in the tissues, releasing carbon dioxide and hydrogen gases. The toxins produced move through the swollen tissue causing further necrosis of neighboring tissue. Gas gangrene is often fatal, spreading throughout the body via the blood.

Ischemic gangrene, which is also known as dry gangrene, occurs when tissues become dehydrated if the blood supply is reduced. It may occur, for example, in the leg if calcification of the arteries is present in the form of arteriosclerosis. The tissues become black, dry, wrinkled, and greasy to the touch. There is also a clearly defined line of separation between the dead and healthy tissue, and there is no infection present. Ischemic gangrene is not uncommon in deaths related to diabetes mellitus.

ADAPTIVE RESPONSES TO CELLULAR INJURY

Although cells are in a constant state of change in relation to fluctuations in their environment, there is a middle ground between the normal, unstressed state of a cell and the overstressed state of an injured cell. Pathological changes in cells are adaptive responses that deviate from the healthy state but allow the cell to avoid injury by altering itself or its environment. There are four adaptive responses to cellular injury: atrophy, hypertrophy, hyperplasia, and metaplasia.

Atrophy

Atrophy is the shrinkage in the size of the cell by the loss of cell substance as illustrated in Figure 3-1. Atrophied cells are not dead; they are an attempt by the cell to adjust to available resources. As the demand placed on cells decreases, or their supply of required resources is reduced, they shrink through the self-digestion of cellular components. There are several causes of cellular atrophy. Cells atrophy during convalescence after recovery from a bone fracture or when workload is diminished during healing. Perhaps an injury has diminished the blood supply to a limb or a nerve has been damaged resulting in paralysis. In both of these examples, pathological atrophy would occur in cells. Atrophy need not result from injury, however. The body's workload is drastically reduced for most people as they age. As people become less active and more sedentary with age, the workload for cells is reduced and the cells shrink. When atrophy occurs as a result of age or a more sedentary lifestyle, it is referred to as *physiological atrophy* because it is not accompanied by a pathological condition.

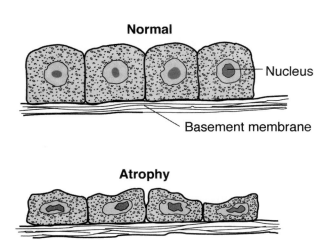

Figure 3-1 Normal cell versus atrophied cell.

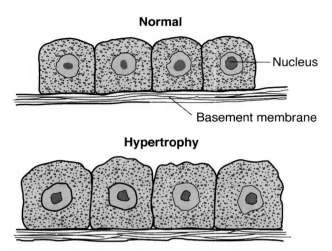

Normal

Nucleus

Basement membrane

Hypertrophy

Figure 3-2 Normal cell versus hypertrophied cell.

Hypertrophy

Another form of cellular adaptation is **hypertrophy**, which is an increase in the size of cells, and consequently, an increase in the size of an organ or tissue. In pure cases of hypertrophy, there is no increase in the number of cells; the cells are just bigger, as indicated in Figure 3-2. There are three types of hypertrophy: physiological, pathological, and compensatory. Bodybuilders exemplify physiological hypertrophy through weightlifting. As the bodybuilder increases stress on the muscle cells, the cells adapt to the increased demand by increasing in size. They must increase in size because neither cardiac muscle cells nor striated muscle cells can replicate.

Pathological hypertrophy occurs when cells have been damaged. For example, a myocardial infarction is a heart attack in which a portion of the heart muscle actually dies. To compensate for the loss of viable cardiac muscle tissue, the remaining cardiac cells may individually increase in size to compensate for the dead cells.

Compensatory hypertrophy differs from pathological hypertrophy due to the absence of disease. For example, if someone is born with only one kidney instead of two, the one viable kidney will hypertrophy to compensate for the absence of the other kidney. A person may live an otherwise healthy life with only one kidney, and the condition may go undiagnosed because the person lacks any signs or symptoms of disease. The absence of a kidney may go unnoticed until the person is examined for some other reason such as a chest x-ray, an ultrasound, or an MRI.

Hyperplasia

Hyperplasia is also an increase in the size of a tissue or organ; however, it differs from hypertrophy in that there is an increase in the number of cells present, not just an increase in the size of individual cells, as indicated in Figure 3-3. Hyper-

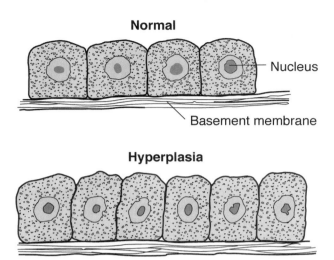

Normal

Nucleus

Basement membrane

Hyperplasia

Figure 3-3 Normal tissue versus hyperplasia.

plasia and hypertrophy often occur in unison. For example, cells in the tissues of the female uterus both increase in number and in size during pregnancy.

Hyperplasia can be either physiological, compensatory, or pathological. Physiological hyperplasia is the result of normal growth. For example, the increase in the number of glandular cells within the female breast at puberty and during pregnancy results from physiological hyperplasia. Compensatory hyperplasia may occur after the removal of part of the liver. Within about 12 hours, the liver will begin to generate cells in an attempt to eventually return to its normal weight. In cases of compensatory hyperplasia, the tissue is responding to an increased workload. Pathological hyperplasia occurs after injury or infection, and it is normally reversible. For example, after a normal menstrual period, hormones are released to develop the lining of the uterus. If these hormone levels become imbalanced, endometrial hyperplasia may ensue, causing abnormal menstrual bleeding. Once the hormone levels are brought back to a normal level, the endometrium typically returns to its normal size.

Metaplasia

Metaplasia is a form of cellular adaptation in which cells regenerate after injury. Basically, during metaplasia, one cell type is replaced by another cell type that is more capable of withstanding a change in environment (see Figure 3-4). Metaplasia is usually reversible.

The healthy epithelial tissues of the trachea, bronchi, and lungs contain ciliated, columnar cells, meaning that they consist of a single layer of column-shaped cells covered with tiny hairs. After habitual cigarette smoking, these healthy cells are replaced with stratified squamous epithelial cells, consisting of multiple layers of cells with a top layer of cells shaped like flat plates. The multiple layers of stratified squamous epithelium are believed to be better able to withstand exposure to cigarette smoke; however, these cells are less capable of

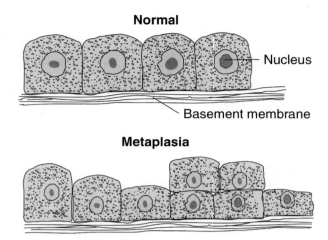

Figure 3-4 Normal tissue versus metaplasia.

removing particles from inhaled air because they do not contain cilia, and they are less effective in the secretion of protective mucous. Most importantly, metaplasia of the epithelium of the respiratory system may induce cancer in smokers. Because metaplasia is normally reversible, in time, the respiratory system may regenerate healthy cells if the smoker stops smoking.

Regeneration

When cells are injured, the body attempts to heal them. There are two processes involved in healing tissues. One is to regenerate damaged tissues with cells of the same type, and the other is to replace tissues with scar tissue originating from connective tissues in the damaged area. The replacement of damaged cells with identical cells is known as **regeneration**.

Small areas of tissue damage can often be repaired through physiological regeneration, which occurs when damaged cells are replaced with identical cells. For example, a small area of skin damage may be repaired through the normal reproduction of skin cells. Dead skin cells cover the area, protecting the newly forming cells from microbiological agents and environmental conditions that may damage them. As the dead skin cells fall away, the new skin cells replace them.

In pathological regeneration, cells other than the originally damaged cells replace the damaged tissue. In the example of damaged skin, a large area of damage may not be repairable through physiological regeneration of normal skin cells, so connective tissues under the skin may reproduce and repair the damaged skin. This process results in scar tissue on the skin. In another example, damaged nerves cannot be repaired through physiological regeneration because neurons do not reproduce. However, there are embryonic cells in the nerves that can reproduce, resulting in a pathological regeneration of damaged nerves.

REVIEW QUESTIONS

Matching

1. _____ atrophy
2. _____ hypertrophy
3. _____ hyperplasia
4. _____ metaplasia
5. _____ amyloid degeneration

a. an increase in the number of cells
b. present in Alzheimer's disease
c. shrinkage of cells
d. regeneration of cells after injury
e. an increase in the size of cells

Multiple Choice

1. Which of the following is not a potential cause of cellular injury?
   a. homeostasis
   b. hypoxia
   c. changes in osmotic pressure
   d. immunological reactions

2. Which of the following is a form of necrosis in which a cheeselike substance is located at the center of an area of pink necrosis surrounded by inflammatory granules?
   a. ischemic necrosis
   b. wet gangrene
   c. caseous necrosis
   d. gas gangrene

3. Which of the following is characterized by cellular swelling, changes in the nature of cellular proteins (denaturation), and the breakdown of cellular organelles in dead cells?
   a. dry gangrene
   b. pathogenesis
   c. necrosis
   d. autolysis

4. Which of the following are examples of pathological hypertrophy?
   i. an increase in upper body muscle in someone with paralysis of the legs
   ii. an increase in the size of the left kidney after damage to the right kidney
   iii. an increase in the size of cells in a damaged area of the right kidney
   iv. an increase in the size of cardiac muscle cells after a heart attack
   a. i and ii
   b. ii and iii
   c. i and iv
   d. iii and iv

5. Which of the following are examples of compensatory hyperplasia?
- i. increase in the size of the left leg after fracturing a bone in the right leg
- ii. increase in the size of the cells surrounding a laceration (cut) on the palm of the right hand
- iii. increase in the size of the lungs after moving from New Orleans, Louisiana, to the less oxygenated air of Denver, Colorado
- iv. a decrease in the size of inflamed nasal tissues after an allergic reaction to pollen
  - a. i and ii
  - b. i and iii
  - c. ii and iii
  - d. ii and iv

Bibliography

Gout (Information from Wellington Regional Rheumatology Unit, Hutt Hospital, Lower Hutt, New Zealand). Retrieved January 19, 2004, from New Zealand Rheumatology Association at http://www.rheumatology.org.nz/nz08003.htm.

Hall, P. (2003). *Metaplasia.* Retrieved May 28, 2003, from Academic Pathology, Queen's University Belfast at http://www.qub.ac.uk/cm/pat/undergraduate/Basiccancer/metaplasia.htm.

Johnson, J. (2003). *Nonspecific defenses.* Retrieved July 26, 2003, from Western Baptist College at http://defiant.wbc.edu/wbc/jjohnson/Pages/InfDis/NonspecificDefenses.html.

Kumar, V., Cotran, R., & Robbins, S. (2003). *Robbins basic pathology* (7th ed.). Philadelphia: Saunders.

Mayer, R. (2000). *Embalming: History, theory, & practice* (3rd ed.). New York: McGraw-Hill.

Neighbors, M., & Tannehill-Jones, R. (2000). *Human diseases.* Clifton Park, NY: Thomson Delmar Learning.

Pathology for funeral service. (1999). Dallas, TX: Professional Training Schools.

Shelton, H. (1992). *Boyd's introduction to the study of disease* (11th ed.). Philadelphia: Lea & Febiger.

Sopher, R. (n.d.). *Cell injury and death.* Retrieved July 24, 2003, from the Department of Pathology, University of North Dakota at http://www.med.und.nodak.edu/depts/path/pathlab/CDI/cdi-index.html.

Thagard, P. (1997). *The concept of disease: Structure and change.* Retrieved May 28, 2003, from the Philosophy Department, University of Waterloo at http://cogsci.uwaterloo.ca/Articles/Pages/Concept.html.

Venes, D. (Ed.). (2001). *Taber's cyclopedic medical dictionary* (19th ed.). Philadelphia: F. A. Davis.

CHAPTER 4

Structural Abnormalities and Birth Defects

Learning Objectives

Upon completion of the chapter, review questions, and case analysis, the reader should be able to:

- Define and contrast amelia, aplasia, phocomelia, and polydactylism.
- Compare cleft palate with cleft lip.
- Describe the different types of color blindness.
- Describe the disease complications of Down syndrome.
- Describe the disease complications of cystic fibrosis.

Key Terms

amelia
aplasia
hernia
hypoplasia

phocomelia
polydactylism
spina bifida

STRUCTURAL ABNORMALITIES AND BIRTH DEFECTS

Human development is a complex process. It may be disrupted by numerous factors at any point from the initial exchange of genetic information between sperm and egg, throughout fetal gestation, to the eventual birth of the infant. In addition, normal development may appear to occur but be accompanied by genetic disorders, which can

Table 4-1 Terminology of Birth Defects

Congenital anomaly	Any development of an organ or structure that is abnormal in form, structure, or position
Malformation	Any anomaly
Hypoplasia	Underdevelopment of a tissue, organ, or the body
Aplasia	Complete failure of a tissue or an organ to develop
Polydactylism	The condition of having more than the normal number of fingers or toes
Phocomelia	A congenital condition in which the proximal portions of the limbs are poorly developed or absent
Amelia	The absence of one or more limbs

ultimately shorten an individual's lifespan. It is, therefore, important for funeral service professionals to be familiar with anatomical anomalies for purposes of embalming, restorative art, communication with medical professionals, and counseling survivors. Table 4-1 includes several terms and their meanings, which are used in conjunction with discussions of structural abnormalities and birth defects.

Spina Bifida

Spina bifida is a structural abnormality that results in the failure of the fetus' spine to close properly during the first month of gestation. It is accompanied by developmental insufficiencies of the brain, spinal cord, or meninges. Infants with spina bifida may have an open lesion on their spine along with damage to the nerves and spinal cord. Even if the opening can be surgically repaired, the nerve damage is usually permanent and results in paralysis of the legs. In cases of spina bifida with no opening of the spinal cord, there may be absent or structurally damaged vertebrae and nerve damage.

In addition to the obvious physical challenges, most children with spina bifida also exhibit mental disability. Bowel and bladder complications often accompany spina bifida, and infants with spina bifida may have a condition known as *hydrocephalus,* in which excessive amounts of cerebrospinal fluid accumulate in the brain.

The three most common types of spina bifida and their characteristics are listed in Table 4-2.

Table 4-2 Types of Spina Bifida

Myelomeningocele	The most severe form of spina bifida and characterized by the protrusion from an opening in the spine of both the malformed spinal cord and the meninges.
Meningocele	Occurs when the spinal cord develops normally but the meninges protrude from a spinal opening.
Occulta	The least severe form, in which one or more vertebrae are malformed and covered by a layer of skin.

There is no cure for spina bifida because the nerve tissue cannot be replaced or repaired, and the prognosis for spina bifida depends on the number and severity of abnormalities. Possible treatments may include surgery, medication, and physical therapy. Ongoing surgery and therapy may be necessary to manage complications throughout the individual's life. Although the prognosis is poorest for infants with complete paralysis, with proper care, most children with spina bifida will live well into adulthood.

Limb Deformities

Amelia is a birth defect resulting in the complete absence of an arm or leg. **Hypoplasia** refers to underdevelopment or incomplete development of tissues due to decreased numbers of cells. Although it can affect any organ or tissue in the body, the term typically applies to the bones and muscles of the lower legs or those of the forearms. When congenital defects of the leg occur, they are often accompanied by deformities of the foot. Hypoplasia of the forearms may be accompanied by missing or shortened thumbs and bones in the wrist. In cases of dentate glenoid anomaly, the end of the scapula is underdeveloped, leading to shortening of the shoulder.

Whereas hypoplasia is the incomplete formation or underdevelopment of a tissue or organ, **aplasia** refers to an absence of cells that leads to incomplete formation of limbs or organs. In cases of aplasia, the most commonly affected bones are the fibula, radius, and ulna. The most common form of aplasia is absence of the fibula bone in the leg. Aplasia can occur in two forms. In the first form of aplasia, the distal end of the bone is missing. In the second form of aplasia, the entire bone is missing. The absence of the bones in the limbs can result in a shortened or bent appearance of the limbs. **Phocomelia** is a congenital condition in which proximal portions of the limbs are poorly developed or missing.

Polydactylism is a fairly common birth defect defined as the presence of one or more extra fingers or toes. The extra digit may appear as a boneless piece of soft tissue that protrudes from the side of a finger or toe, or the extra digit may be fully formed resulting in six or more fingers or toes on one hand or foot. Polydactylism can normally be repaired surgically by removing the extra digit and reconstructing or realigning any missing or excess bone. With modern surgical techniques, even complex cases of polydactylism are often corrected, resulting in a normally appearing and functioning hand or foot.

Cleft Palate and Lip

According to the Cleft Palate Foundation (*About cleft lip and palate* [n.d.]), 1 of every 700 newborns is affected by cleft lip or cleft palate. A cleft lip is a separation of the two sides of the lip, which may include the bones of the upper jaw (the maxillae). In contrast, a cleft palate occurs when the two sides of the palate fail to fuse during fetal development, resulting in an opening between the palatine bones that form the roof of the mouth. Color Plate 8 pictures a child with a cleft lip, and Color Plate 9 pictures a cleft palate.

Both cleft lip and cleft palate are fetal birth defects and can occur on one side or on both sides. A one-sided cleft is known as a unilateral cleft lip or a unilateral cleft palate, while clefts occurring on both sides are known as bilateral cleft lip or bilateral cleft palate. Because the lip and the palate develop separately, individuals may have a cleft lip, a cleft palate, or both cleft lip and cleft palate. The majority of clefts appear to be due to genetic factors. Treatment for cleft lip and cleft palate may include surgery, dental/orthodontic care, and speech therapy.

Color Blindness

Color blindness, or color deficiency, refers to a condition in which individuals have difficulties identifying various colors and shades of colors. The term *color blind* is misleading because color-blind people are not blind at all; instead, they cannot distinguish between some colors, and some may not see colors at all. Color blindness is due to defects in specialized cells in the retina of the eye, called *cones*, that enable humans to see in color, as opposed to many nonhuman animals that have no color perception. There are three basic types of color blindness, and they are described in Table 4-3.

Although color blindness can be acquired, most cases are inherited, and it affects males almost exclusively. Illnesses that can lead to color blindness include Alzheimer's disease, diabetes, glaucoma, leukemia, liver diseases, chronic alcoholism, macular degeneration, multiple sclerosis, Parkinson's disease, and sickle cell anemia. Some medications may cause color blindness, including antibiotics, barbiturates, antituberculosis drugs, high blood pressure medications, and medications used to treat nervous disorders and psychological problems. Chemical causes of color blindness include carbon monoxide, carbon disulfide, fertilizers, styrene, and lead-based chemicals. There is no treatment or cure for congenital color blindness, but acquired color blindness may be temporary.

Table 4-3 Types of Color Blindness

Red/green color blindness	People with red/green color blindness can distinguish between red and green when comparing the two side by side; however, they cannot determine if a color is red or green when shown only one of the two colors.
Blue color blindness	Individuals with blue color blindness cannot distinguish between blue and yellow. They see instead only white or grey. Blue color blindness usually occurs due to physical disorders, such as liver disease or diabetes mellitus.
Achromatopsia	Total color blindness; an extremely rare, hereditary disorder. Individuals with achromatopsia cannot see any colors, and their vision is limited to black, white, and shades of gray. Achromatopsia results in poor visual acuity and extreme sensitivity to light.

Vascular Nevus

A vascular nevus is a type of birthmark, also known as a strawberry mark, in which superficial blood vessels are enlarged. Vascular nevi vary in size and shape, are slightly elevated from the surface of the skin, and normally have a red or purple color. Although they may appear anywhere on the skin, vascular nevi typically appear on the face, head, neck, and arms.

Down Syndrome

Down syndrome is named after J. Langdon Down, a 19th-century British physician. It is also goes by the name of trisomy 21. It received its alternate name because people with Down syndrome have an extra chromosome, usually number 21 or 22. The typical number of chromosomes in the healthy human DNA is 46—23 from the male sperm and 23 from the female egg. Mental retardation occurs in Down syndrome to varying degrees. (*Note:* the term *mental retardation* is being used here in its medical sense, which is a suggestion of a slowed function of the brain. The term *mentally disabled* is preferable to retarded in social settings.) The following signs of Down syndrome are observable in the child in Color Plate 10:

- Sloped forehead
- Small ear canals
- Gray or light yellow spots around the iris of the eyes
- Flat nose or absent bridge
- Low-set ears
- Dwarfed physical appearance
- Short broad hands with a single palmar crease

Down syndrome is the result of a genetic mutation. Although it has not been related to environmental factors, it has been linked to mothers' age. According to the National Institute of Child Health and Human Development (*Facts about Down syndrome* 2003), mothers who become pregnant by the age of 30 have less than a 1 in 1,000 chance of having a baby with Down syndrome, in comparison to mothers over the age of 49 who have a 1 in 12 chance.

Cystic Fibrosis

Cystic fibrosis (CF) is the most common fatal genetic disease in the United States. According to the National Human Genome Research Institute (2003), about 30,000 people in the United States have the disease. Cystic fibrosis is caused by mutations in the cystic fibrosis transmembrane regulator gene. The protein associated with this gene should allow cells to release chloride and other ions, but in CF, the cells are defective and do not release the chloride. The lack of chloride results in a salt imbalance in the cells. The defective cells produce a thick, sticky mucus that clogs the lungs, leads to infection, and blocks the pancreas. In addition, the presence of this thick mucous stops digestive enzymes from reaching the intestine, where they are required for proper digestion. Diabetes mellitus is frequently found in cases of cystic fibrosis. Researchers are focusing on ways to cure CF by correcting the defective gene or the defective protein. Cystic fibrosis is a terminal disease, in most cases at an average age of 20.

Sudden Infant Death Syndrome

According to the Centers for Disease Control and Prevention (*Vaccine fact sheet* 2001), sudden infant death syndrome (SIDS) is the diagnosis given for the sudden death of an infant under one year of age that remains unexplained after a thorough case investigation. By definition, therefore, SIDS, also known as cot death or crib death, is not the result of structural abnormalities or birth defects, it is an idiopathic disorder. Although it is not included in the ABFSE Pathology Curriculum Outline, it is an important cause of death for funeral service practitioners to understand to avoid stigmatizing families of SIDS victims, as SIDS is not due to child abuse or neglect.

Cases of SIDS include an autopsy, a death scene investigation, a review of the infant's health status, and a review of other family members' medical histories. Most SIDS deaths occur between the ages of two and four months, and approximately 3,000 SIDS deaths occur in the United States annually. Death occurs during sleep without any apparent struggle. Although the cause of SIDS is unknown, there are certain risk factors associated with babies who die from SIDS:

- Babies who sleep in a prone position (on their stomach).
- Babies whose mothers smoked during pregnancy.
- Babies exposed to second-hand smoke after birth.
- Babies born to mothers less than 20 years old.
- Babies born to mothers who had inadequate prenatal care.
- Babies born to mothers who abused drugs during pregnancy.
- Babies who are premature or of low birth weight.
- Babies who sleep on soft surfaces (soft mattresses, sofas, cushions, waterbeds, sheep skins).
- Babies who sleep with fluffy or loose bedding (pillows, quilts, stuffed toys).
- Babies who are male.
- Babies who are African American or Native American.

Evidence suggests that some SIDS babies are born with abnormalities in the part of brainstem that controls breathing during sleep by regulating carbon dioxide and oxygen levels. A large number of babies who die from SIDS have respiratory or gastrointestinal infections prior to their deaths. Other SIDS babies have excess immune system cells and proteins that interact with the brain to alter heart rate, slow breathing during sleep, or induce deep sleep. It is also believed by some scientists that SIDS is a manifestation of an inborn error of fatty acid metabolism associated with a deficiency of an enzyme known as acetyl coenzyme A.

Hernias

Although hernias may appear at any time in life, some people are born with congenital hernias. A **hernia** is the protrusion of an organ through the wall normally containing it. Two common sites of hernias are in the groin and in the diaphragm. Hernias tend to occur in the groin because the abdominal organs place a great deal of pressure on the muscular wall of the superior aspect of the pelvic cavity. If the abdominopelvic wall is weak at birth, a hernia known as an inguinal hernia, may occur. Hernias also tend to occur in the diaphragm. The diaphragm separates the thorax from the abdomen, and if the diaphragm is weak at birth, organs such as the stomach may protrude superiorly into the thoracic cavity. Hernias in which the stomach protrudes through the esophageal hiatus of the diaphragm are referred to as hiatal hernias. Both inguinal and hiatal hernias can be treated surgically.

REVIEW QUESTIONS

Matching

1. _____ phocomelia
2. _____ polydactylism
3. _____ achromatopsia
4. _____ trisomy 21
5. _____ hiatal

a. extra fingers or toes
b. hernia in which a portion of the stomach protrudes through the diaphragm
c. Down syndrome
d. absence of the proximal portion of a limb
e. total color blindness

Multiple Choice

1. Which of the following refers to the underdevelopment of a tissue, organ, or the body?
   a. malformation
   b. aplasia
   c. hypoplasia
   d. amelia
2. Which of the following is the most severe form of spina bifida?
   a. congenital
   b. myelomeningocele
   c. meningocele
   d. occulta

3. Which of the following is the most common form of aplasia?
   a. underdevelopment of the humerus
   b. presence of an extra finger
   c. extreme curvature of the radius
   d. absence of the fibula
4. Which of the following is a genetic disease characterized by the presence of an extra chromosome?
   a. Down syndrome
   b. cystic fibrosis
   c. vascular nevus
   d. cleft palate
5. During what range of age do most SIDS deaths occur?
   a. one and three weeks
   b. one and two months
   c. two and four months
   d. two and three years

Putting Learning to Work!

The purpose of the following case analysis is to allow you to apply the information you have learned in a real-world situation. Read the case carefully and try to answer the following questions:

What disorder do you suspect the person had at the time of death?

What potential embalming complications do you anticipate?

What precautions should you take as the embalmer to limit the effects of these complications?

Case Analysis

During the embalming of a twelve-year-old boy, you notice an ulcer on the bottom of his left foot. On aspiration of the thoracic cavity, you notice the presence of thick mucous containing fibrous strains. The boy wears a colostomy bag on his abdomen, and he appears emaciated and underweight for his age and height.

Bibliography

About cleft lip and palate. (n.d.). Retrieved May 30, 2003, from the Cleft Palate Association at http://www.cleftline.org/aboutclp.

Aplasia. (2003). In *The encyclopedia of medical imaging* (Vol. III:1). Retrieved January 19, 2004, from Amersham Health at http://www.amershamhealth.com/medcyclopaedia/volume%20iii%201/aplasia.asp?SearchType=0&CiResultsSize=on&SearchString=aplasia.

Facts about Down syndrome. (2003). Retrieved May 30, 2003, from the National Institutes of Health, National Institute for Child Health and Human Development at http://www.nichd.nih.gov/publications/pubs/downsyndrome/down.htm#DownSyndrome.

Hypoplasia. (2003). In *The encyclopedia of medical imaging* (Vol. III:1). Retrieved January 19, 2004, from Amersham Health at http://www.amershamhealth.com/medcyclopaedia/Volume%20III%201/HYPOPLASIA.asp.

Kumar, V., Cotran, R., & Robbins, S. (2003). *Robbins basic pathology* (7th ed.). Philadelphia: Saunders.

Mayer, R. (2000). *Embalming: History, theory, & practice* (3rd ed.). New York: McGraw-Hill.

Neighbors, M., & Tannehill-Jones, R. (2000). *Human diseases*. Clifton Park, NY: Thomson Delmar Learning.

National Human Genome Research Institute. (2003). Retrieved January 8, 2005, at http://www.genome.gov/10001213.

NINDS spina bifida information page. (2001). Retrieved May 30, 2003, from the National Institutes of Health, The National Institute of Neurological Disorders and Stroke at http://www.ninds.nih.gov/health_and_medical/disorders/spina_bifida.htm.

Pathology for funeral service. (1999). Dallas, TX: Professional Training Schools.

Shelton, H. (1992). *Boyd's introduction to the study of disease* (11th ed.). Philadelphia: Lea & Febiger.

Steefel, L. (1999). Color blindness. In *The Gale encyclopedia of medicine*. Retrieved May 30, 2003, from http://www.findarticles.com/cf_dls/g2601/0003/2601000336/p1/article.jhtml.

Vaccine fact sheet: Facts about SIDS. (2001). Retrieved May 30, 2003, from the Centers for Disease Control and Prevention, National Vaccine Program Office at http://www.cdc.gov/od/nvpo/fs_tableVII_doc5.htm.

Venes, D. (Ed.). (2001). *Taber's cyclopedic medical dictionary* (19th ed.). Philadelphia: F. A. Davis.

Color Plate 8 Cleft lip. (Courtesy of Dr. Joseph Konzelman, School of Dentistry, Medical College of Georgia.)

Color Plate 9 Cleft palate. (Courtesy of Dr. Joseph Konzelman, School of Dentistry, Medical College of Georgia.)

Color Plate 10 Down Syndrome (Copyright Marijane Scott, Marijane's Designer Portraits, C.P.P., Indiana; Down Right Beautiful 1996 Calendar.)

CHAPTER 5

Inflammation

Learning Objectives

Upon completion of the chapter and review questions, the reader should be able to:

- Describe the function of inflammation.
- Define each of the cardinal signs and symptoms of inflammation, being sure to include how the process of inflammation causes each.
- Explain the process of inflammation.
- Identify inflammatory exudates by their physical appearance.
- Differentiate between the outcomes of inflammation.

Key Terms

abscess	purulent
carbuncle	pus
chemotaxis	pustule
exudates	resolution
furuncle	ulcer
hemorrhage	vasoconstriction
inflammation	vasodilation
phagocytosis	vesicle

FUNCTION OF INFLAMMATION

The causes of cellular injury elicit a complex process of defense and repair within the tissues known as inflammation. **Inflammation** is an immunological defense against injury, infection, or allergy, marked by increases in regional blood flow, immigration of white blood cells, and release of chemical toxins. Inflammation is one mechanism the body

Table 5-1 Cardinal Signs and Symptoms of Inflammation

Scientific Name	Common Name	Cause
Tumor	Swelling	Increased permeability of vessels
Calor	Heat	Vasodilation
Rubor	Redness	Vasodilation
Dolor	Pain	Nervous stimulation and swelling
Functio laesa	Altered function	Swelling and pain

uses to protect itself from invasion by foreign organisms and to repair tissue trauma. It may produce systemic fevers, joint and muscle pains, organ dysfunction, and exhaustion.

In a nutshell, inflammation is the body's attempt to contain and eliminate the initial cause of injury to cells. In addition, the inflammation processes is essential in the removal of dead and necrotic tissues resulting from the original injury. The inflammation process has as its goal the ultimate repair of injured tissues. If the injury cannot be repaired, the inflammation processes is an integral part of the formation of scar tissues. Although inflammation is a first line of defense against injury to cells, and it is the backbone of tissue repair, it can also be harmful to the body. Inflammatory responses are the basis of anaphylactic allergic reactions to such events as bee stings or taking penicillin. Other harmful effects of inflammation include rheumatoid arthritis and atherosclerosis.

Table 5-1 includes the five cardinal signs and symptoms of inflammation. Most of the signs and symptoms associated with inflammation are the result of increases in the volume of fluids present in the tissues. One way that the body increases the amount of fluid in the inflamed tissues is through **vasodilation**, which is the increase in the diameter of vessels.

 ## CAUSES OF INFLAMMATION

Inflammation can be caused by physical irritants, chemical irritants, infectious agents, or immunological reactions typical of autoimmune diseases. Table 5-2 describes the various types of inflammation. Each of these types of inflammation begins as acute inflammation. Acute inflammation is characterized by being short in duration, lasting only a few minutes to a few days. Acute inflammatory processes attempt to regenerate tissues and restore them to normal function with no residual effects.

If complete resolution is not possible due to the extent of the injury, scar tissue may form to fill the void left by the damaged tissue. Acute inflammation may progress into chronic inflammation. Chronic inflammation differs from acute inflammation in that chronic inflammation can last from days to years.

Table 5-2 Types of Inflammation and Their Characteristics

Serous inflammation	Exudation of clear fluid with few cells
Fibrinous inflammation	Fibrin-rich exudate
Purulent inflammation	Exudate rich in pus
Ulcerative inflammation	Loss of epithelium resulting in ulcerous lesion
Pseudomembranous inflammation	Ulceration and a pseudomembrane over the ulcer
Chronic inflammation	Active inflammation, tissue destruction, and the presence of an inflammatory exudate containing lymphocytes and macrophages
Granulomatous inflammation	Specialized form of chronic inflammation characterized by the formation of granulomas (accumulation of chronic inflammatory cells), e.g., tuberculosis

PROCESS OF INFLAMMATION

The inflammatory processes is quite complex, involving multiple stages and sequences of events. Although the events depicted in Figure 5-1 are an oversimplification of the processes of inflammation, they provide an insight into the attainment of the three basic goals of the inflammatory process: to isolate, eliminate, and regenerate.

Stepping on a dirty, rusty nail would cause an inflammatory response. After the nail has punctured the skin and driven pieces of sock, shoe, soil, and rust, as well as microorganisms deep into the tissues, inflammation begins. First, vasoconstriction of the venules surrounding the puncture wound occurs. **Vasoconstriction** is a decrease in the diameter of a vessel. These tiny veins (venules) constrict for about 15 to 30 minutes to isolate the contaminants within the site of injury to protect other surrounding tissues.

Second, chemicals like histamine are released within the injury site initiating vasodilation that increases blood flow, causing swelling, redness, and heat. The increased blood flow flushes the wound of foreign matter. Following the increase in permeability of the blood vessels due to chemotaxis, blood flow slows, and leukocytes migrate to the vessel walls. **Chemotaxis** is the movement of white blood cells to an area of inflammation in response to the release of chemical mediators by neutrophils, monocytes, and injured tissues. The leukocytes mix with the platelets along the edges of the vessel wall within the site of injury. The different cells work together to recognize foreign cells, engulf those cells, and destroy them in a process known as phagocytosis (Figure 5-2). **Phagocytosis** is a process in which phagocytes (i.e., neutrophils, monocytes, and macrophages) engulf and destroy microorganisms, other foreign antigens, and cell debris.

At the same time, a blood clot forms to stop the initial bleeding, and a scab forms to wall off the inflammatory process. After the tissue is repaired, the scab falls away, and any tissue that could not be replaced is repaired with scar tissue. Besides scar tissue, there are several possible lesions that may develop as a result of the inflammatory response.

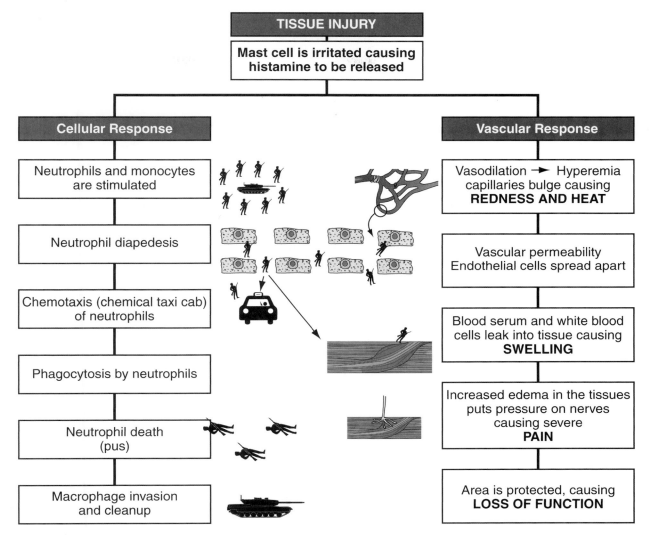

Figure 5-1 Acute inflammation—cellular and vascular responses.

Inflammatory Lesions

A lesion is a specific pathologic structural or functional change brought about by disease. Table 5-3 presents a list of frequently encountered inflammatory lesions and a description of each.

During the processes of inflammation, an abscess may form. An **abscess** is an inflamed area of pus that is walled off by a membrane. Abscesses wall off the inflammatory processes within a fibrous capsule to protect surrounding tissues from further damage. **Ulcers** are open sores or lesions of skin or mucous

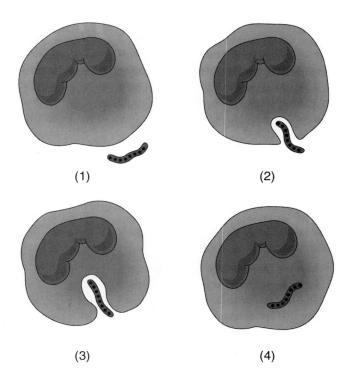

(1)   (2)

(3)   (4)

Figure 5-2 Phagocytosis of a bacteria by a white blood cell. Phagocytosis can occur in the bloodstream, or white cells squeeze through capillary walls and destroy bacteria in the tissues.

Table 5-3 Descriptions of Inflammatory Lesions

Abscess	A localized accumulation of pus
Ulcer	An open sore or lesion of skin or mucous membrane accompanied by sloughing of inflamed necrotic tissue
Vesicle	Blisterlike elevation of skin containing serous fluid
Furuncle (boil)	An abscess or pustular infection of a sweat gland or hair follicle
Carbuncle	Several communicating boils of the skin and subcutaneous tissues that produces and discharges pus and dead tissue
Pustule	A small elevation of the skin containing pus

membranes accompanied by sloughing of inflamed necrotic tissue. A **vesicle** is a blisterlike elevation of skin containing serous fluid. A **furuncle**, which is also known as a boil, is an abscess or pustular infection of a sweat gland or hair follicle. A **pustule** is a small elevation of the skin containing pus. A **carbuncle** is an abscess of the skin formed by the merger of two or more furuncles.

Pus

Pus is protein-rich fluid containing white blood cells, especially neutrophils, and cell debris produced during inflammation. Pus commonly is caused by infection with pus-forming (pyogenic) bacteria such as streptococci, staphylococci, gonococci, and pneumococci (all described in detail in Part Two of this book). Normally, pus is white or yellow, but red pus may also occur if small blood vessels rupture. Brown pus, which is known as chocolate pus, and bluish-green pus may also occur depending on the type of microorganism involved in the inflammatory process. Pus that has been walled off by a membrane leads to an abscess.

INFLAMMATORY EXUDATES

Inflammation often is accompanied by the production and secretion of inflammatory exudates. An **exudate**, which is any fluid released from the body with a high concentration of protein, cells, or solid debris, oozes through the tissues into a cavity or to the surface. Escape of blood from the blood vascular system is known as **hemorrhage**, and hemorrhagic exudates contain blood. Serous exudates are rich in proteins and contain white blood cells, while a **purulent** exudate is primarily composed of pus resulting from infections. Purulent exudates may also be known as suppurative exudates. Exudates result from the numerous cells involved in the inflammatory response pictured in Figure 5-3 and listed in Table 5-4 (see Appendix C for a review of the function of these cells in the blood).

OUTCOMES OF INFLAMMATION

The ultimate goal of inflammation is **resolution**, which is defined as the termination of the inflammatory response with the affected part returning to its normal state. Once the inflammatory process ends, the body attempts to repair the injured tissues, returning the body to its original, healthy state if possible. The process of healing wounds is complex and orderly, with only a few outcomes based on the extent of the damage to the tissues and the type of tissue.

First, the tissue may simply undergo regeneration, in which damaged cells are replaced with identical new cells. Not all tissue has the same capacity for regeneration, and certain diseases interfere with the healing process. A common complication of diabetes is the inability of the body to heal wounds in a timely fashion. It is particularly important for individuals with diabetes to check their feet and other body parts for ulcers that may not heal without medical intervention. In the absence of disease conditions, connective tissue and epithelial tissue are capable of regeneration if not too severely damaged. Muscle tissue, however, tends not to regenerate readily, and destroyed nerve cell bodies are typically incapable of regeneration.

If regeneration is not possible, the tissue may repair itself, which is defined as the restoration of damaged tissue by the growth of new, healthy cells not necessarily of the same type as the original tissue. A scar, which is also known as a *cicatrix*, is a form of repaired tissue consisting of connective tissue. Scars contain no blood vessels, hair follicles, oil or sweat glands, or nerve endings.

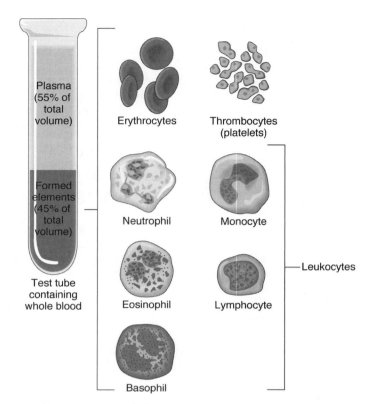

Figure 5-3 Major components of blood.

Table 5-4 Cellular Components of Inflammation

Neutrophils	First cells to enter site of injury; able to kill bacteria and engulf material (phagocytosis); produce chemicals to attract other cells (chemotaxis); short lived
Eosinophils	Kill bacteria; involved in allergic reactions and parasitic infections; longer lived; present in chronic inflammation
Basophils/mast cells	Release histamine, causing blood vessel dilation (vasodilation); known as basophils in blood, as mast cells in tissue
Macrophages	Enter site of injury within 3–4 days; able to kill bacteria and engulf material (phagocytosis); present in chronic inflammation
Lymphocytes	White blood cells; have surface proteins specific for antigens (any molecule that can stimulate an immune response); memory lymphocytes can "remember" a previously encountered antigen

REVIEW QUESTIONS

Matching

1. _____ dolor
2. _____ rubor
3. _____ abscess
4. _____ vesicle
5. _____ ulcer

a. redness
b. a localized accumulation of pus
c. blisterlike elevation of skin containing serous fluid
d. pain
e. an open sore or lesion of skin or mucous membrane accompanied by sloughing of inflamed necrotic tissue

Multiple Choice

1. Which of the following exudates contains pus?
   a. hemorrhagic exudate
   b. purulent exudate
   c. serous exudate
   d. inflammatory exudate
2. Which of the following is true of an abscess?
   i. It is a localized area of infection.
   ii. It contains pus.
   iii. It is the cause of scar tissue formation.
   iv. It protects surrounding tissue from further damage by walling off the infection.
      a. i, ii, and iii
      b. i, ii, and iv
      c. i, iii, and iv
      d. ii, iii, and iv
3. Which of the following statements describes the purpose of vasoconstriction of the venules surrounding a puncture wound?
   a. Vasoconstriction of the venules stops swelling.
   b. Vasoconstriction of the venules attracts chemical defenses of the body to the injury site.
   c. Vasoconstriction of the venules prevents the initial spread of the infection.
   d. Vasoconstriction of the venules stops excessive bleeding.
4. Which of the following is a specific pathological structural or functional change brought about by a disease?
   a. inflammatory exudates
   b. chronic inflammation
   c. function laesa
   d. lesion

5. Which of the following are short-lived cells that are the first to enter an injury site?

    a. neutrophils

    b. eosinophils

    c. basophils

    d. lypmphocytes

Bibliography

Kumar, V., Cotran, R., & Robbins, S. (2003). *Robbins basic pathology* (7th ed.). Philadelphia: Saunders.

Mayer, R. (2000). *Embalming: History, theory, & practice* (3rd ed.). New York: McGraw-Hill.

Neighbors, M., & Tannehill-Jones, R. (2000). *Human diseases*. Clifton Park, NY: Thomson Delmar Learning.

Pathology for funeral service. (1999). Dallas, TX: Professional Training Schools.

Shelton, H. (1992). *Boyd's introduction to the study of disease* (11th ed.). Philadelphia: Lea & Febiger.

Sopher, R. (n.d.). *Inflammation*. Retrieved July 24, 2003, from the Department of Pathology, University of North Dakota at http://www.med.und.nodak.edu/depts/path/pathlab/Inflammation/Inf-Index.html.

Venes, D. (Ed.). (2001). *Taber's cyclopedic medical dictionary* (19th ed.). Philadelphia: F. A. Davis.

CHAPTER 6

Disturbances in Circulation

Learning Objectives

Upon completion of the chapter, review questions, and case analysis, the reader should be able to:

- Discuss the causes of edema.
- Describe physiological, pathological, active, and passive hyperemia.
- Define anasarca, ascites, hydrothorax, hydrocele, and hydropericardium.
- Discuss the causes of thrombi.
- Discuss the different types of emboli and how they enter the bloodstream.
- Explain the consequences of the presence of emboli in the body.
- Describe the types and causes of hemorrhage.
- Discuss the differences between hypoxia and ischemia.
- Describe the postmortem conditions associated with disturbances in circulation.

Key Terms

anasarca	hemoptysis
ascites	hydropericardium
ecchymosis	hydrothorax
edema	hyperemia
embolus	hypoxia
epistaxis	ischemia
exsanguination	melena
hematemesis	petechiae
hematoma	thrombus
hematuria	

CAUSES OF EDEMA

Edema, which used to be known as dropsy, is a local or generalized condition in which the body tissues contain an excessive amount of tissue fluid. Edema may result from four primary causes:

1. Increased permeability of capillary walls
2. Increased capillary pressure due to venous obstruction or heart failure
3. Inflammatory conditions
4. Fluid and electrolyte disturbances

Edema can be caused by increased permeability of capillary walls, which allows excess fluid to leach out into the extravascular tissues. Obstruction in veins can also cause edema, due to an associated increase in capillary blood pressure. Other causes of edema include heart failure, lymphatic obstruction, kidney failure, inflammation, electrolyte disturbances, malnutrition, starvation, and toxins. Table 6-1 describes different types of edema. **Anasarca** is severe, generalized edema. **Ascites** is the accumulation of fluid in the abdomen. **Hydrothorax** is edema in the pleural cavity, and **hydropericardium** is accumulation of fluid in the pericardial sac that surrounds the heart.

Figure 6-1 depicts a person with edema of the leg, and Figure 6-2 shows pitting edema.

HYPEREMIA

Hyperemia is increased flow of blood in an area of the body. Its two forms are active hyperemia and passive hyperemia. Active hyperemia is increased arterial blood supply to an organ for physiologic reasons. It occurs during exercise when

Table 6-1 Types of Edema

Anasarca	Severe, generalized edema.
Ascites	The accumulation of fluid in the abdomen. May be caused by interference in venous return as occurs in congestive heart failure; obstruction of the vena cava or portal vein; obstruction in lymphatic drainage; cirrhosis of the liver; cancer; electrolyte imbalance; or infections of the peritoneum.
Hydrothorax	A collection of fluid in the pleural cavity causing shortness of breath (dyspnea). May be caused by lung cancers, lung infections, and pleurisy.
Hydrocele	Edema of the scrotum.
Hydropericardium	Edema of the pericardial sac that surrounds the heart. It is characterized by chest pain or discomfort, diminished cardiac function with signs of heart failure, and difficulty swallowing (dysphagia) and shortness of breath (dyspnea).
Pitting edema	Edema usually of the skin of the extremities. When pressed firmly with a finger, the skin maintains the depression produced by the finger.
Pulmonary edema	A potentially life-threatening accumulation of fluid in the lungs. The fluid may inhibit the exchange of oxygen and carbon dioxide.

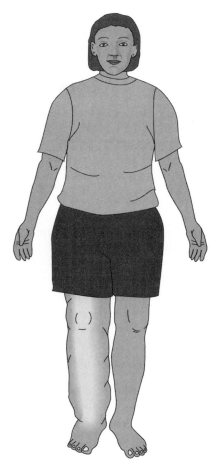

Figure 6-1 Lymphedema in the right lower extremity.

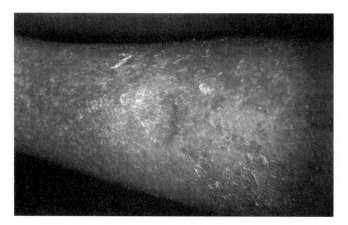

Figure 6-2 Pitting edema. (Courtesy of Robert A. Silverman, MD, Pediatric Dermatology, Georgetown University.)

the blood flow increases to the muscles. Active hyperemia may also be pathological, however, as in acute inflammatory diseases. In these cases, the redness, loss of function, heat, swelling, and pain associated with inflammation result from hyperemia.

Passive hyperemia is the engorgement of an organ or tissues with venous blood resulting from inadequate venous drainage. The presence of excess blood in the liver and other abdominal organs is an example of passive hyperemia associated with congestive heart failure. Passive hyperemia causes a reddish-blue discoloration of the affected parts because venous return is impaired. As the venous blood becomes deoxygenated, the discoloration, which is known as *cyanosis,* is accentuated. The congestion of capillary beds due to severe cases of passive hyperemia is related to the development of both edema and microscopic hemorrhaging.

Cyanosis of the fingernail bed can be observed by gently squeezing the finger at the base of the fingernail to prevent the blood from draining from the tip of the finger. As the blood fills the capillaries under the fingernail, they become congested due to the mild pressure on the venous blood vessels causing cyanosis under the fingernail. The cyanosis becomes more pronounced as the blood becomes more deoxygenated. The fingernail beds, the palms of the hands, the soles of the feet, and the sclera, or the whites, of the eyes are good places to look for discolorations because in those locations the discolorations are present regardless of race or skin complexion.

ISCHEMIA AND HYPOXIA

Ischemia is a deficiency of arterial blood flow to an organ or tissue, while **hypoxia** is a decrease in the level of oxygen within a tissue. Examples of sometimes fatal ischemia include ischemic heart disease, which can cause myocardial infarctions, and transient ischemic attacks in the flow of blood to the brain, which can be as mild as fainting or as severe as a fatal stroke.

Although ischemia and hypoxia are often related, they indicate two different pathological conditions. Ischemia, which is too little blood flow, will eventually result in hypoxia, which is too little oxygen; however, hypoxia need not occur only as a result of ischemia. Hypoxia may occur for any reason in which the blood does not contain enough oxygen. For example, in cases of carbon monoxide poisoning, there is ample blood flow, but the hemoglobin is bound with carbon monoxide and cannot transport sufficient amounts of oxygen.

Thrombi and emboli can block the flow of blood within arterial blood vessels causing ischemia of the tissues distal to the blockage.

THROMBOSIS

Thrombosis is the formation of a blood clot, and the blood clot is referred to as a **thrombus**. A thrombus is a stationary blood clot and has the potential to fragment in the blood stream. There are four common causes of blood clots:

1. Injuries to blood vessels
2. A reduced rate of blood flow
3. Alterations in the composition of blood
4. Certain diseases of the blood

One of the most common reasons for blood to become prone to excessive clotting is damage to the endothelial lining of the blood vessels. When the lining of the blood vessels is damaged, thrombocytes aggregate on the rough, damaged endothelium, instead of slipping past on its otherwise smooth surface. Stasis of blood, which means that the blood flows too slowly through the vessels, also causes blood clotting as a result of the slow blood flow. For example, after a small cut, the blood settles along the edges of the cut and on the surface of the skin, which signals the clot to form in order to stop the loss of blood. Blood composition changes, increasing the likelihood of clot formation as well. A person who is dehydrated is more likely to experience excessive clotting because the clotting agents in the blood are closer together and the blood flows more slowly. In addition, the change in the fluid levels of the blood's composition result in more clots. Some of the most obvious causes of blood clot formation are diseases of the blood that affect clotting. For example, in cases of thrombocytosis, there is an excess in the number of platelets in the blood. The extra platelets cause excessive clotting.

Blood clots in the heart and arterial circulation are typically due to damage to the endothelial lining of the vessels or the lining of the chambers of the heart. Thrombi may form in cases of hypertension, in scarred vascular or cardiac valves, or in the presence of certain toxins present in bacterial infections of the blood. The presence of atherosclerotic plaque may attract platelets, causing them to form clots on the plaque. These clots may obstruct the flow of blood through the vessels. Similarly, any blood flow stasis allows the thrombocytes to come into contact with the endothelium, which starts the process of clot formation.

Besides inherited genetic mutations of clotting agents in the blood, clotting disorders may also be associated with prolonged bed rest, myocardial infarction, surgery, bone fractures, burns, cancer, sickle cell anemia, and oral contraceptive use. In addition to the damage to surrounding and distal tissues to the blood clot, thrombi often fragment and enter the flow of blood.

There are a variety of consequences that may be associated with blood clots, including sudden death. Excessive blood clotting may cause a severe reduction in the flow of blood to an area, which is known as ischemia. For example, strokes may be caused by a blood clot in one of the arteries in the brain. Blood clots may also cause a condition known as passive hyperemia. In passive hyperemia, a blood clot forms in a vein, which causes blood to pool in the tissues, potentially leading to moist gangrene. The excess fluids in the tissues serves as a breeding ground for microorganisms that cause the gangrene. Blood clots in the blood vessels of the heart, primarily the coronary artery, may lead to myocardial infarction (MI). An infarct occurs when the supply of nutrients to the tissues is prevented due to a blockage of the arteries leading to the tissue. During a myocardial infarct, the area of the heart muscle affected dies, which may lead to acute cardiac failure. An acute MI is commonly referred to as a heart attack, and it is frequently caused by a blood clot in the coronary artery.

EMBOLISM

An embolism is the sudden obstruction of a vessel by debris. An embolism is caused by an **embolus**, which is a free-floating object in the bloodstream, such as blood clots, cholesterol-containing plaques, bacteria, cancer cells, amniotic fluid, fat from the marrow of broken bones, and injected substances like air bubbles. Embolisms can be life-threatening conditions; emboli that block the flow of blood to the heart or brain can result in sudden death. Table 6-2 lists and describes some of the more common forms of emboli.

Regardless of the type of embolism, the consequences are quite similar. An embolism can result in the blockage of blood flow to the tissues, which is known as ischemia. An embolism may also result in the death of tissues distal to the blockage, which is known as infarction. An embolism may spread infection and may cause more systemic death of tissues if the blockage is not complete. Necrosis of tissues due to emboli typically results from the gradual starvation of the tissues of necessary blood for nutrients and the removal of wastes resulting from cellular respiration.

Table 6-2 Common Emboli

Fragments of thrombi	One of the most common forms of embolism occurs when a blood clot (thrombus) breaks apart, fragmenting into small pieces of the clot that travel throughout the bloodstream where they may become lodged in smaller vessels and block the flow of blood.
Microorganisms	Many microorganisms spread throughout the body by multiplying in the blood, which is known as septicemia. For example, bacteremia, which occurs when bacteria multiply in the blood, can cause congestion of the tissues and death due to blood poisoning.
Tumor cells	Metastasis is the process in which cancer cells spread throughout the body. For example, a single tumor cell may break off of a larger tumor in the lung and spread through the blood to the liver, where a new, secondary tumor grows. It is also possible for tumor-cell emboli to block blood vessels, preventing the flow of blood.
Animal parasites	A variety of animal parasites are capable of spreading through the blood and causing emboli. (Some parasites require a stage of growth in a blood cell in their lifecycle to mature and replicate.)
Fat	During crushing injuries, fat globules in the tissues may enter damaged blood vessels. This occurrence is particularly common in fractures of bone, where fat globules from the yellow bone marrow are able to enter the blood vessels. If a fat embolus occludes an artery of the heart or brain, it can cause sudden death.
Gas	Bubbles may enter the blood during chest injuries, surgery, or a simple inoculation (a shot). In another example, divers may experience a condition known as "the bends" in which nitrogen that is dissolved in the blood forms nitrogen bubbles that cause serious illness or death.
Foreign bodies	Emboli can be formed of any free-floating object in the blood; therefore, any foreign object small enough may become an embolus. Examples of foreign body emboli include bullet fragments, microscopic glass shards, and grains of sand.

HEMORRHAGE

One of the most common forms of injury to the circulatory system is bleeding, which is known as hemorrhaging. A hemorrhage is defined as the escape of blood from the blood vascular system. Four common causes of hemorrhage include trauma, vascular diseases, high blood pressure (hypertension), and diseases of the blood.

Petechiae

Petechiae (singular = petechia) are antemortem pinpoint-size hemorrhages of small capillaries in the skin or mucous membranes (see Color Plate 11). Petechiae result from areas of superficial bleeding into the skin, appearing as round, pinpoint-size dots that are not raised. The dots may range from red to purple as they age and disappear. Petechiae are usually found on the lower legs, but may be distributed all over the body. The treatment and outcome of petechiae depends on the underlying cause. Petechiae in the deceased remains are not removed during the injection of arterial embalming fluids because postmortem petechiae cause a permanent, extravascular stain.

Common causes of petechial hemorrhage include:

- Blunt force trauma
- Allergic reactions to medications
- Autoimmune disorders
- Liver disorders such as cirrhosis
- Infections such as typhus and endocarditis
- Deficiencies in vitamins C, K, or B_{12}
- Deficiency of platelets in the blood
- Blood transfusions
- Blood thinners
- Blood infections
- Radiation and chemotherapy for cancer
- Violent vomiting or coughing

Ecchymosis

Ecchymosis is the scientific name for a common bruise (see Color Plate 12). Large areas of ecchymoses are associated with blood clotting disorders. They may also occur during prolonged usage of nonsteroidal anti-inflammatory drugs (NSAIDs), which reduce inflammation in chronic inflammatory disorders such as arthritis, lupus erythematosis, and any number of autoimmune disorders. Ecchymosis is often present in the hands and arms of the deceased due to the introduction of intravenous drugs and fluids. In the deceased, the discolorations due to ecchymosis are permanent and extravascular, so they will not be removed during the injection of arterial embalming fluids.

Epistaxis

Epistaxis is the scientific name for blood coming from the nose. Epistaxis typically originates from the nasal septum, when the nasal mucosa overlying a dilated blood vessel is injured. However, a so-called bloody nose may signal a more serious underlying condition, such as a blood clotting disorder or cancer. Most nosebleeds stop within a few minutes with or without pressure to the forehead, nose, or upper lip. Sports-related trauma and various other causes make epistaxis a common condition in active and apparently healthy people.

In the deceased, blood or any body fluid appearing in the nose, mouth, or ears is known as *purge*. Frothy, red blood is a sign of purge from the lungs. Purge that is dark and has the appearance of coffee grounds is from the stomach. A pink or clear fluid in the nose or ears indicates purge from the brain.

Pressure in the thorax or abdomen due to microbial growth and gas formation is a likely cause of purge. Edema associated with swelling of the brain and tissues surrounding the brain can cause purge from the cranium. It is important not only to remove the purging fluid, but to treat the cause of the purge. If the cause of the purge is not treated, the purge may reoccur during funeralization.

Hemoptysis

The word *hemoptysis* comes from the Greek *haima,* which means "blood," and *ptysis,* which means "spitting." **Hemoptysis** is the coughing of bloody sputum from the respiratory tract. Sputum can derive from anywhere within the respiratory tract, and it may contain mucus, cellular debris, pus, caseous material, or microorganisms.

Most cases of hemoptysis are not severe, being caused by the rupturing of a small blood vessel during coughing or due to respiratory infection. Nonetheless, hemoptysis may be a sign of serious illnesses including cancers, chronic dilation and infection of the bronchioles and bronchi, pulmonary emboli, pneumonia, tuberculosis, cystic fibrosis, or occupational diseases.

Hematemesis

Hematemesis is the vomiting of blood. The bleeding is usually from the upper gastrointestinal (GI) tract, including the upper small intestine (duodenum), the stomach, or the esophagus. A common cause of hematemesis results from scars in cases of liver cirrhosis. However, the most common cause of upper GI bleeding is an ulcer in the stomach or small intestine.

Inflammation of the stomach, which is known as gastritis, or inflammation of the esophagus, which is known as esophagitis, can also cause bloody vomit. The veins around the esophagus become swollen, and they may bleed for no apparent reason. The esophagus may bleed due to tearing after severe coughing or vomiting. Such vomiting may be caused by drinking too much alcohol. Large amounts of bloody vomit usually are not due to stomach or esophageal cancers, although small amounts of bright, red blood or dark brown material that resembles coffee grounds may be present in vomit in association with esophageal and stomach cancers.

Melena

Melena is black, tarry feces caused by the digestion of blood in the gastrointestinal tract, and it is common in the newborn. Melena is usually caused by gastrointestinal bleeding from the esophagus, stomach, or proximal small intestine in adults, but the ingestion of black licorice, lead, Pepto-Bismol, or blueberries can also cause black stools or false melena. It requires at least 2 tablespoons of blood, or 60 milliliters, to cause melena. Maroon-colored stools suggest that the blood is coming from the middle portion of the intestinal tract, and bright red discolorations originate in the colon. Bright red stool may indicate hemorrhoids, inflammatory bowel disease, viral intestinal infections, necrotizing enterocolitis, colon polyps, or colon cancer. While maroon stool may be caused by diverticulosis, intestinal infections, inflammatory bowel disease, or tumors, melena is typically a sign of bleeding ulcers or gastritis.

Hematuria

Hematuria is the presence of blood in the urine, and it indicates that something is causing bleeding in the genitourinary tract, which may be occurring in the kidneys, the ureters, the prostate gland, the bladder, or the urethra. There are two types of hematuria, microscopic and gross. In microscopic hematuria, the amount of blood in the urine is so small that it cannot be seen without a microscope, while in cases of gross hematuria the urine is pink, red, or brown and may contain small blood clots. The amount of blood in the urine, however, is not necessarily an indicator of the severity of disease.

Other possible symptoms of hematuria include abdominal pain; reduced urinary output; fever; frequent urination (polyuria); inability to empty, or void, the bladder when urinating; or urgency to urinate. There are also nonpathological causes that may turn the urine pink or red, including excessive consumption of beets, berries, rhubarb, food coloring, certain laxatives, and some pain medications. Some of the pathological conditions related to hematuria are:

- Enlargement of the prostate gland in men
- Kidney stones
- Kidney diseases
- Medications such as quinine, rifampin, phenytoin
- Blunt force trauma to the urinary system
- Benign or malignant tumors in the urinary system
- Urinary tract blockages
- Viral infections of the urinary tract
- Sexually transmitted diseases
- Sickle cell anemia
- Systemic lupus erythmatosus

Exsanguination

Exsanguination is massive bleeding from anywhere in the body. Typically, the term *exsanguinate* refers to the loss of blood to the point of death. It would be appropriate to describe the rupture of an aortic aneurysm that led to someone's death as exsanguination. If someone were in an automobile accident that led to rupture of the spleen, and that person died from the loss of blood, the bleeding would be referred to as exsanguination. Extreme trauma such as severing of limbs and other forms of mutilation may occur due to the occupational use of heavy equipment on farms or in factories. Such extreme trauma can result in sudden death due to exsanguination. In addition, traumas such as stabbings, gun shot wounds, or other penetrating injuries associated with homicide may also cause sudden death due to exsanguination.

POSTMORTEM CONDITIONS ASSOCIATED WITH DISTURBANCES IN CIRCULATION

The arterial embalming of the deceased is contingent on proper distribution of arterial embalming fluids through the blood vascular system. If the deceased died due to complications associated with circulatory disturbances, it is important for the embalmer to recognize the possible effects such disorders may have on the embalming processes. There are eight postmortem conditions that may have implications on the embalming of persons who die due to circulatory disturbances:

1. Diminished circulation
2. Edema
3. Abscess
4. Hemorrhage
5. Emaciation
6. Dehydration
7. Rapid decomposition
8. Discoloration

Diminished circulation is one of the most important challenges for the embalmer to overcome. The presences of blood clots, tumors, and emboli can occlude blood vessels that are necessary for the distribution of embalming fluid throughout the deceased. If death occurred due to diminished blood flow, the distribution of embalming fluid will also be inhibited. Disturbances in blood flow may also cause different portions of the human remains to be dehydrated and emaciated prior to death.

Edema in the tissues, accompanied by decreased blood flow, results in a breeding ground for infectious agents. These conditions also inhibit the immune system from defending the body from microorganisms. The combination of a good environment for bacterial growth and a weakened immune response may result in abscess formation.

Bleeding disorders may cause internal bleeding, resulting in discolorations of the tissues of the deceased. The presence of hemorrhaging may be accompanied by bruising and hematomas. The introduction of intravenous (IV) medications typically results in ecchymoses on the hands or forearms. A **hematoma** is a swelling consisting of a mass of extravascular blood, which is usually clotted and confined to an organ, tissue, or space (see Color Plate 13).

Any significant hemorrhages can cause embalming fluid to enter the extravascular tissues, where it may cause localized swelling and distention of the tissues. This condition is especially significant in cases of head trauma. Persons who die due to sudden head trauma may not live long enough for the heart to pump blood out of the blood vessels. The vessels may still be torn, and the pressure associated with the introduction of embalming fluids may cause swelling of the delicate tissues that surround the eyes. As blood is forced out of the blood vessels into the tissues that surround the eyes during arterial embalming, they may become discolored and swollen.

Finally, decomposition of human remains is largely due to a process known as hydrolysis, which is the chemical reaction of a compound with water, usually resulting in the formation of one or more new compounds. In the case of the decomposing human remains, water decomposes tissues through hydrolysis. The presence of edema in the tissues results in rapid decomposition.

REVIEW QUESTIONS

Matching

1. _____ anasarca
2. _____ ascites
3. _____ hematuria
4. _____ melena
5. _____ hemoptysis

a. blood in the urine
b. blood in the sputum
c. generalized edema
d. digested blood in the feces
e. edema in the abdomen

Multiple Choice

1. Which of the following results from the slowing of blood flow?
   a. the blood transports large proteins into the interstitial fluids
   b. the blood becomes less viscous
   c. the blood warms
   d. the blood clots
2. Which of the following is a hemorrhage characterized by pinpoint bleeding?
   a. petechia
   b. ecchymosis
   c. hemoptysis
   d. epistaxis

3. Which of the following is edema of the scrotum?
   a. hydrothorax
   b. hydrocele
   c. hydropericardium
   d. hemoptysis

4. The presence of an embolus in the coronary artery, which supplies blood to the myocardium, might cause which of the following?
   i. ischemia leading to a myocardial infarction
   ii. eventual hypoxia of the cells in the myocardium
   iii. passive hyperemia in the myocardium
   iv. immediate hydropericardium
      a. i and ii
      b. ii and iii
      c. iii and iv
      d. i and iv

5. Maroon-colored stool indicates that bleeding is occurring in which portion of the digestive tract?
   a. esophagus
   b. stomach
   c. ileum or jejunum
   d. rectum

Putting Learning to Work!

The purpose of the following case analysis is to allow you to apply the information you have learned in a real-world situation. Read the case carefully and try to answer the following questions:

   What disorder do you suspect the person had at the time of death?

   What potential embalming complications do you anticipate?

   What precautions should you take as the embalmer to limit the effects of these complications?

Case Analysis

A 21-year-old man died on his birthday in his college dorm room. His friends took him out to celebrate his birthday, and he became severly intoxicated. The man's blood alcohol level was over 0.40, which resulted in a lethal alcohol intoxication. Prior to convulsions and coma, he spent the night vomiting. During your class analysis, you notice that the man's face is covered with small red dots under the skin. He also has some blood in his mouth and nose, and the whites of his eyes have red dots similar to those on his face.

Bibliography

Kumar, V., Cotran, R., & Robbins, S. (2003). *Robbins basic pathology* (7th ed.). Philadelphia: Saunders.
Mayer, R. (2000). *Embalming: History, theory, & practice* (3rd ed.). New York: McGraw-Hill.
Neighbors, M., & Tannehill-Jones, R. (2000). *Human diseases*. Clifton Park, NY: Thomson Delmar Learning.
Pathology for funeral service. (1999). Dallas, TX: Professional Training Schools.
Shelton, H. (1992). *Boyd's introduction to the study of disease* (11th ed.). Philadelphia: Lea & Febiger.
Venes, D. (Ed.). (2001). *Taber's cyclopedic medical dictionary* (19th ed.). Philadelphia: F. A. Davis.

CHAPTER 7

Neoplasms and Cysts

Learning Objectives

Upon completion of the chapter, review questions, and case analysis, the reader should be able to:

- Compare and contrast benign tumors and malignant tumors.
- List the benign tumors that arise from each of the four basic tissues of the body.
- List the malignant tumors that arise from each of the four basic tissues of the body.
- Describe ovarian and sebaceous cysts.
- Explain the potential embalming complications associated with neoplasms.
- Discuss the meanings of the suffixes -oma, -sarcoma, and carcinoma as related to the naming of tumors.
- Differentiate between neoplastic and nonneoplastic growths.

Key Terms

benign
cachexia
cyst
emaciation

malignant
metastasis
neoplasms

 ## CANCER

The second leading cause of death in the United States is cancer. Only cardiovascular deaths occur with more frequency than deaths related to cancer. Despite its high mortality, cancer is not well understood. Before a cure for cancers can ever be discovered, scientists need to learn more about the causes and pathogenesis of cancers. However, great strides forward have been made in the study of cancer. In fact, in many circumstances, cancers like Hodgkin's lymphoma are curable, and the molecular basis of cancer is better understood now than ever.

CHARACTERISITCS OF BENIGN AND MALIGNANT TUMORS

The word *neoplasia* literally means "new growth," from *neo* (new) and *plasia* (growth). The study of tumors, or **neoplasms**, is called *oncology* from *oncos* (tumor) and *logos* (study). Unlike hyperplasia, which is an increase in the number of cells and overall size of tissue, neoplasia is abnormal growth. Neoplasms, which are commonly referred to as tumors, are not abnormal in the sense that they are too large or too small; they are abnormal growths because they should not be present at all. A neoplasm is an abnormal mass of tissue that, unlike normal tissue, exhibits an uncoordinated and excessive growth, as illustrated in Figure 7-1. Basically, neoplasms do not respond to normal growth controls and act as parasites that compete with normal cell growth.

Oncologists, or scientists who study tumors, divide neoplasms into two broad categories: benign and malignant. Not all tumors are cancers, and those that are not are referred to as **benign**. A benign tumor is not recurrent or progressive and may be referred to as nonmalignant. Benign tumors do not spread but remain localized. Typically they do not recur after surgical removal, and they do not cause extensive tissue damage. Benign tumors resemble surrounding tissues and do not result in whole-body changes. However, it should be noted that benign tumors can be responsible for serious diseases and can be fatal depending on their size and location.

A malignant tumor, in contrast, exhibits all the opposite features of benign tumors. **Malignant** tumors are known as cancers—derived from the Latin word for "crab"—because they infiltrate tissues with crablike extensions causing severe tissue destruction as they grow. In addition to their destructive growth patterns, cancers spread throughout the body. The spread of cancer is referred to as

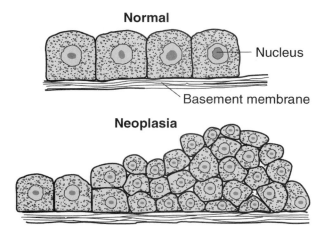

Figure 7-1 Normal tissue versus neoplasia.

Table 7-1 Comparison of Benign and Malignant Neoplasms

	Benign	Malignant
Growth	Grow by expansion	Grow by infiltration
Metastasis (spread)	Do not metastasize	Metastasize creating secondary foci
Surgical removal	Do not usually return	Can recur after removal
Tissue damage	Not extensive	Extensive
Tissue involvement	Localized changes	Whole-body changes
Appearance	Resemble tissue of origin	Do not resemble surrounding tissues
Survivability	Generally are not fatal	Fatal if not treated

metastasis. Table 7-1 provides a comparison of the characteristics of both benign and malignant neoplasms.

Although many cancers are fatal, all cancers are not lethal—assuming they are discovered early and treated successfully. The combination of high mortality and tissue destruction results in the need for restorative art skills on the part of the embalmer in cancer-related deaths. Treatments for cancer often involve amputation and the use of prosthetic devices, which require further restorative efforts by mortuary science professionals. Systemic changes to the body can result in numerous other potentially complicating factors (e.g., blood clotting changes, damage to blood vasculature, edema, dehydration) that can affect embalming.

TISSUE ORIGINS OF TUMORS

This chapter focuses on the histological comparison of tumors by classifying tumors based on the tissues from which they stem. Other texts may classify tumors based on their clinical manifestations—the tumors' behaviors and characteristics (e.g., how they spread or their appearance).

All neoplasms are composed of two portions: the transformed tumor cells and supporting connective tissues. Just like all living tissues, tumors have a blood supply embedded in their connective tissue layer. Tumors are outgrowths of basic body tissues, except they do not adhere to the mechanisms of proper growth regulation. For example, a melanocytic nevus is a benign tumor that is commonly known as a mole. The skin cells divide to replace dead cells that slough off the surface of the body, but for some as yet unexplained reason, the new skin cells do not form as they should. Instead, they grow into a mole. If they were to form a malignant tumor, it would be called skin cancer. The difference between skin cancer and a mole is that skin cancer destroys tissues, does not resemble other skin cells, and spreads throughout the body causing death, while a mole remains localized causing no damage to the body as a whole.

The four basic body tissues from which neoplasms originate are epithelial tissue, connective tissue, muscle tissue, and nervous tissue. Epithelial tissue may be a single layer (simple epithelium) or have multiple layers (stratified epithelium). It is found primarily within mucous membranes, serous membranes, and the epidermis of the skin. Additionally, a specialized type of epithelial tissue known as endothelium lines the blood vessels in the body. Epithelial tissue allows for the absorption, secretion, movement of substances, and general protection of the body from microorganisms.

 ## NAMING TUMORS

All neoplasms are divided into either benign tumors or malignant tumors, and their names are derived from their tissue of origin and whether or not they are cancerous. In almost all cases, benign tumors end with the suffix –*oma*. This suffix is attached to the name of the tissue from which the tumor originates. For example, a fibroma is a benign tumor of fibrous connective tissue. A chondroma is a benign tumor of cartilage. A lipoma is a benign tumor of fat. For a list of some of the more significant benign tumors, their tissue of origin, and their names, see Table 7-2.

Malignant tumors follow the same general naming structure as benign tumors with few exceptions. Instead of ending in the suffix –*oma,* the names of cancers generally end in either the suffix –*sarcoma* or –*carcinoma*. Generally speaking, sarcomas arise from connective tissues, while carcinomas originate in epithelial tissues. For example, a malignant tumor arising from fibrous connective tissue is known as a fibrosarcoma, and a malignant neoplasm composed of cartilaginous cells is a chondrosarcoma. Table 7-3 lists examples of malignant tumors, their tissue type, and their tissue of origin.

Although the following three tumors end with the suffix –*oma,* they are not benign, but, rather, they are malignant tumors: a glioma, a lymphoma, and a melanoma. A glioma is a form of brain cancer, a lymphoma is a cancer of the lymphatic system, and a melanoma is a skin cancer. Although they do not follow

Table 7-2 Benign Neoplasms

Tissue Type	Tissue of Origin	Tumor Name
Epithelial tissue	Epithelial lining of glands or ducts	Adenoma
	Epithelial lining of glands or ducts	Papilloma
	Tumor of melanocytes	Nevus
	Mucous membranes	Polyp
	Blood vessel endothelium	Hemangioma
Connective tissue	Bone	Osteoma
	Cartilage	Chondroma
	Fat	Lipoma
	Fibrous connective tissues	Fibroma
Muscle tissue	Striated muscle	Rhabdomyoma
	Smooth muscle	Leiomyoma
Nervous tissue	Nerves	Neuroma

Table 7-3 Malignant Neoplasms

Tissue Type	Tissue of Origin	Tumor Name
Epithelial tissue	Melanocytes	Melanoma
	Stratified squamous cells	Squamous cell carcinoma
	Epithelial lining of glands or ducts	Adenocarcinoma
	Urinary tract epithelium	Transitional cell carcinoma
	Basal cells of skin	Basal cell carcinoma
	Blood vessel endothelium	Hemangiosarcoma
Connective tissue	Bone	Osteosarcoma
	Cartilage	Chondrosarcoma
	Fat	Liposarcoma
	Fibrous connective tissue	Fibrosarcoma
	Lymph vessels	Lymphangiosarcoma
Muscle tissue	Striated muscle	Rhabdomyosarcoma
	Smooth muscle	Leiomyosarcoma
Nervous tissue	Brain	Glioma

the standard naming structure, these names are firmly entrenched in medical terminology.

SIGNIFICANT BENIGN TUMORS

Although there are too many benign tumors to describe in the pages of this textbook, the following section offers a brief description of some significant benign neoplasms. The purpose in describing these tumors is to provide a fuller understanding of the wide range of disease complications attributable to benign tumors. Most importantly, although benign tumors imply a certain level of innocent existence, they can be serious pathological disorders.

Benign Tumors of Epithelial Tissue

Adenomas. Pituitary adenomas typically are slow growing, benign neoplasms of epithelial origin. In most circumstances they arise from the anterior lobe of the pituitary gland and are capable of producing systemic disorders. In female, pituitary adenomas can cause the loss of menstruation, the spontaneous flow of milk from the breast, and infertility. In males, they can cause underdevelopment of the testicles, decreased sex drive, and impotence. Adenomas that secrete excess growth hormone can cause gigantism in children and acromegaly in adults.

Adenomas of the adrenal glands, which set atop the kidneys, can result in a disorder known as Cushing's disease in which cortisol is overproduced. Although symptoms vary from person to person, most patients have upper-body obesity, severe fatigue and muscle weakness, high blood pressure, backache, elevated blood sugar, easy bruising, and bluish-red stretch marks on the skin. In women, there may be increased growth of facial and body hair, and menstrual periods may become irregular or stop completely.

Papillomas. Papillomas are wartlike tumors caused by the human papilloma virus, which can cause abnormal tissue changes on the feet, hands, vocal cords, face, and genitals (see Color Plate 14). Papilloma lesions of the larynx can grow large enough to interfere with breathing and be fatal. The main treatment for laryngeal papilloma is surgical removal. Since the tumors are confined to the surface of the vocal folds, patients often retain their voice after surgery because the underlying vocal fold tissues are not damaged.

Genital warts are growths found on the external sex organs, as illustrated in Figure 7-2. They are usually painless, but may cause itching, burning, or slight bleeding. Warts can also be found around the urethra and anus. Inside the vagina and on the cervix, warts are usually flat and can be identified by a pap smear. There are two kinds of abnormal tissue caused by human papilloma virus: condyloma (warts) and dysplasia (precancer). Dysplasia is the presence of abnormal cells on the surface of the skin. Dysplasia is not cancer, but may progress into cancer over a period of years if it is not treated. The only way to tell if dysplasia is present on the skin of the genital organs is by a pap smear or biopsy.

Little is known about the spread of human papilloma virus, although it is mainly spread through sexual contact. Women may be exposed to human papilloma virus and not develop dysplasia or genital warts for many years. Both men and women can be infected with the virus and not know it. Interestingly, a link between human papilloma virus and cigarette smoking has been established. Smoking increases the chance of developing dysplasia, while stopping smoking may reduce the reappearance of dysplasia after treatment.

Polyps. Polyps can be found on the lining of the intestinal tract, trachea, esophagus, stomach, small intestine, or colon. Polyps can range in size from a few

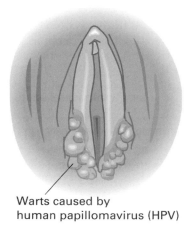

Warts caused by
human papillomavirus (HPV)

Figure 7-2 Genital warts.

millimeters to several centimeters in diameter. Inflammatory polyps occur with acute or chronic inflammation and are present by the dozen in cases of chronic ulcerative colitis. Polyps often require removal due to bleeding or blockage of the bowel. Some polyps are precancerous, meaning that they have a potential to develop into cancers over time.

Benign Tumors of Connective Tissue

Osteomas. An osteoma is a benign tumor originating in or consisting of bone tissue. Osteomas are found mostly on the bones of the face and skull, but may develop on the clavicle, pelvis, eye, tongue, or extremities. Typically, they cause no symptoms and are not treated. The presence of osteomas in the auditory canals of individuals who swim in cold water suggests that they may result from an inflammatory reaction.

Chondromas. Chondromas are rare, benign tumors that tend to arise at the base of the skull near the pituitary gland. This slow-growing tumor may be present but asymptomatic for a long time. Chondromas are composed of cartilage formed by the meninges that surround the brain and spinal cord. Because it is usually accessible and has well-defined margins, surgical removal is not uncommon.

Lipomas. Lipomas are benign tumors composed of fat cells, and they may occur in any fat tissues. They are common soft tissue lesions but are unusual in bone. Lipomas may grow within or between muscles, and, occasionally, they may be associated with nerve paralysis, bone deformity, and carpal tunnel syndrome. Lipomas of soft tissue are likely to be present in the tissues of the back, extremities, and thorax. Synovial lipomas are round or oval masses of fat covered with a synovial membrane in the knee.

Angiomas. An angioma is a benign tumor that consists of vessels. These tumors can be located anywhere on the body (see Color Plate 15). Some of the different types include spider angiomas, cherry angiomas, and senile angiomas. Benign tumors of blood vessels are known as hemangiomas, while benign tumors of lymph vessels are known as lymphangiomas. Port-wine stains, or birthmarks, are hemangiomas of the capillaries. Although they are not generally treated due to disease symptoms, they may be treated for cosmetic reasons. They may be removed through electrification or liquid nitrogen may be sprayed on the skin. Although infrequent, angiomas may recur after removal.

Fibromas. Fibromas are a category of benign tumor composed of fibrous tissue. Ossifying fibromas are firm and gritty and often involve the maxilla and mandible. A particularly aggressive form of ossifying fibroma, known as aggressive juvenile ossifying fibroma, can destroy the maxilla and adjacent structures. Fibromas also occur in the ovaries, and some forms are capable of synthesizing both male and female sex hormones in the ovary.

Benign Tumors of Muscle Tissue

Rhabdomyomas.   Rhabdomyomas are benign tumors that are the most common primary cardiac tumors in the fetus, neonate, and young child. Rhabdomyomas are the result of excessive growth of muscle elements within the muscular walls of the heart. In 50 percent of the cases, rhabdomyoma is associated with tuberous sclerosis. Tuberous sclerosis is a genetic disease that affects different family members at different rates. The prognosis depends on the number, size, and location of the tumors. About one-third of infants with tuberous sclerosis die, and most experience seizures and mental disability.

Leiomyomas.   Leiomyomas are benign tumors that arise from smooth muscle and may develop wherever smooth muscle is present. For example, leiomyomas may originate from the tunica media within the walls of arteries and veins, muscle of the male scrotum or the labia majora of the vagina, or the erectile muscles of the nipple. Uterine leiomyomas are the most common neoplasms of the female genital tract. They are frequent in women over 30, rare in women younger than 18, and they are less likely after menopause. They are one of the most frequent reasons for major surgery during women's reproductive years.

Benign Tumor of Nervous Tissue

Neuromas.   A benign tumor of nervous tissue is known as a neuroma. Acoustic neuromas usually grow slowly on the eighth cranial nerve leading from the brain to the inner ear over a period of years. The brain is not invaded by the growing tumor, but the tumor pushes the brain as it enlarges. Acoustic neuromas may affect balance, hearing, and facial muscles. Neuromas can also press on the trigeminal nerve, affecting facial sensation. Although it is rare, when neuromas cause severe pressure on the brainstem and cerebellum, they may be fatal.

Neuromas may also occur on the peripheral nerves of the feet. Even though a neuroma can occur at any site in the foot, the most common place is between the third and fourth toes. Almost 90 percent of the cases occur in women, and the most common complaint is a sharp pain in the ball of the foot with tingling and numbness traveling to the toes. When the foot is squeezed, a clicking sound may be heard called Mulder's Sign. This sign is frequently, but not always, present with neuromas in the foot.

SIGNIFICANT MALIGNANT TUMORS

This section offers a brief description of some important malignant neoplasms. The purpose in describing these tumors is to provide a fuller understanding of the effects that cancer has on the entire body as an organism. Unlike benign tumors that simply have the potential to initiate disease complications, malignant tumors almost always manifest in severe disease conditions and death if not treated.

Malignant Tumors of Epithelial Tissue

Melanomas. Melanoma is a serious form of skin cancer that begins in the melanocytes, which are the cells that make skin pigment called melanin (see Color Plate 16). Although melanoma accounts for only about 4 percent of all skin cancer cases, it causes most skin cancer–related deaths. Melanoma is often curable if detected and treated in its early stages. The chance of developing melanoma increases with age, but it affects all age groups and is one of the most common cancers in young adults. The occurrence of melanoma is exacerbated by exposure to sunlight. Melanoma may occur in the skin, in the eye, and, rarely, in other areas where melanocytes are found, such as the digestive tract, meninges, or lymph nodes. Melanoma may metastasize, spreading cancer cells to the lymph nodes, liver, lungs, or brain. The signs of melanoma are:

- A growth that increases in size and appears brown, black, red, pink, or multicolored.
- A mole that changes color, texture, or shape, or grows larger than a pencil eraser.
- A spot or growth that itches, hurts, crusts, scabs, erodes, or bleeds.
- A sore that lasts for more than four weeks, or heals and then reopens.
- A scaly bump that grows a projection similar to a small horn.

Squamous Cell Carcinomas. Squamous cell carcinoma is the second most common skin cancer. It arises from the epidermis and resembles the squamous cells in the outer layers of the skin (see Color Plate 17). Although squamous cell carcinomas may remain isolated in the epidermis, they eventually penetrate the underlying tissues if not treated. In a small percentage of cases, squamous cell carcinoma will metastasize.

Squamous cell carcinoma is most common on sun-exposed parts of the body, leading scientists to believe that chronic exposure to sunlight causes squamous cell carcinoma. However, some researchers believe that squamous cell carcinoma may be inherited as well. This form of skin cancer is likely to appear on the ear, lower lip, face, neck, bald scalp, hands, shoulders, arms, or back. Individuals with dark skin complexion are less likely than fair-skinned individuals to develop skin cancer.

More than two-thirds of the skin cancers that do develop are squamous cell carcinomas, usually arising on the sites of preexisting inflammatory skin conditions or burns. Any changes in a preexisting skin growth such as a mole, or the presence of an open sore that fails to heal, should prompt an individual to seek medical attention. Early treatment of precancerous lesions may prevent them from developing into squamous cell carcinoma.

Adenocarcinomas. The World Health Organization defines adenocarcinoma as a malignant epithelial tumor with tubular, acinar, or papillary growth patterns, or mucus production by the tumor cells. Basically, this definition implies that adenocarcinomas look like the tissues of a gland, and they can produce fluids. Many forms of cancer can produce fluids, which may cause edema in the abdomen or chest, calling for thorough aspiration of the deceased to retard decomposition. Adenocarcinomas are most likely to occur in the lungs, esophagus, colon, or the parotid salivary glands. Color Plate 18 is a photograph of an ulcerated adenocarcinoma of the colon.

Adenocarcinoma is the most common type of lung cancer, especially among women and nonsmokers. It is among a family of cancers known as non-small cell carcinomas. Oncologists refer to the three Ps of adenocarcinomas—peripheral, pigmented, and puckered. The majority of adenocarcinomas occur at the periphery of the lung, and often cause no symptoms until they are well developed. Patients, therefore, may have no idea that they have cancer, until it has spread throughout their body and is already beyond treatment and, therefore, fatal. They frequently lie just below the membranes that surround the lungs, which are known as the pleura. The pleural surface is retracted (puckered) over the neoplasm. The combination of the black pigmentation and the mucus secreted by the tumor gives it a glistening, pale gray color. Adenocarcinomas may result from scars caused by previous diseases and trauma to the lungs.

Transitional Cell Carcinomas. Although transitional cell carcinoma can occur anywhere that transitional cells are present, it is the most common cancer of the urinary system. It arises from the transitional epithelium lining the urinary system, and it is fatal unless treated. Upper-urinary-tract tumors may be present bilaterally, meaning that they are found in both kidneys at the same time. Transitional cell carcinoma in the urinary system is twice as common among Caucasians as African Americans, with men being affected two to three times more frequently than women. Symptoms of renal cancer include bloody urine and a dull pain caused by the gradual obstruction of the urinary collecting system. People who work in the chemical, petrochemical, aniline dye, and plastics industries, and those exposed to coal, coke, tar, and asphalt are at increased risk for transitional cell carcinoma of the urinary system.

Basal Cell Carcinomas. Basal cell carcinoma is not only the most common form of skin cancer, it is the most common of all cancers; one out of every three new cancers is a skin cancer. Basal cell carcinomas are most common in older men who have spent a majority of their lifetime outdoors. However, the average age of onset of the disease has steadily decreased, and more women are developing basal cell carcinomas. Chronic exposure to sunlight is believed to be the cause of almost all basal cell carcinomas. Occasionally, however, contact with arsenic, exposure to radiation, and complications of burns, scars, vaccinations, and tattoos have been suspected as causes of basal cell carcinoma. Basal cell carcinoma occurs most frequently on the face, ears, neck, scalp, shoulders, and back, and arises from the basal cells in the epithelial tissues of the skin (see Color Plate 19). Following are important warning signs of basal cell carcinoma:

- An open sore that bleeds, oozes, or crusts and remains open for three or more weeks.
- A reddish patch that crusts, itches, or hurts, located on the chest, shoulders, arms, or legs.
- A shiny bump that is translucent or pink, red, white, black, or brown.
- A pink growth with an elevated border and a crusted indentation in the center.

- The appearance of tiny blood vessels on the surface of a growth as it enlarges.
- A scarlike area that is white, yellow, or waxy with poorly defined borders.
- Shiny and taut skin around a growth.

Malignant Tumors of Connective Tissue

Osteosarcomas. Osteosarcoma is an aggressive, rapid growing tumor that often spreads to the lungs in its early stages. This form of bone cancer appears as a hard, white tissue with scattered areas of fleshlike tissue that bleeds. Osteosarcomas are painful, enlarging masses that can invade joints by growing along the path of surrounding ligaments. Survival rates are good when tumors respond to chemotherapy and surgery. A high percentage of osteosarcoma respond to chemotherapy, which is useful to suppress and treat metastases. Chemotherapy is responsible for a dramatic increase in survival rates and a decrease in the need for amputation. When the tumor is not responsive to chemotherapy, amputation is necessary to contain the spread of this cancer of the bone.

Chondrosarcomas. Chondrosarcoma is a type of bone cancer that primarily affects the cartilage cells of the femur, arm, pelvis, knee, and spine. Although less frequent, other areas such as the ribs may be affected. Chondrosarcoma is the second most common cancer of bone and it is most common between the ages of 50 and 70. Although the exact cause of chondrosarcoma is not known, scientists believe this form of bone cancer may be inherited. Treatment for chondrosarcomas may include surgery, radiation therapy, physical therapy, and chemotherapy. Following are characteristic signs and symptoms of chondrosarcoma:

- Presence of a large mass on the affected bone.
- Feelings of pressure around the mass.
- Pain that is worse at night.
- Pain that is not relieved through rest.
- Pain that may be present for years but increases gradually over time.

Liposarcomas. Liposarcoma is a fatty, cancerous tumor that grows in deep connective tissue spaces—primarily behind the knee (popliteal space), in the medial thigh, behind the digestive organs (retroperitoneal region), and in the shoulder area. Although liposarcoma is one of the least frequent soft tissue sarcomas occurring in childhood, when it does occur in children, it favors the lower extremities. Surgical excision is the treatment of choice for these tumors; however, their location may make complete removal difficult. Even after surgical removal, local recurrences are common, and metastases often are observed in the lung and liver, resulting in high mortality rates. Almost two-thirds of children with liposarcoma are boys. The cancer appears in infancy at an average age of 14 months, and in early adolescence at an average age of about 13.

Angiosarcomas. Angiosarcomas are uncommon, malignant neoplasms that grow rapidly, arising from cells derived from vessels. They are aggressive, spreading throughout lymph nodes and the rest of the body. They are more frequent in skin and soft tissue but may occur in any region of the body, including the liver, breast, spleen, bone, or heart. Angiosarcomas have a high mortality rate owing to their biological properties and their misdiagnosis. Often, the cancer is advanced by the time signs and symptoms appear. Malignant vascular tumors can be aggressive, difficult to treat, and fatal. Angiosarcoma of the liver and bone are more frequent in males, and angiosarcoma of the breast is most common in premenopausal women between 30 and 50 years old. Malignant tumors of blood vessels are known as hemangiosarcomas, and malignant tumors of lymph vessels are known as lymphangiosarcomas.

Fibrosarcomas. Fibrosarcomas of bone are large, destructive, infiltrating malignant tumors consisting of fibrous tissue. They occur most often in the extremities and result in pathologic bone fractures because the tumor infiltrates the surrounding soft tissues and bones as it grows and spreads. Recurrence after surgery is common, and bone cancer due to fibrosarcoma is fatal if not treated.

Lymphomas. Lymphoma is a malignant tumor that results from a mutation during lymphocyte production. Cancerous lymphocytes can grow in many parts of the body, including the lymph nodes, spleen, bone marrow, blood, or other organs. Hodgkin's disease and non-Hodgkin's lymphoma are the two main types of cancer of the lymphatic system. Following are some typical symptoms of lymphoma:

- Painless swelling of the lymph nodes in the neck, axillary space, or groin
- Swelling in the legs or ankles
- Abdominal discomfort or bloating
- Fever
- Weight loss
- Night sweats
- Chills
- Lack of energy
- Itching (pruritis)

Malignant Tumors of Muscle Tissue

Rhabdomyosarcomas. Rhabdomyosarcoma is a rare, fast-growing, malignant tumor that accounts for over half of the soft tissue sarcomas in children. Although it also affects adolescents between the ages of 13 and 15, it is more common among children ages 1 to 5. The most common sites of rhabdomyosarcomas are the head, neck, urogenital tract, and the extremities. Rhabdomyosarcoma often causes a noticeable lump on a child's body, but other signs may also be present. For example, tumors in the nose or throat may cause bleeding, congestion, swallowing problems, or neurological problems if they extend into the brain.

Diagnosis of rhabdomyosarcoma is often delayed due to a lack of symptoms, and it is usually diagnosed during examinations associated with other injuries. Surgery and radiation therapy are used to treat the primary site of the tumor, while chemotherapy is used to treat the spread of rhabdomyosarcoma throughout the body. The mortality rate of this form of cancer is high, with only 50 percent of children with rhabdomyosarcoma surviving five years.

Leiomyosarcomas. A leiomyosarcoma is a malignant neoplasm of smooth muscle that commonly metastasizes to the lungs, although leiomyosarcomas in the digestive system are more likely to spread to the liver. Smooth muscle is the muscle tissue found in the walls of muscular organs like the heart and stomach as well as the walls of blood vessels. Although leiomyosarcomas can develop at any site in the body, the most common sites are the uterus and the stomach. Leiomyosarcomas usually start as a rapidly growing, painless, swellings in the wall of an organ or a blood vessel. The treatment for leiomyosarcoma is surgery, radiation therapy, and chemotherapy.

Malignant Tumor of Nervous Tissue

Gliomas. Glioma is a form of brain cancer that arises from supporting cells in the brain called glial cells. There are three types of glioma named after the cells from which they originate: astrocytomas, ependymomas, and oligodendrogliomas, all of which occur in the frontal and temporal lobes of the cerebrum of the brain and spread through the cerebrospinal fluid to the spinal cord. Brain tumors, like all tumors, are graded from one through four depending on their malignancy and rate of growth. Grade one is the least advanced and grade four the most. Grade one and two tumors may be referred to as low grade tumors, and three and four as high grade.

The symptoms of gliomas are caused by the blockage of the ventricles of the brain, leading to increased intracranial pressure due to the buildup of cerebrospinal fluid and the swelling of brain tissue. Treatment for brain cancers includes surgery, radiation therapy, and chemotherapy. Depending on the location and extent of the glioma, it may be inoperable. Mortality for gliomas is high, and for unknown reasons, they are more common in men than women.

Gliomas are characterized by:

- Headaches
- Vomiting
- Visual impairment
- Changes in mood, behavior, and personality
- Paralysis and problems with coordination, speech, and memory

CYSTS

A **cyst** is defined as a sac within or on the body surface containing air or fluid, although a cyst may also be defined as a closed pocket or pouch of tissue that can be filled with air, fluid, pus, or other material. Two of the most common forms of cysts are ovarian cysts and sebaceous cysts.

Ovarian Cysts

An ovarian cyst is a fluid-filled sac that develops in the ovary and consists of one or more chambers. Although they are not malignant, ovarian cysts may have to be removed surgically because of twisting of part of the ovary, which may lead to gangrene. Another reason to remove ovarian cysts is the pressure they may exert on surrounding tissues as they grow.

Ovarian cysts may be present at birth, or they may occur late in women's lives. Most ovarian cysts occur during women's childbearing years, and, although they are usually benign, they may mask the presence of other conditions, such as cancer, ectopic pregnancy, or appendicitis.

Ovarian cysts frequently occur and resolve without treatment during women's menstrual cycle. Normally, women experience no symptoms or signs of ovarian cysts. When they rupture, however, they can lead to sharp, severe abdominal pain, which is experienced by 25 percent of menstruating women (Kazzi and Roberts 2001). Ovarian cysts may also become inflamed and cause spontaneous bleeding. Sometimes, ovarian cysts can lead to more complicated cyst formation, which can result in infection, blood clots in the ovarian vessels, emboli in the lungs, blood poisoning, and death. Ovarian cysts may also be associated with infertility and irregular menstrual bleeding. In infants, ovarian cysts can cause abdominal edema (ascites) and insufficient development of the lungs or kidneys. Ovarian cysts occur in 30 percent of women with regular menstrual cycles and 50 percent of women with irregular menstrual cycles.

Sebacious Cysts

A sebaceous cyst is a closed sac found just under the skin containing a cheeselike material formed from skin secretions (Lehrer 2003). Sebaceous cysts, which are also known as epidermal cysts, keratin cysts, or epidermoid cysts, are the product of swollen hair follicles or trauma to the skin. A sac of cells is created when a protein known as keratin is secreted from sebaceous sweat glands.

Sebaceous cysts are commonly found on the face, neck, and trunk of the body. Color Plate 20 is a photograph of an epidermoid cyst in the urethra of the penis. They are usually slow-growing, painless, lumps under the skin; however, they may become inflamed and painful. They may be accompanied by redness and a grayish white, cheesy, foul smelling material that drains from the cyst. Typically, sebaceous cysts do not require treatment, although they may be excised by a healthcare provider if they form an abscess. It is not uncommon for sebaceous cysts to return after they are surgically removed.

NONNEOPLASTIC CHANGES

It is important to remember that not all changes in body tissues are neoplastic in nature. Cells adapt to their environment through hypertrophy, hyperplasia, and metaplasia, and none of these changes necessarily signals the presence of neoplasms. When cells increase in size during hypertrophy, there is no increase in the number of cells, as there is in neoplasia. Similarly, during hypertrophy, the increase in the number of cells present does not necessarily signal the presence of tumors. For example, cells in the tissues of the female uterus both increase in number and in size during pregnancy, which is a form of nonneoplastic change. And when one cell type is replaced by another cell type during reversible metaplasia during the healing process, no neoplasms are necessarily present. However, it should be noted that nonneoplastic changes in body tissues may potentially mask the presence of an underlying neoplasm.

POSTMORTEM CONDITIONS ASSOCIATED WITH NEOPLASMS

As a leading cause of death, embalmers will frequently encounter person's who have died due to malignant neoplasms. It is important for the embalmer to be familiar with seven common postmortem conditions associated with neoplasms:

1. Emaciation
2. Dehydration
3. Cachexia
4. Discoloration
5. Hemorrhage
6. Tissue Deformation
7. Extravascular Obstruction

One aspect of most cancers is that they are debilitating. Besides the direct effect of the tumors themselves on the body, there are a variety of iatrogenic disorders related to radiation therapy, chemotherapy, and the surgical excision of malignant tissues. Although the severity of debilitation varies from one person to the next, the embalmer can expect cancer deaths to include excess fluids near tumors, loss of hair (alopecia), jaundice, blood clotting disorders, and prosthetic devices.

Long periods of debilitation may also be associated with the presence of bedsores, dehydration, and cachexia. **Emaciation** is the state of being extremely lean, and debilitating diseases are associated with atrophy of tissues resulting in emaciation. Chronic diseases like cancer often result in **cachexia**, which refers to malnutrition and a general wasting of the body. The deceased child pictured in Figure 7-3 is cachexic due to starvation. Emaciation and cachexia may necessitate the hypodermic injection of tissue builder in the shallow or sunken areas of the face such as the temples or the orbits of the eyes.

The method of growth of both benign and malignant neoplasms can complicate the embalming process. Because benign tumors grow by expansion, they may compress neighboring blood vessels, inhibiting the distribution of embalming fluids. Malignant neoplasms grow by infiltration, causing extensive tissue damage and deformation. Entire areas of the body may require surface embalming and sectional embalming techniques. Deformations of the deceased will likely require restorative art techniques as well.

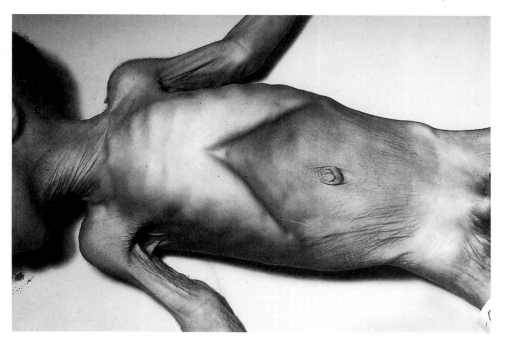

Figure 7-3 Cachexia and emaciation due to starvation. (Reprinted with permission from Vincent J. DiMaio and Dominick DiMaio, 2001, *Forensic pathology*, 2nd ed. Copyright CRC Press, Boca Raton, FL.)

REVIEW QUESTIONS

Matching

1. _____ fibrosarcoma
2. _____ emaciation
3. _____ leiomyosarcoma
4. _____ papillomas
5. _____ basal cell carcinoma

a. a malignant neoplasm of smooth muscle that commonly metastasizes to the lungs

b. the state of being extremely lean

c. large, destructive, infiltrating malignant tumors consisting of fibrous tissue

d. the most common form of skin cancer

e. wartlike tumors

Multiple Choice

1. Which of the following is true of benign tumors?
    a. They grow by expansion.
    b. They metastasize, creating secondary foci.
    c. They cause whole-body changes.
    d. They cause extensive tissue damage.
2. Which of the following is another name for a melanocytic nevus?
    a. wart
    b. plaque
    c. mole
    d. birthmark
3. Which of the following is a benign tumor?
    a. glioma
    b. lymphoma
    c. melanoma
    d. osteoma
4. Which of the following tumors originates from epithelial tissue?
    a. neuroma
    b. squamous cell carcinoma
    c. fibrosarcoma
    d. Hodgkin's lymphoma
5. Which of the following tumors is found in the urinary tract?
    a. chondrosarcoma
    b. angiosarcoma
    c. rhabdomyosarcoma
    d. transitional cell carcinoma

Putting Learning to Work!

The purpose of the following case analysis is to allow you to apply the information you have learned in a real-world situation. Read the case carefully and try to answer the following questions:

What disorder do you suspect the person had at the time of death?

What potential embalming complications do you anticipate?

What precautions should you take as the embalmer to limit the effects of these complications?

Case Analysis

An 81-year-old woman is found dead in her apartment. She lived alone in a government housing project. She was found on the bathroom floor by her neighbor. It was widely known in the apartment complex that the woman frowned on medical treatment in favor of home remedies. The neighbor knew she needed medical care because she had heard the woman vomiting on several occasions, and the woman asked her to read a letter from her son because she was having headaches that made it hard for her to see well enough to read. The neighbor also thought that the woman might have had Alzheimer's disease because she could not remember the neighbor about a month earlier in the hallway. The woman also developed a problem with her speech, and she seemed to have trouble with her coordination.

Six months earlier her personality was that of a different woman. She was always outside on the steps talking with her neighbors and watching the children play. Recently, the neighbor states that she almost never saw the woman out of the apartment. When the neighbor offered help two weeks earlier, the woman was belligerent and told her to leave.

Bibliography

About squamous cells. (n.d.). Retrieved May 29, 2003, from The Skin Cancer Foundation at http://www.skin cancer.org/squamous/index.php.

Carsi, B., & Sim, F. (2001). Angiosarcoma. Retrieved May 29, 2003, from eMedicine at http://www.emedicine. com/med/topic138.htm.

Chondrosarcoma. (2001). Retrieved May 29, 2003, from ViaHealth at http://www.viahealth.org/disease/ bone_disorders/chondrosar.htm.

Corno, A., de Simone, G., & Catena, G. (1984). Cardiac rhabdomyoma: Surgical treatment in the neonate. *Journal of Thoracic Cardiovascular Surgery, 87*, 725.

DeGroot, H. (2003). *Osteoma*. Retrieved May 29, 2003, from http://bonetumor.org/tumors/pages/page12.html.

Donegan, W., Spratt, J., & Orsini, J. (Eds.). (2002). *Cancer of the breast*. Philadelphia: Saunders.

Enneking, W. (1995). Osteosarcoma. In *Musculoskeletal pathology*. Retrieved May 29, 2003, from http://www.med.ufl.edu/medinfo/ortho/ostsarc.html#A1.

Fibrosarcoma. (n.d.). In *The encyclopedia of medical imaging* (Vol. III). Retrieved May 29, 2003, from Amersham Health at http://www.amershamhealth.com/medcyclopaedia/Volume%20III%201/ FIBROSARCOMA.asp.

Fretz, P., & Hughes, J. (2003). *Adenocarcinoma: Lung tumors*. Retrieved May 29, 2003, from the Virtual Hospital, University of Iowa Health Care at http://www.vh.org/adult/provider/radiology/LungTumors/ PathologicTypes/Text/Adenocarcinoma.html.

Hall, P. (2003). *Metaplasia*. Retrieved May 28, 2003, from Academic Pathology, Queen's University Belfast at http://www.qub.ac.uk/cm/pat/undergraduate/Basiccancer/metaplasia.htm.

Howard, S. (2002). Rhabdomyosarcoma. In *Medical Encyclopedia*. Retrieved May 29, 2003, from MedlinePlus, the U.S. National Library of Medicine and the National Institutes of Health at http://www.nlm.nih.gov/ medlineplus/ency/article/001429.htm.

Human papilloma virus. (1997). Retrieved May 29, 2003, from the Department of Gynecology and Obstetrics, University of Iowa at http://obgyn.uihc.uiowa.edu/Patinfo/Adhealth/hpv.htm.

Interstitial cystitis. (2002). Retrieved June 9, 2003, from the National Kidney and Urologic Diseases Information Clearinghouse, National Institutes of Health at http://www.niddk.nih.gov/health/urolog/pubs/cystitis/cystitis.htm.

Kazzi, Amine A., & Roberts, Robin. (2001). Ovarian cysts. Retrieved March 14, 2004, from eMedicine at http://www.emedicine.com/EMERG/topic352.htm.

Knopf, K. (2002). Endometrial cancer. In *Medical Encyclopedia*. Retrieved July 25, 2003, from MedlinePlus, the U.S. National Library of Medicine and the National Institutes of Health at http://www.nlm.nih.gov/medlineplus/ency/article/000910.htm.

Knowles, D. (2002). Leydig cell tumors. In *Medical Encyclopedia*. Retrieved July 25, 2003, from MedlinePlus, the U.S. National Library of Medicine and the National Institutes of Health at http://www.nlm.nih.gov/medlineplus/ency/article/000409.htm.

Konety, B., & Pirtskhalaishvili, G. (2002). *Transitional cell carcinoma, renal*. Retrieved May 29, 2003, from eMedicine at http://www.emedicine.com/med/topic2003.htm.

Konstantakos, A., & Dudgeon, D. (2002). *Liposarcoma*. Retrieved May 29, 2003, from eMedicine at http://www.emedicine.com/ped/topic1317.htm.

Kumar, V., Cotran, R., & Robbins, S. (2003). *Robbins basic pathology* (7th ed.). Philadelphia: Saunders.

Learning about lymphoma. (2002). Retrieved May 29, 2003, from the Lymphoma Research Foundation at http://www.lymphoma.org/site/PageServer?pagename=lymphoma.

Lehrer, Michael. (2003). Sebaceous cysts. In *Medical Encyclopedia*. Retrieved March 14, 2004, from MedlinePlus, the U.S. National Library of Medicine and the National Institutes of Health at http://www.nlm.nih.gov/medlineplus/ency/article/000842.htm.

Lipoma. (n.d.). In *The encyclopedia of medical imaging* (Vol. III:1). Retrieved May 29, 2003, from Amersham Health at http://www.amershamhealth.com/medcyclopaedia/Volume%20III%201/LIPOMA.asp.

Lung cancer: Hard to cure, easy to prevent. (2003). In *Physicians desk reference series*. Retrieved July 23, 2003, from Thomson Learning at http://www.gettingwell.com/content/lifelong_health/chapters/fgac30.shtml.

Lymphoma.com. (n.d.). Retrieved June 5, 2003, from http://www.lymphoma.com.

Mayer, R. (2000). *Embalming: History, theory, & practice* (3rd ed.). New York: McGraw-Hill.

Miethke, M., & Raugi, G. (2003). *Leiomyoma*. Retrieved May 29, 2003, from eMedicine at http://www.emedicine.com/DERM/topic217.htm.

Mixed giomas: The cancer BACUP factsheet. (2001). Retrieved May 29, 2003, from the British Association of Cancer United Patients at http://www.cancerbacup.org.uk/info/mixedglioma.htm.

Neighbors, M., & Tannehill-Jones, R. (2000). *Human diseases*. Clifton Park, NY: Thomson Delmar Publishing.

Ovarian cyst. (2003). Retrieved July 25, 2003, from the American Academy of Family Physicians at http://familydoctor.org/handouts/279.html.

Papilloma. (2002). Retrieved May 29, 2003, from The Voice Disorders Center at the Massachusetts Eye and Ear Infirmary, Harvard Medical School Teaching Hospital at http://www.voicedisordercenter.meei.harvard.edu/disorders/papilloma.html.

Pathology for funeral service. (1999). Dallas, TX: Professional Training Schools.

Peckham, M., Pinedo, H., & Veronesi, U. (Eds.). (1995). *Oxford textbook of oncology*. New York: Oxford University Press.

Raghavan, D., Brecher, M., Johnson, D., Meropol, N., Moots, P., & Thigpen, J. (Eds.). (1999). *Textbook of uncommon cancer*. New York: Wiley.

Rhabdomyosarcoma. (2002). Retrieved May 29, 2003, from the Pediatric Oncology Resource Center at http://www.acor.org/diseases/ped-onc/diseases/rhabdo.html.

Sachdeva, K., & Makhoul, I. (2002). *Renal cell carcinoma*. Retrieved June 9, 2003, from eMedicine at http://www.emedicine.com/MED/topic2002.htm.

Shelton, H. (1992). *Boyd's introduction to the study of disease* (11th ed.). Philadelphia: Lea & Febiger.

Sowaka, J., Gurwood, A., & Kabat, K. (2001). Pituitary adenoma. In *Handbook of ocular disease management*. Jobson Publishing. Retrieved May 29, 2003, from http://www.revoptom.com/handbook/SECT54a.HTM.

Steinberg, G., & Kim, H. (2002). *Bladder cancer*. Retrieved June 9, 2003, from eMedicine at http://www.emedicine.com/med/topic2344.htm.

Testicular cancer. (2003). Retrieved July 25, 2003, from MedlinePlus, the U.S. National Library of Medicine and the National Institutes of Health at http://www.nlm.nih.gov/medlineplus/testicularcancer.html.

Vanni, R. (2002). Uterus: Leiomyoma. In *Atlas of genetics and cytogenetics in oncology haematology*. Retrieved May 29, 2003, from http://www.infobiogen.fr/services/chromcancer/Tumors/leiomyomID5031.html.

Venes, D. (Ed.). (2001). *Taber's cyclopedic medical dictionary* (19th ed.). Philadelphia: F. A. Davis.

What is leiomyosarcoma? (2001). Retrieved May 29, 2003, from the British Association of Cancer United Patients at http://www.cancerbacup.org.uk/questions/specific/sarcomas/sts/leiomyosarcoma.htm.

What is liver cancer? (n.d.). Retrieved June 7, 2003, from the American Cancer Society at http://www.cancer.org/docroot/cri/content/cri_2_2_1x_what_is_liver_cancer_25.asp.

What you need to know about cancer of the colon and rectum. (2002). Retrieved June 7, 2003, from the National Cancer Institute, National Institutes of Health at http://www.cancer.gov/cancerinfo/wyntk/colon-and-rectum.

What you need to know about cancer of the pancreas. (2002). Retrieved June 7, 2003, from the National Cancer Institute, National Institutes of Health at http://www.cancer.gov/cancerinfo/wyntk/pancreas.

CHAPTER 8

Diseases of the Blood

Learning Objectives

Upon completion of the chapter, review questions, and case analysis, the reader should be able to:

- Describe leukocytosis and leukopenia along with their associated disease complications.
- Define anemia and explain the differences in primary anemia and secondary anemia.
- Compare and contrast the hemopoietic disorders leukemia and polycythemia vera.
- Differentiate between the bleeding disorders hemophilia, thrombocytopenia, and purpura.
- Explain the pathogenesis of hemolytic disease of the newborn.

Key Terms

anemia
erythrocytosis
hemophilia
leukemia

leukocytosis
leukopenia
purpura
thrombocytopenia

 ## DISORDERS OF THE BLOOD

There are numerous disorders of the blood, but they generally can be divided into one of three categories: diseases of the red blood cells, diseases of the white blood cells, or bleeding disorders. Diseases of the red blood cells are usually associated with anemia. Diseases of the white blood cells are normally associated with a disorder of the growth of white blood cells. Because the blood is present throughout the body, diseases involving the blood may present in several anatomic locations, affecting multiple organs and tissues. While reading this chapter, the reader may review the components of blood by referring to Appendix C.

Leukocytosis

Leukocytosis is an increase in the number of white blood cells in the blood. It is a condition associated with a reactive change within the blood. Leukocytosis should not be confused with leukemia, which is a form of white blood cell cancer associated with the excessive malformation of white blood cells. Leukocytosis does not usually occur in viral infections and may be caused by any of the following:

- Hemorrhage
- Extensive surgeries
- Coronary occlusions
- Cancer
- Pregnancy
- Chemical intoxication
- Toxemias (poisons)

Leukopenia

A reactive change in the composition of blood, **leukopenia** is a disease condition in which there are a decreased number of white blood cells in the blood. It may be caused by a wide variety of pharmaceutical agents, as well as a failure of bone marrow to produce white blood cells. Leukopenia is common after both chemotherapy treatments and radiation therapy in treating cancer, as well as in some viral diseases like HIV, which affect the immune system.

Anemia

Anemia is a blood disorder in which the capacity of the blood to transport oxygen is decreased, usually because the total number of red blood cells is diminished. The two broad categories of anemia are primary anemia and secondary anemia. Primary anemia includes those types of anemia in which there is a decrease in the production of red blood cells, while secondary anemia includes those anemias in which there is an increased loss or destruction of red blood cells. There is a wide variety of types of anemia, and each is treated by its cause. Generally speaking, anemia results from bleeding or from decreased levels of red blood cells, due to either their increased destruction or decreased production in the body.

Aplastic Anemia. Aplastic anemia is caused by improper growth or impaired function of bone marrow. Chemicals such as benzene and arsenic may cause destruction of bone marrow. X-rays and ionizing radiation are physical agents that may damage the bone marrow as well. In cases of aplastic anemia, the red bone marrow is unable to produce adequate amounts of red blood cells to transport hemoglobin.

Hemolytic Anemia. Hemolytic anemia results from the hemolysis, or rupturing, of red blood cells prematurely. Hemolytic anemia may be a congenital disorder, or it may be due to the effects of toxic agents. In this form of anemia, the hemoglobin separates into heme and globin prematurely, reducing the available amount of hemoglobin in the blood to transport the oxygen.

Pernicious Anemia. Pernicious anemia is caused by a failure of the body to produce enough intrinsic factor, an intestinal chemical, to absorb vitamin B_{12} in the intestine. Vitamin B_{12} is required for the process of absorbing iron in the diet. Sufficient levels of iron ingestion in the diet are important for red blood cell production because red blood cells are capable of transporting oxygen in their hemoglobin. The binding site for oxygen within the hemoglobin is the heme, which consists primarily of iron. Green, leafy vegetables like spinach are an excellent source of iron. Remember, however, that pernicious anemia is not due to a lack of iron in the diet, it is due to a lack of intrinsic factor, which allows the proper absorption of iron from digesting food. Eating more iron-containing foods, therefore, does not resolve cases of pernicious anemia.

Sickle Cell Anemia. Sickle cell anemia is a hereditary, chronic anemia, characterized by the presence of a large number of crescent- or sickle-shaped red blood cells. To inherit sickle cell anemia, both parents must have possessed the recessive gene for hemoglobin S. Inheriting the trait for hemoglobin S from only one parent results in other forms of sickle cell anemia, which are not discussed here (i.e., sickle cell-b0 thalassemia, hemoglobin SC disease, or sickle cell-b + thalassemia). Figure 8-1 describes the chain of events associated with malformed red blood cells, and the disorders sickle cell anemia can cause.

The alteration in the hemoglobin of these deformed red blood cells is due to a single amino acid substitution in one of the chains of amino acids from which hemoglobin is produced, resulting in hemoglobin S. Because people with sickle trait were more likely to survive malaria outbreaks in Africa than those with normal hemoglobin, it is believed that hemoglobin S is a genetic alteration that evolved as a protection against malaria.

Sickle cell anemia is usually present after about six months of age. It continues throughout life with sudden exacerbated episodes known as crises. The most serious crises involve severe pain emanating from damaged bone marrow, which leads to necrosis of the bone marrow. Fat emboli can spread from the necrotic bone marrow, causing sudden death by stroke or heart failure. Around the world, sickle cell anemia occurs almost exclusively among African-Americans, native Africans, and Mediterranean populations.

Leukemia

Leukemia is a cancer of the white blood cells or the tissues which synthesize white blood cells. The primary sign of leukemia is a white blood cell count elevated 10 to 100 times that of the normal range. Leukemia is more frequent in combination with Down syndrome, overexposure to radiation, or among persons being treated aggressively with chemotherapy. It is categorized by its acute or chronic nature and by the type of white blood cell affected. The four

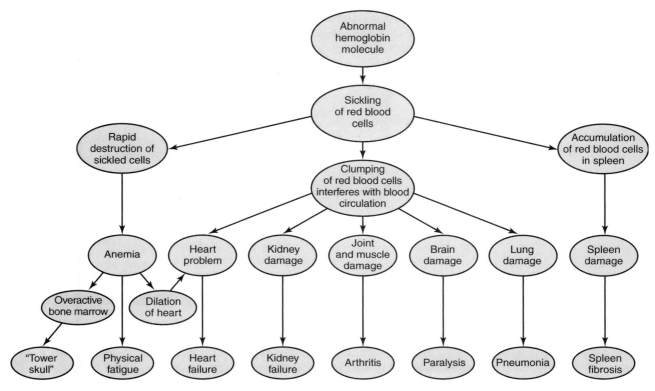

Figure 8-1 A series of damages and effects caused by sickle cell anemia.

major forms of leukemia are acute myelocytic leukemia (AML), acute lympho-cytic leukemia (ALL), chronic myeloid leukemia (CML), and chronic lymphocytic leukemia (CLL).

 ## Polycythemia Vera

Polycythemia vera, which is also known as **erythrocytosis**, is an idiopathic disorder of the blood. As its name suggests, erythrocytosis is an abnormally high red blood cell count. Polycythemia vera is a chronic, life-shortening disorder involving bone marrow. In addition to a high red blood cell count, which increases the viscosity of the blood causing thrombi and clotting, there is a noted increase in the concentration of hemoglobin in the blood. The characteristics of polycythemia vera are:

- Weakness
- Fatigue
- Vertigo (dizziness)
- Tinnitus (ringing in the ears)
- Irritability

- Enlarged spleen
- Congestion of the face causing a ruddy discoloration
- Redness and pain in the extremities
- Black-and-blue spots on the skin
- Coma
- Stroke

Of importance to the embalmer is the utilization of radioactive phosphorus (^{32}P) in the treatment of this disease. When embalming the remains of persons treated with radioactive materials, it is always important to contact the hospital radiation protection officer to ensure the safety of the embalmer and the public.

Hemophilia

The oldest known hereditary bleeding disorder, **hemophilia** is a hemorrhagic disease characterized by a tendency toward excessive and sometimes spontaneous bleeding. There are two types of hemophilia, A and B. Both types are caused by low levels or complete absence of a blood protein essential for blood clotting to take place. Hemophilia A is due to a lack of the blood clotting protein factor VIII, and hemophilia B (also known as Christmas disease) is due to a lack of factor IX. Interestingly, females transmit the disease, but almost always, only males exhibit the disease complications. Although it is possible for hemophiliacs to die from internal bleeding, the administration of blood clotting factors has proven to be an effective method of resolving this disorder.

Thrombocytopenia

Thrombocytopenia refers to a severely reduced platelet (thrombocytes) count in the blood. It typically occurs when the bone marrow fails to produce platelets as quickly as they are used, or when platelets are removed too quickly from the blood. Platelets typically last about ten days in the blood, and there are between 150 million and 400 million platelets per milliliter of blood (Harrison and Machin 2001). When the platelet count falls below 100 million, in the case of thrombocytopenia, the platelets are less efficient at forming clots, and the risk of spontaneous bleeding increases. Thrombocytopenia can cause several bleeding disorders. In particular, it can cause bleeding from the nose and gums, and it may be fatal if spontaneous bleeding inside the head or digestive tract occurs.

In diagnosing thrombocytopenia many causes are possible. One is the presence of immune system antibodies in the blood of some people that bind to their platelets. These antibodies may bind to the chemicals in the test tube used to count the platelets, giving a false indication of thrombocytopenia. Other causes include impairment of the bone marrow that produces platelets and increased platelet destruction in the blood, which can result from infections like meningitis, complications of pregnancy, cancers like leukemia or prostate cancer, or blood diseases related to food poisoning. The treatment of thrombocytopenia depends entirely on the cause, but it is aimed at controlling spontaneous bleeding and restoring proper thrombocyte levels in the blood.

Purpura

Spontaneous bleeding in the subcutaneous tissues such as that associated with thrombocytopenia, is known as **purpura**. All forms of purpura have the symptoms of hemorrhaging into the skin, leaving discolorations that are red, darkening into purple, and that usually disappear in two to three weeks (see Color Plate 21). Purpura is common after either chemotherapy or radiation therapy in cancer treatment. In the deceased, the discolorations due to purpura are permanent and extravascular, so they will not be removed during the injection of arterial embalming fluids.

Hemolytic Disease of the Newborn

Hemolytic disease of the newborn—formerly known as erythroblastosis fetalis—occurs when a child is conceived of an Rh-positive father and an Rh-negative mother. The disorder only occurs if the child inherits the Rh-positive factor from the father, rather than the Rh-negative factor from the mother. Although the blood of the fetus and the mother do not mix, occasionally leakage can occur. When the fetus' Rh-positive blood mixes with the Rh-negative blood of the mother, the mother produces antibodies against the Rh factor. During the pregnancy, usually not enough time will pass to allow the development of Rh factor antibodies, which might cause harm to the fetus. However, if a second Rh-positive fetus is conceived the Rh factor antibodies can cross the placental barrier and endanger the fetus. After the birth of her first Rh-positive infant, the administration of a drug to the mother prevents her from making the anti-Rh antibodies, protecting any future fetuses.

REVIEW QUESTIONS

Matching

1. _____ phosphorus 32
2. _____ ecchymosis
3. _____ tinnitis
4. _____ intrinsic factor deficiency
5. _____ vertigo

a. pernicious anemia
b. ringing in the ears
c. bruise
d. dizziness
e. sometimes used to treat erythrocytosis

Multiple Choice

1. Which of the following disorders is caused by the premature rupture of red blood cells?
   a. sickle cell anemia
   b. hemolytic anemia
   c. erythrocytosis
   d. hemophilia
2. Which of the following diseases is characterized by a significant decrease in the number of white blood cells?
   a. leukemia
   b. leukocytosis
   c. erythroblastosis fetalis
   d. leucopenia
3. Which of the following is a hemorrhagic disorder caused by a decrease in the number of circulating blood platelets?
   a. thrombocytopenic purpura
   b. hemophilia
   c. thrombosis
   d. melena
4. Which of the following is due to a lack of the blood clotting protein factor VIII?
   a. aplastic anemia
   b. hemophilia B
   c. Christmas disease
   d. hemophilia A
5. Which of the following diseases is believed to have evolved through a genetic alteration to protect the body against malaria?
   a. leukemia
   b. thrombocytopenia
   c. sick cell anemia
   d. hemophilia

Putting Learning to Work!

The purpose of the following case analysis is to allow you to apply the information you have learned in a real-world situation. Read the case carefully and try to answer the following questions:

> What disorder do you suspect the person had at the time of death?

> What potential embalming complications do you anticipate?

What precautions should you take as the embalmer to limit the effects of these complications?

Case Analysis

A 63-year-old woman died in the intensive care unit of a local hospital. She had been in the intensive care unit for the past week, in a coma, after a sudden stroke. Approximately six weeks before, she complained to her daughter of feeling weak and tired. She also had spells of dizziness, and she noticed a ringing in her ears. During your case analysis, you notice that she has a ruddy color to her face, and that her extremities are slightly red. She is also covered with what appears to be small bruises.

Bibliography

Anemia. (2003). Retrieved July 24, 2003, from MedlinePlus, the U.S. National Library of Medicine and the National Institutes of Health at http://www.nlm.nih.gov/medlineplus/anemia.html.

Bleeding disorders. (2003). Retrieved July 24, 2003, from MedlinePlus, the U.S. National Library of Medicine and the National Institutes of Health at http://www.nlm.nih.gov/medlineplus/bleedingdisorders.html.

Harrison, C., & Machin, S. (2001). *Thrombocytopenia (reduced platelet count).* Retrieved March 14, 2004, from http://www.netdoctor.co.uk/diseases/facts/thrombocytopenia.htm.

Hematuria. (2001). Retrieved June 5, 2003, from the Urology Channel at http://www.urologychannel.com/hematuria/index.shtml.

Hemophilia. (n.d.). Retrieved June 5, 2003, from MEDCEU at http://www.medceu.com/tests/hemophilia.htm.

Hemoptysis. (2001). Retrieved June 5, 2003, from the Pulmonary Channel at http://www.pulmonologychannel.com/hemoptysis.

Hendrickson, G. (2001). Petechia. In *Diseases and conditions encyclopedia.* Retrieved June 5, 2003, from http://health.discovery.com/diseasesandcond/encyclopedia/972.html.

Kumar, V., Cotran, R., & Robbins, S. (2003). *Robbins basic pathology* (7th ed.). Philadelphia: Saunders.

Levy, A. (2002). Sickle cell anemia. In *Medical Encyclopedia.* Retrieved June 5, 2003, from MedlinePlus, the U.S. National Library of Medicine and the National Institutes of Health at http://www.nlm.nih.gov/medlineplus/ency/article/000527.htm.

Mayer, R. (2000). *Embalming: History, theory, & practice* (3rd ed.). New York: McGraw-Hill.

Neighbors, M., & Tannehill-Jones, R. (2000). *Human diseases.* Clifton Park, NY: Thomson Delmar Learning.

Pathology for funeral service. (1999). Dallas, TX: Professional Training Schools.

Shelton, H. (1992). *Boyd's introduction to the study of disease* (11th ed.). Philadelphia: Lea & Febiger.

Sopher, R. (n.d.). *Hematopathology.* Retrieved July 24, 2003, from the Department of Pathology, University of North Dakota at http://www.med.und.nodak.edu/depts/path/pathlab/h-html/h.html.

Venes, D. (Ed.). (2001). *Taber's cyclopedic medical dictionary* (19th ed.). Philadelphia: F. A. Davis.

CHAPTER 9

Diseases of the Heart and Blood Vessels

Learning Objectives

Upon completion of the chapter, review questions, and case analysis, the reader should be able to:

- List the predisposing factors for heart and blood vessel diseases.
- Describe the etiology and pathogenesis of congestive heart failure, myocardial infarction, and coronary artery disease.
- Define and describe the inflammatory disorders of the heart.
- Explain the disease complications associated with defects causing valvular insufficiency, valvular stenosis, and valvular prolapse.
- Describe the etiology and pathogenesis of rheumatic heart disease, heart dilatation, and hypertensive heart disease.
- Compare and contrast arteriosclerosis, atherosclerosis, arteritis, and phlebitis.
- Differentiate between aneurysms and varicose veins.
- Explain the relationship between hypertension and hypertrophy of the heart.

Key Terms

aneurysm
angina
arrhythmia
atherosclerosis
dilatation
dyspnea

endocarditis
fibrillation
hypertension
infarction
pericarditis

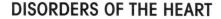

DISORDERS OF THE HEART

For both sexes and among all racial groups in the United States, cardiovascular disease is a leading killer. However, the risk for heart disease, stroke, and other cardiovascular disorders is not the same for all individuals. Predisposing factors for cardiovascular diseases include high blood pressure, drug abuse, high cholesterol levels, tobacco use, physical inactivity, poor nutrition, obesity, and diabetes. Cardiovascular diseases are believed to be inherited as well. While reading this chapter, the reader may review the anatomy of the heart by referring to Appendix D.

Congestive Heart Failure

Congestive heart failure (CHF) is a common cause of death listed by physicians on death certificates. It is a disorder affecting multiple body systems, in which the heart is unable to pump as much blood as the venous system supplies. Instead of pumping out all of the blood from the ventricles during systole, some amount of residual blood remains in the ventricles after diastole. Therefore, blood becomes congested in the ventricles and throughout the venous system, at the same time, an insufficient amount of blood enters the arterial system. Fluids accumulate in the venous system, and associated tissues become edematous. The overburdened heart gradually weakens and undergoes both anatomical and physiological changes. Congestive heart failure may result in cardiac failure and involve either the left side, the right side, or the entire heart.

The most common cause of right-sided cardiac failure is a disorder of the left ventricle. Right-sided heart failure leads to anasarca, which is severe generalized edema, especially in the hands, feet, and abdomen. Chronic right-sided heart failure also leads to enlargement of abdominal organs such as the liver, which is a condition known as hepatomegaly. Figure 9-1 illustrates some of the most common signs of congestive heart failure.

The most common causes of left-sided cardiac failure include high blood pressure, mitral or aortic valve diseases, coronary artery disease, and diseases of the myocardium. Congestive heart failure on the left side of the heart causes the development of pulmonary edema in the chest because the heart cannot remove the excess fluid from the lungs as part of pulmonary circulation, which is illustrated in Figure 9-2.

Individuals with left-sided heart failure commonly experience shortness of breath, which is also known as **dyspnea**. Decreased left-sided cardiac output eventually results in less blood entering the kidneys. The kidneys respond by reabsorbing more sodium and water into the blood vascular system. The increase in blood volume adds to the congestion and causes the heart to work that much harder. Congested blood quickly becomes clotted and can result in embolisms that can cause stroke or blockage of the coronary artery.

Congestive heart failure eventually leads to failure of the heart to beat properly. Sudden death occurs when the weakened heart undergoes fibrillation and arrhythmia. **Fibrillation** is a quivering or spontaneous contraction of the individual cardiac cells, while the loss of the normal beating rhythm of the heart is known as **arrhythmia**. Chronic heart failure also results in neurological changes

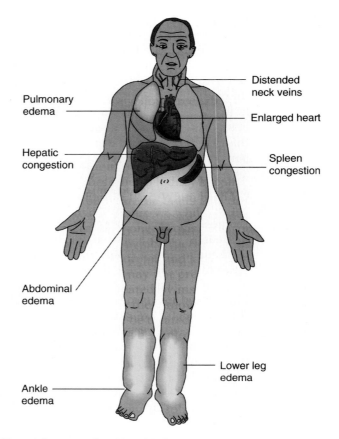

Distended
neck veins

Pulmonary
edema

Enlarged heart

Hepatic
congestion

Spleen
congestion

Abdominal
edema

Lower leg
edema

Ankle
edema

Figure 9-1 Signs of congestive heart failure.

that cause the heart rate to increase and the contractions of the heart to become more forceful, both of which contribute to the gradual decline associated with congestive heart failure.

Hypertrophy and Dilatation

The heart changes anatomically in cases of congestive heart failure due to its physiological inability to pump a sufficient amount of blood to clear venous congestion. It may also enlarge in relationship to other diseases such as diabetes. The two types of enlargement of the heart are cardiac hypertrophy and cardiac **dilatation** (dilation).

Although laypeople may use the terms *cardiac hypertrophy* and *cardiac dilatation* interchangeably, there is a difference in the two conditions. Cardiac *hypertrophy* refers to an increase in the size of the heart or an increase in the size of part of the heart due to an increase in the size of the muscle fibers. It is an enlargement of the heart that is initially a positive, adaptive response to an increased cardiac workload by allowing the heart to pump more blood, as experi-

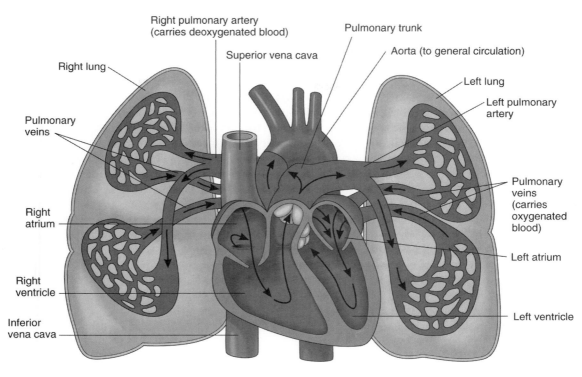

Right pulmonary artery
(carries deoxygenated blood)

Pulmonary trunk

Superior vena cava

Aorta (to general circulation)

Right lung

Left lung

Left pulmonary
artery

Pulmonary
veins

Right
atrium

Pulmonary
veins
(carries
oxygenated
blood)

Left atrium

Right
ventricle

Inferior
vena cava

Left ventricle

Figure 9-2 Cardiopulmonary circulation.

enced by conditioned athletes. However, the long-term effects of pathological enlargement are detrimental. Cardiac *dilatation* is a pathological condition in which the heart or a chamber of the heart increases in size due to a stretching of the muscle fibers in the walls of the chamber. The chambers of the heart can become stretched when one or more of them routinely becomes overfilled with blood.

In both the athletic and the pathological heart, the oxygen demand of cells increases as the cells of the heart muscle increase in size. Unlike the athlete's heart, however, the capillary beds of the diseased myocardium do not increase in size in response to the increased size of the heart. The result is that the heart muscle slowly becomes starved of oxygen. Additionally, the cells of the pathologically enlarged heart do not contract as efficiently as healthy cardiac cells. Ultimately, the stretched muscle fibers in the chambers of the heart can result in damage to the cardiac septum or the heart valves, allowing the backflow of blood in the heart.

Myocardial Infarction

A myocardial infarction (MI) is commonly referred to as a heart attack. An **infarction** is the formation of an area of necrosis in a tissue caused by obstruction in the artery supplying the area, although an infarct may also occur if the vein that drains the area of tissue becomes occluded. Most heart attacks are the result of a blood clot within the coronary artery that blocks the flow of blood to the heart muscle, which is also known as a thrombosis. Myocardial infarction indicates that necrosis has occurred in an area of the heart muscle as a result of the reduced blood flow through the coronary artery. Men are much more likely than women to experience an MI, and about half of all cases of MI are fatal due to acute cardiac failure. When a portion of the coronary artery is blocked, but blood is still allowed to flow to the myocardium, chronic cardiac failure ensues. In contrast, if the coronary artery becomes entirely occluded, acute cardiac failure occurs.

The chest pain associated with heart attacks is referred to as **angina** pectoris. The pain is not usually described as stabbing or sharp, and it is not usually exacerbated by taking deep breaths, coughing, or swallowing. Angina pectoris may occur for days or weeks before an acute myocardial infarction, at which point, the pain is more severe and is exacerbated during physical activity, after eating a large meal, or during exposure to cold weather.

Myocardial infarctions may include any or all of the following signs and symptoms:

- Sensation of a crushing pressure behind the breastbone
- Chest pain radiating to the neck, jaw, abdomen, shoulder, or left arm
- Nausea
- Vomiting
- Difficulty breathing
- Anxiety or fear

Inflammatory Diseases of the Heart and Blood Vessels

There are several terms associated with inflammation of structures within the cardiovascular system. They are defined in Table 9-1 for easy reference.

Endocarditis. An inflammation of the endocardium of the heart, which may include the heart valves or the cardiac septum, is known as **endocarditis**. Endocarditis may occur when the surface of the lining of the heart is damaged due

Table 9-1 Inflammation of the Heart and Blood Vessels

Endocarditis	Inflammation of the lining of the heart or the heart valves, often due to infection
Pericarditis	Inflammation of the tissues that surround the heart
Myocarditis	Inflammation of the heart muscle
Carditis	Inflammation of the heart
Arteritis	Inflammation of the arteries
Phlebitis	Inflammation of the veins

to blood clots that traumatize the tissues. Bacteria may then infect the damaged tissue. In this form of endocarditis, the heart valves may become involved, resulting in damage to the structure of the valves. Damaged heart valves may disrupt the flow of blood through the heart because the heart valves are unable to properly function. Endocarditis may also result from an infection after the implantation of artificial heart valves, and endocarditis is commonly associated with the use of intravenous drugs. The infections associated with endocarditis may spread to the kidneys, inflaming the lining of the renal blood vessels.

Pericarditis.   The pericardium serves as a protective barrier to the spread of infection. The tough, fibrous outer layer is a sac that surrounds the heart and attaches to the diaphragm, sternum, and the cartilage attached to the ribs. The inner layer of the pericardium lines the surface of the heart. If the area between the two layers of the pericardium becomes inflamed, the condition is referred to as **pericarditis**. Two common causes of pericarditis include infections and blunt force trauma, such as that resulting from the chest striking the steering wheel during an automobile collision.

There is a small amount of fluid normally present between the two layers of the pericardium. If, during the inflammatory process, an excessive amount of fluid accumulates within the pericardial sac, a fatal condition known as *cardiac tamponade* may ensue. The excess fluid results in a disturbance of the electrolyte and protein balance in the pericardial sac, and the pressure inside the sac increases as the fluid accumulates. The result of these changes is that the heart is unable to expand fully and has less force when it contracts, so it cannot pump as much blood. The blood pressure drops, and more fluid accumulates around the heart. Pericarditis is the inflammation of the pericardial sac that surrounds the heart, while cardiac tamponade is the decrease in blood pressure due to the accumulation of fluids in the pericardial sac associated with pericarditis.

Cardiomyopathy

Cardiomyopathy is a disease of the heart muscle due to a variety of causes. Alcoholic cardiomyopathy is due to excessive alcohol consumption. Hypertrophic cardiomyopathy is enlargement of the infant cardiac septum. Hypertrophic cardiomyopathy may lead to congestive heart failure but is often asymptomatic, with the exception of a heart murmur. Although hypertrophic cardiomyopathy may go unnoticed for a lifetime, it may also result in acute cardiac failure during exercise. Parasitic cardiomyopathy is an infection in the myocardium associated with parasitic organisms, while restrictive cardiomypathy results from a lack of flexibility of the walls of the heart's chambers.

Primary and secondary cardiomyopathy differ in that primary cardiomyopathy is idiopathic, while secondary cardiomyopathy has a known cause or is associated with another disease. Secondary cardiomyopathy may be associated with toxic chemicals, metabolic disorders such as diabetes mellitus, or inherited cardiac disorders.

Valvular Defects

The primary function of the heart valves is to prevent the backflow of blood between the chambers of the heart. Diseases of the heart valves can be both acquired and congenital, and they can occur either singularly or in association with other diseases. Although the tricuspid valve and the pulmonic valve may become diseased, deformities are much more common in the aortic and mitral valves. There are two mechanisms by which deformed cardiac valves may cause disease. Valvular defects can cause obstruction of the blood flow and deformed valves are more susceptible to infection.

There are three ways that valves typically disrupt blood flow: insufficiency, stenosis, and prolapse. Valvular insufficiency, which is also referred to as incompetence, is a congenital condition, in which the valves of the heart fail to form properly in the fetus. In contrast, both valvular stenosis, which is also known as a stricture, and valvular prolapse are acquired disorders. A valvular stenosis is characterized by a narrowing of the valvular orifice, causing disruption in the flow of blood. Valvular prolapse is due to excessive stretching of the valves, causing extension of the inner layers of the valve and stretching the valve out of shape, preventing it from closing properly. Severe defects of the heart valves can be fatal.

Rheumatic Heart Disease

Sometimes an infectious disease like rheumatic fever can cause valvular defects. Rheumatic fever is characterized by severe arthritis in multiple joints in the body. It results from a bacterial infection that originates as strep throat and spreads to the heart. The bacteria that cause the initial rheumatic fever may remain dormant in the body for years before they damage the heart valves. Rheumatic heart disease causes damage to the mitral valve in most cases, which can lead to endocarditis and infection of multiple layers of the heart. If the valvular defect is severe enough, rheumatic heart disease can eventually lead to cardiac failure.

Hypertensive Heart Disease

Uncontrolled blood pressure can result in several severe disorders within the body's organs, specifically the brain, kidneys, and heart. High blood pressure is technically referred to as hypertension. **Hypertension** is high blood pressure based on three readings spread out over several weeks in which blood pressure is higher than 140 millimeters of mercury systolic or 90 millimeters of mercury diastolic. When the left ventricle of the heart hypertrophies in combination with a history of high blood pressure, the individual is diagnosed with hypertensive heart disease. As the wall of the left ventricle increases in size, its demand for nutrients also increases; however, the ability of the heart to deliver nutrient-rich blood diminishes as the heart enlarges. As the wall of the left ventricle hypertrophies, it becomes tighter and less efficient at pumping, reducing the overall cardiac output of blood. Chronic hypertension also predisposes individuals to atherosclerosis, which can cause coronary artery disease.

Atrial Septal Defect

Occasionally, the foramen ovale fails to properly close at birth, which is a condition referred to as atrial septal defect. The hole in the interatrial septum causes too much blood to bypass the right ventricle and the lungs of the newborn infant. The blood does not reach the lungs and is not sufficiently oxygenated. This condition results in a "blue baby" due to the cyanotic discoloration of the infant's tissues, which are deficient in oxygen. In some babies, this condition is mild and will correct itself, while others require immediate surgical intervention.

VASCULAR DISORDERS

In the United States, cardiovascular diseases contribute significantly to sudden deaths. There is a link between diseases of the blood vessels and both cardiac failure and stroke. Chronic conditions such as arteriosclerosis and hypertension, as well as inflammatory conditions such as arteritis and phlebitis, can all lead to the disruption of proper circulation of the blood. Tissues must have a continuous supply of nutrients, and the waste created by cellular respiration must be continuously removed from the tissues. Failures in the blood vascular system to supply nutrients and remove waste can lead to death of the tissues and, eventually, death of the body.

Coronary Artery Disease

Coronary artery disease, which is also known as ischemic heart disease or coronary heart disease, is the most common cause of death in economically developed countries, including the United States. Coronary artery disease is characterized by the narrowing of the lumen of the coronary arteries due to atherosclerosis, as represented in Figure 9-3. There are three changes that can contribute to the severity of coronary artery disease: acute plaque changes, blood clots in the coronary artery, and spasms of the coronary artery.

A waxy substance called plaque—which is made of cholesterol, fatty compounds, calcium, and a blood-clotting material called fibrin—reduces the flow of blood in the coronary artery. The presence of plaque may result in blood clot formation within the coronary artery. Thickening of the arterial walls may also lead to spasms in the muscularis layer of the coronary artery. The coronary artery then cannot supply blood to the myocardium adequately. The loss of oxygen-rich blood starves the heart muscle and leads to its death, which is referred to as myocardial infarction.

Arteriosclerosis

Arteriosclerosis is a general term that literally means "hardening of the arteries." It is a disease of the arterial vessels marked by thickening, hardening, and loss of elasticity in the arterial walls. There are three forms of arteriosclerosis: atherosclerosis, sclerosis of arterioles, and calcification of the medial layer of the arteries, which is a rare disorder known as Mönckeberger's calcification. The

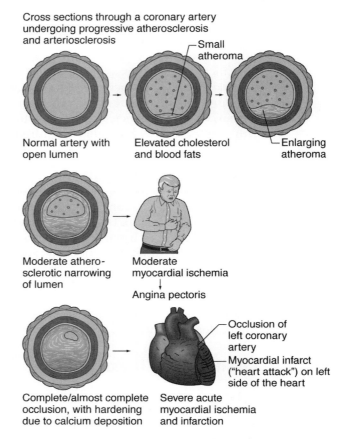

Cross sections through a coronary artery undergoing progressive atherosclerosis and arteriosclerosis

Normal artery with open lumen

Elevated cholesterol and blood fats — Small atheroma

Enlarging atheroma

Moderate athero-sclerotic narrowing of lumen

Moderate myocardial ischemia
↓
Angina pectoris

Complete/almost complete occlusion, with hardening due to calcium deposition

Severe acute myocardial ischemia and infarction

Occlusion of left coronary artery

Myocardial infarct ("heart attack") on left side of the heart

Figure 9-3 Pathogenesis of coronary artery disease.

most prominent of these forms of arteriosclerosis is atherosclerosis, which is a leading cause of disease throughout the Western world.

Arteriosclerosis is typically found in the large and medium-size arteries in the body, which include the aorta, carotid arteries, iliac arteries, coronary arteries, and the femoral arteries. The presence of a large quantity of plaque causes the artery to be hard, inelastic, and brittle. During the process of raising the artery for the injection of arterial embalming fluids, the embalmer may have difficulty inserting the arterial tube due to the presence of plaque. Additionally, large pieces of plaque lining the endothelium of the inner arterial wall may be visible.

Arteriosclerosis is commonly present in the femoral arteries because the blood pressure is lower in the femoral arteries than it is in the carotid arteries. It is also possible that the slow occlusion of the femoral arteries would not result in death as quickly as the occlusion of the carotid arteries. There would, therefore, be a longer period in which plaque could form within the femoral arteries without being life threatening.

Atherosclerosis

Coming from the Greek words *athero* (porridge) and *sclerosis* (hardness), **atherosclerosis** is a process in which deposits of fatty substances—cholesterol, cellular waste, calcium, and other substances—build up in the inner lining of an artery, forming plaque (see Color Plate 22). It usually affects large and medium-size arteries and is common among the elderly. Although plaque can become large enough to occlude arteries, where it reduces blood flow, it is most dangerous when its integrity is challenged, allowing the possibility of fragmentation.

If fragile plaque ruptures, the pieces of plaque each become a floating embolus that can stimulate the formation of blood clots. If the embolism blocks an artery that supplies blood to the heart, the resulting acute cardiac failure can lead to sudden death. If the artery leads to the brain, a stroke may occur that may also lead to sudden death. Obstruction of the arteries of either the upper or lower extremities can lead to gangrene.

Atherosclerosis is a slow, complex disease, which typically starts in childhood and progresses with age. It is believed to be caused by damage to the endothelium lining the arteries. Potential causes of damage to the arterial walls are believed to include elevated levels of cholesterol and triglyceride in the blood, high blood pressure, smoking tobacco, and diabetes. Hypertension, obesity, family history of cardiovascular diseases, and physical inactivity all predispose individuals to atherosclerosis.

Aneurysm

An **aneurysm** is the abnormal enlargement or bulging of an artery caused by damage to or weakness in the blood vessel wall. Although aneurysms can occur in any blood vessels, they almost always form in an artery. Aneurysms are not unlike a weak spot in the side of a bicycle tire's inner tube. As more air is forced into the inner tube, the pressure eventually causes the weak spot to rupture. Figure 9-4 is a photograph of a ruptured aortic aneurysm.

There are several areas in which aneurysms are more common in the body than others. Although most fatal aneurysms occur in the abdominal aorta or in cerebral arteries of the brain, aneurysms may occur in the thoracic aorta of the chest or in the large arteries of the lower extremities, where they are known as peripheral aneurysms. The rupture of an aneurysm can cause life-threatening bleeding and may lead to sudden death.

Most people are unaware that they have an aneurysm because in most cases they are asymptomatic. Some symptoms may include pain in the back, abdomen, or groin. Most aneurysms are detected during a physical exam for other health reasons. Small aneurysms rarely rupture and can be treated by medications like beta blockers that lower blood pressure, which reduces the pressure of the blood against the arterial walls. However, large aneurysms may require surgical removal. During surgery, the damaged portion of the artery is replaced with a flexible tube called a graft.

The symptoms of a cerebral aneurysm differ from the symptoms of an aortic aneurysm. Although a ruptured aneurysm can heal when the bleeding stops, in more serious cases, the bleeding may cause brain damage resulting in

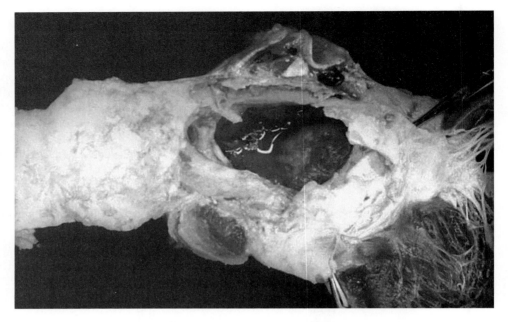

Figure 9–4 A ruptured aortic aneurysm. (Courtesy of the Centers for Disease Control and Prevention, Atlanta, GA, Susan Lindsley.)

paralysis, coma, or death. Brain aneurysms can be detected by imaging tests such as magnetic resonance imaging (MRI), computed axial tomography (CAT scans), and angiograms. An angiogram is an X-ray used to produce images of the inside of blood vessels. The following disease characteristics are commonly associated with cerebral aneurysms:

- Headaches
- Drowsiness
- Neck stiffness
- Nausea
- Vomiting
- Mental confusion
- Vertigo (dizziness)
- Loss of consciousness

Hypertension

Hypertension, which is commonly referred to as high blood pressure, can contribute to coronary artery disease, strokes, kidney failure, and sudden rupture of the aorta. In addition, chronic high blood pressure associated with hypertensive heart disease can cause acute cardiac failure and result in sudden death. Although there are no rigid rules for determining high blood pressure, a sustained systolic pressure of over 140 or a sustained diastolic pressure of over 90 is considered hypertension. Normal blood pressure should be near 120 over 80. Reduction of hypertension greatly reduces the incidence and death rates from coronary artery disease, heart failure, and stroke.

There are several reasons why scientists believe that individuals develop high blood pressure, although 90 to 95 percent of the cases of hypertension have no known cause. These idiopathic cases of high blood pressure are believed to be related to social factors such as stress, obesity, smoking, physical inactivity, and diets high in salt. Of these factors, high salt intake has consistently been linked to hypertension. Besides its other detrimental effects, high blood pressure ultimately damages the lining of blood vessels. This damage to the blood vessels increases risk for both rupture of blood vessels in the brain, causing stroke, and rupturing the aorta, causing uncontrolled internal bleeding.

Arteritis

Arteritis is an idiopathic, inflammatory disease that affects the arteries of the body. The most common causes are direct infections caused by agents such as bacteria, fungi, and viruses. For example, arteritis may accompany infectious respiratory diseases like aspergillosis, pneumonia, and tuberculosis. Lesions may appear in the inflamed arteries of the respiratory system in relation to these infections.

Arteritis is also present in diseases in which the body's immune system attacks its own tissues. These diseases are known as autoimmune diseases, and arteritis may accompany autoimmune diseases like systemic lupus erythematosus, rheumatoid arthritis, and inflammatory bowel disease. Two diseases characterized by idiopathic arteritis include Takayasu's arteritis and giant cell arteritis, which is also known as temporal arteritis.

Takayasu's Arteritis. Takayasu's arteritis is an inflammatory disease of the aorta and the arteries that branch from it. It is especially prevalent among young, Asian women, and women in general are eight times more likely than men to develop Takayasu's arteritis. The typical age of onset of the disease is between 15 and 30. Disruption in the distribution of blood may result in problems with chewing or speaking. Muscles in the face and arms may atrophy, and vision loss is common. Heart failure is likely, stemming from severe hypertension. Takayasu's arteritis can also cause weakness of the arterial walls resulting in aneurysms. In some cases, Takayasu's arteritis is fatal, while others experience long-term survival.

Following are some of the most typical indicators of Takayasu's arteritis:

- Anemia
- Fever
- Night sweats
- Weight loss
- Joint pain
- Fatigue
- Impaired speech and chewing
- Vision loss
- Atrophy of extremities

Temporal Arteritis. Temporal arteritis is the most common form of arterial inflammation and is also known as giant cell arteritis. The disorder receives its name because it is usually first diagnosed in the temporal artery in the side of the head in association with complaints of headaches. The cause of the disease is unknown, but the affected vessels are infiltrated by immune cells like lymphocytes and plasma cells. Loss of some vision is present in about half the cases of temporal arteritis. If blindness is to be prevented, it is crucial to recognize and treat temporal arteritis early in its progression because it spreads from the temporal arteries to other arteries, such as the ophthalmic arteries of the eye, the carotid arteries, and the aorta.

Phlebitis

Phlebitis is an inflammatory condition of the veins of the legs, in which blood clots form along the walls and valves of the veins. The valves within the veins help prevent gravity from causing the blood to reverse its flow, as illustrated in Figure 9-5.

In a condition known as deep venous thrombosis, the inflammation of the veins of the legs can spread throughout the pelvis. The most common characteristic of phlebitis is pain and redness along the involved veins of the lower leg.

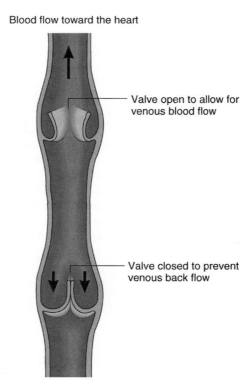

Blood flow toward the heart

Valve open to allow for venous blood flow

Valve closed to prevent venous back flow

Figure 9-5 Valves in the veins.

Phlebitis can be caused by changes in the blood's ability to form clots, pooling of the blood in the veins of the legs due to pregnancy or immobility, or even cancer.

Most cases of phlebitis occur in the calf muscle region, and the clots that form there can travel to the lungs blocking the pulmonary artery. The pulmonary artery transports blood to the lungs to be replenished with oxygen, and if it becomes occluded, the body may go into acute cardiac failure. Chronic phlebitis may cause ulcers in the skin, usually by the ankles and lower shin bones, that are slow to heal due to the pooling of nutrient-depleted venous blood. The lower legs often swell, and the skin becomes hard and thick.

Varicose Veins

The name varicose veins comes from the Latin word *varix* meaning "twisted." Varicose veins are enlarged veins, which are close to the skin's surface, most commonly found in the legs and feet. However they may also occur in other areas of the body such as the veins of the esophagus. Varicose veins are caused by excessive venous blood pressure that deforms the veins. Certain cancers may also cause varicose veins. In most cases, varicose veins are only of cosmetic concern, while others experience aching pain. The most positive indicator of varicose veins is the presence of dilated, elongated, and scarred veins that appear through the skin. Predisposing factors for varicose veins include age, pregnancy, obesity, being female, and sitting or standing for long periods. The characteristics of varicose veins of the legs are:

- Sensation of pressure in the legs and feet
- Throbbing, burning, muscle cramps
- Edema in the legs and feet
- A brownish-gray discoloration of the ankles
- Itching around a particular vein
- Ulcers of the legs or feet

POSTMORTEM CONDITIONS ASSOCIATED WITH DISEASES OF THE HEART AND BLOOD VESSELS

Since the blood vessels are used to introduce embalming fluid into the deceased, diseases of the heart and blood vessels are of extreme importance to the embalmer. Many of the diseases discussed in this chapter result in intravascular resistance to the flow of arterial embalming fluids, due to damaged vascular walls and the lumen of the vessels. In addition, diseased blood vessels can be predisposed to fragility and rupture, the presence of blood clots, and increased blood viscosity due to slowed blood flow. The use of pre-injection and co-injection chemicals help prepare the blood vessels and alter the blood composition to accept the preservative fluids. It is always important to cautiously monitor injection pressures and the rate of flow of arterial embalming fluid to prevent swelling of tissues, but it is especially important in the presence of diseased or damaged blood vessels.

REVIEW QUESTIONS

Matching

1. _____ endocarditis
2. _____ fibrillation
3. _____ arrhythmia
4. _____ hypertensive heart disease
5. _____ atrial septal defect

a. quivering or spontaneous contraction of the individual cardiac cells
b. inflammation of the lining of the heart or the heart valves, often due to infection
c. high blood pressure leading to enlargement of the heart
d. cause of "blue babies"
e. the loss of the normal beating rhythm of the heart

Multiple Choice

1. Which of the following is not considered to be a predisposing factor for cardiovascular diseases?
   a. obesity
   b. chemical agents
   c. tobacco use
   d. hypertension

2. Which of the following may occur when the surface of the lining of the heart is damaged due to blood clots that traumatize the tissues?
   a. endocarditis
   b. pericarditis
   c. atrial septal defect
   d. rheumatic heart disease

3. Which of the following begins with excess fluid accumulation that disturbs the electrolyte and protein balance in the pericardial sac?
   a. cardiomyopathy
   b. myocardial infarction
   c. cardiac dilatation
   d. cardiac tamponade

4. Which of the following is an abnormal enlargement or bulging of an artery caused by damage to or weakness in the blood vessel wall?
   a. arteriosclerosis
   b. atherosclerosis
   c. aneurysm
   d. endocarditis

5. Which of the following is an inflammatory condition of the veins of the legs, in which blood clots form along the walls and valves of the veins?
   a. phlebitis
   b. Takayasu's arteritis
   c. giant cell arteritis
   d. temporal arteritis

Putting Learning to Work!

The purpose of the following case analysis is to allow you to apply the information you have learned in a real-world situation. Read the case carefully and try to answer the following questions:

What disorder do you suspect the person had at the time of death?

What potential embalming complications do you anticipate?

What precautions should you take as the embalmer to limit the effects of these complications?

Case Analysis

A 52-year-old man died this morning at the emergency room. He is 5′ 8″ tall and weighs approximately 265 pounds. He collapsed in his driveway in the middle of January. He had been shoveling snow for about an hour, when he came inside to warm himself. He told his wife he did not care for any hot chocolate to drink because he had indigestion. He also stated that his shoulder and left arm were sore from shoveling snow. He paced anxiously around the kitchen before he returned to shoveling snow. As he paced, he unbuttoned his shirt and complained that he felt like someone was sitting on his chest. He collapsed about 20 minutes after returning to shoveling.

Bibliography

About cardiovascular disease. (2002). Retrieved June 4, 2003, from the National Center for Chronic Disease Prevention and Health Promotion, Centers for Disease Control and Prevention at http://www.cdc.gov/cvh/aboutcardio.htm.

Aneurysms. (1998). Retrieved June 4, 2003, from the Cleveland Clinic Health Information Center at http://www.clevelandclinic.org/health/health-info/docs/0300/0391.asp?index=3930.

Atherosclerosis. (n.d.). Retrieved June 4, 2003, from the American Heart Association at http://www.americanheart.org/presenter.jhtml?identifier=4440.

Chua, P. S. (n.d.). *On phlebitis and DVT*. Retrieved June 4, 2003, from Heart to Heart Talk, CEBU Cardiovascular Center at http://www.cdc-cdh.edu/hospital/cardio/art100.html.

Egland, A. (2001). *Temporal arteritis*. Retrieved June 4, 2003, from eMedicine at http://www.emedicine.com/EMERG/topic568.htm.

Enlarged heart. (n.d.). Retrieved June 4, 2003, from the American Heart Association at http://www.americanheart.org/presenter.jhtml?identifier=4517.

Hemorrhoids. (2002). Retrieved June 7, 2003, from the National Digestive Diseases Information Clearing-house, National Institutes of Health at http://www.niddk.nih.gov/health/digest/pubs/hems/hemords.htm.

Internet Stroke Center. (2003). Retrieved July 25, 2003, from the University of Washington in St. Louis at http://www.strokecenter.org/prof/index.html.

Kumar, V., Cotran, R., & Robbins, S. (2003). *Robbins basic pathology* (7th ed.). Philadelphia: Saunders.

Marill, K. (2001). *Endocarditis*. Retrieved June 4, 2003, from eMedicine at http://www.emedicine.com/EMERG/topic164.htm.

Mayer, R. (2000). *Embalming: History, theory, & practice* (3rd ed.). New York: McGraw-Hill.

Neighbors, M., & Tannehill-Jones, R. (2000). *Human diseases*. Clifton Park, NY: Thomson Delmar Learning.

NINDS vasculitis including temporal arteritis information page. (2001). Retrieved June 4, 2003, from the National Institute of Neurological Disorders and Stroke, National Institutes of Health at http://www.ninds.nih.gov/health_and_medical/disorders/vasculitis_doc.htm.

Pathology for funeral service. (1999). Dallas, TX: Professional Training Schools.

Riaz, K., & Forker, A. (2003). *Hypertensive heart disease*. Retrieved June 4, 2003, from eMedicine at http://www.emedicine.com/med/topic3432.htm.

Shelton, H. (1992). *Boyd's introduction to the study of disease* (11th ed.). Philadelphia: Lea & Febiger.

Takayasu's Arteritis Foundation. (n/d). Retrieved June 4, 2003, from http://www.takayasu.org.

Valley, V., & Fly, C. (2002). *Pericarditis and cardiac tamponade*. Retrieved June 4, 2003, from eMedicine at http://www.emedicine.com/EMERG/topic412.htm.

Varicose veins. (2003). Retrieved June 4, 2003, from the Mayo Clinic at http://www.mayoclinic.com/invoke.cfm?id=DS00256.

Venes, D. (Ed.). (2001). *Taber's cyclopedic medical dictionary* (19th ed.). Philadelphia: F. A. Davis.

CHAPTER 10

Diseases of the Digestive System

Learning Objectives

Upon completion of the chapter, review questions, and case analysis, the reader should be able to:

- Describe the inflammatory digestive disorders.
- Compare and contrast pharyngitis and esophagitis.
- Explain the etiology and pathogenesis of peptic ulcers and ulcerative colitis.
- Compare and contrast cholelithiasis, cholecystitis, and cholangitis.
- Explain the role of bilirubin in the presence of jaundice.
- Compare and contrast hepatitis, cirrhosis of the liver, bronze diabetes, and liver cancer.
- Discuss the impact of digestive system diseases on the deceased.

Key Terms

adhesion	intussusception
autolysis	paralysis
colostomy	stenosis
icterus	volvulus

DISORDERS OF THE DIGESTIVE SYSTEM

While reading this chapter, the reader may review the anatomy of the digestive system by referring to Appendix E. There are numerous inflammatory diseases of the digestive system, and Table 10-1 lists some of the most common.

Table 10-1 Inflammatory Disorders of the Digestive System

Gingivitis	Inflammation of the gums
Pharyngitis	Inflammation of the pharynx (soar throat)
Esophagitis	Inflammation of the esophagus
Gastritis	Inflammation of the stomach
Enteritis	Inflammation of the lining of the intestines
Colitis	Inflammation of the colon
Appendicitis	Inflammation of the vermiform appendix
Hemorrhoids	Inflammation of the blood vessels of the rectum
Cholecystitis	Inflammation of the gall bladder
Cholelithiasis	Gallstones
Cholangitis	Inflammation of the bile duct
Pancreatitis	Inflammation of the pancreas
Peritonitis	Inflammation of the membrane surrounding the abdominal cavity

Gingivitis

Gingivitis is a periodontal disease of the gums involving inflammation and infection that can result in destruction of the gums, which are also known as the gingiva. As it progresses, it may involve the tooth sockets. Gingivitis is caused by the long-term effects of plaque, which is a sticky material that develops on the exposed portions of the teeth. Plaque may consist of bacteria, mucus, or particles of food. In time, plaque mineralizes into a hard deposit known as tartar. Gingivitis is more common in cases of uncontrolled diabetes, due to hormonal changes associated with pregnancy, and among those with poor dental hygiene.

Pharyngitis

Pharyngitis is an inflammation of the pharynx that results in a sore throat. Pharyngitis is caused by a variety of microorganisms, but most cases are caused by a virus (Hurtado 2003). The most frequent viral causes of pharyngitis include the common cold, flu, adenovirus, mononucleosis, and HIV. Bacterial causes of pharyngitis include streptococcus, corynebacterium, *Neisseria gonorrhoeae*, and *Chlamydia pneumoniae*.

Esophagitis

Esophagitis is a condition caused by gastroesophageal reflux, which occurs when gastric contents are passively regurgitated into the esophagus. Gastric acid irritates the squamous epithelium of the esophagus, leading to the formation of ulcers in the esophageal mucosa. Eventually, a columnar epithelial lining may develop that can become malignant. The most common complaint of esophagitis is heartburn, which is also known as dyspepsia. Symptoms are more severe when lying down, when bending over, when wearing tight clothing, or after large meals. Other common symptoms include upper abdominal discomfort, nausea, bloating, and fullness.

Gastritis

Gastritis is inflammation of the stomach lining, and it can be caused by excessive alcohol consumption, prolonged use of nonsteroidal anti-inflammatory drugs (NSAIDs), pernicious anemia, autoimmune disorders, or the bacteria that cause ulcers. It may develop after major surgery, traumatic injury, burns, or severe infections. The most common symptoms are abdominal pain, belching, bloating, nausea, or vomiting.

Ulcerative Colitis

Ulcerative colitis is a disease that causes ulcers in the lining of the rectum and lower part of the colon, but it may affect the entire large intestine. Figure 10-1 illustrates the appearance of ulcers in conjunction with colitis. Ulcerative colitis rarely affects the small intestine except for the ileum. The inflammation

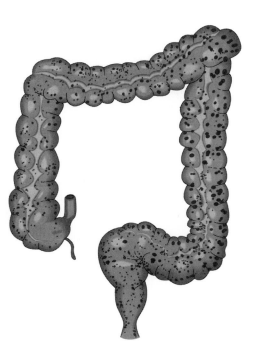

Figure 10-1 Ulcerative colitis.

causes diarrhea, and the ulcers bleed and produce pus in the lining of the colon where the inflammation has killed the epithelial cells. Ulcerative colitis is an inflammatory bowel disease, which is a general name for inflammatory diseases of the small intestine and colon.

Ulcerative colitis may be misdiagnosed because its symptoms are similar to other intestinal disorders such as Crohn's disease. Crohn's disease causes inflammation deeper within the intestinal wall than ulcerative colitis, and Crohn's disease usually occurs in the small intestine, although it can also occur in the mouth, esophagus, stomach, duodenum, large intestine, appendix, and anus.

Ulcerative colitis is an idiopathic disorder, although the most popular theory of its etiology is that the body's immune system reacts to a virus or a bacterium by causing ongoing inflammation in the intestinal wall. Ulcerative colitis can cause arthritis, inflammation of the eye, liver disease, osteoporosis, skin rashes, and anemia. Scientists think these complications may occur when the immune system triggers inflammation in other parts of the body. Ulcerative colitis can include any or all of the following:

- Weight loss
- Loss of appetite
- Rectal bleeding
- Loss of body fluids and nutrients
- Frequent fever
- Bloody diarrhea
- Nausea
- Severe abdominal cramps

About 25 percent to 40 percent of ulcerative colitis patients must eventually have their colons removed because of massive bleeding, severe illness, rupture of the colon, or risk of cancer. Surgery to remove the colon and rectum is known as a proctocolectomy, and may be followed by a colostomy.

During a **colostomy**, the surgeon creates a small hole in the abdomen about the size of a quarter called a stoma (Figure 10-2). The intestine is separated and attached to the stoma. Feces travels through the small intestine and exits the body through the stoma instead of the anus. A pouch is worn over the opening to collect waste, and the patient empties the pouch as needed. A stoma may be located almost anywhere on the abdomen, depending on the degree of removal of the colon. The site of the colostomy determines the characteristics of the feces that passes through the stoma (Figure 10-3).

Peptic Ulcers

An ulcer is a localized area of necrosis on the skin or mucous membranes. Ulcers are due to an erosion of the lining of the stomach or small intestine. The dead tissue in an ulcer sloughs off, eventually leaving behind a hole in the damaged area of tissue. Peptic ulcers occur in the stomach and duodenum of the small intestine. In the stomach, they are known as gastric ulcers, and in the duodenum they are known as duodenal ulcers.

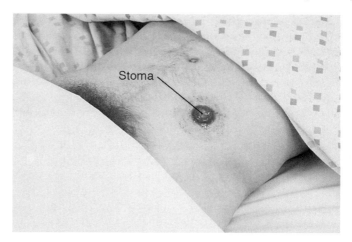

Figure 10-2 Typical colostomy stoma.

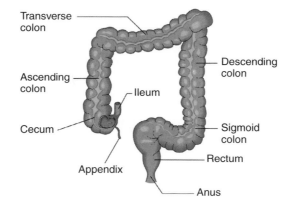

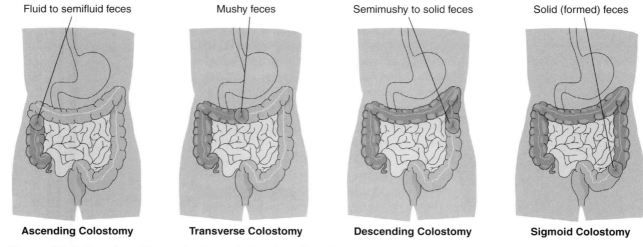

Figure 10-3 The site of the colostomy determines the characteristics of the feces.

The most common symptom of peptic ulcers is abdominal pain, especially occurring two to three hours after eating or after skipping a meal. The pain may abate with the use of antacids or by drinking milk. Other symptoms of peptic ulcers include nausea, vomiting, weight loss, fatigue, heartburn, indigestion, belching, chest pain, vomiting blood, or blood in the feces.

One complication of ulcers is the possibility of hemorrhaging. Although the loss of blood due to hemorrhaging may be serious, the potential for perforation is of more concern. If an ulcer perforates, the contents of the digestive tract are able to pass through the ulcer into the abdominal cavity. Microorganisms in the digestive tract may then infect the abdominal cavity and cause peritonitis, which is an inflammation of the membrane that lines the abdominal cavity. Peritonitis can be fatal.

If peptic ulcers occur in the pyloric region of the stomach, which leads to the duodenum of the small intestine, scar tissue may form. The accumulation of scar tissue in the pyloric region of the stomach may narrow the opening through which the food passes into the small intestine, which is known as a pyloric **stenosis**.

Although it was once believed that stress and spicy foods caused ulcers, it is now know that ulcers are due to a bacterial infection. Stress does not cause ulcers. The bacteria that causes most peptic ulcers is *Helicobacter pylori*. One factor that may contribute to the formation of peptic ulcers is the use of aspirin, ibuprofen, or naproxen. These medications, and others like them, can irritate the lining of the stomach, contributing to ulcer formation (Hart 2003b). A rare cause of peptic ulcers may be Zolliger-Ellison syndrome, in which the presence of a tumor in the pancreas causes peptic ulcers in the stomach and duodenum.

Crohn's Disease

Crohn's disease is an inflammatory bowel disease, which is the general name for diseases that cause inflammation in the intestines. It may also be called ileitis or enteritis, and its cause is unknown. The most common complication is blockage of the intestine, which occurs due to swelling and scar tissue formation in the intestinal wall. Ulcers that tunnel through the affected area into surrounding tissues such as the bladder, vagina, or skin may also be present. The tunnels, which are known as fistulas, are common and often become infected. Other complications associated with Crohn's disease include arthritis, skin problems, inflammation in the eyes or mouth, kidney stones, gallstones, and diseases of the liver and biliary system. The characteristics of Crohn's disease are:

- Abdominal pain in the lower right region
- Diarrhea
- Rectal bleeding
- Weight loss
- Fever
- Ulcers in the intestines

Enteritis

Enteritis is an inflammation of the intestine caused by microorganisms, which typically involves the stomach and intestines. The microorganisms are usually ingested in contaminated food or water. There are a variety of microorganisms that can cause enteritis, but some of the more common include staphylococcus, salmonella, shigella, campylobacter, and *Escherichia coli*. Symptoms of enteritis may include abdominal pain, cramping, diarrhea, fever, and dehydration. Vomiting is rarely associated with enteritis (Stone 2003). These symptoms may appear soon after exposure, or they may take several days to manifest. Enteritis is most dangerous to infants and the elderly. It is most common after traveling to areas with untreated or contaminated water.

Colitis

Colitis is an inflammation of the large intestine. There are a variety of types of colitis including pseudomembranous colitis, Crohn's disease, ulcerative colitis, ischemic colitis, irritable bowel syndrome, necrotizing enterocolitis, cryptosporidium enterocolitis, and cytomegalovirus colitis (Muir 2002). Colitis may be caused by both acute and chronic infections, and it may also be caused by disease processes associated with disorders such as ulcerative colitis and Crohn's disease. A lack of blood flow to the large intestine may cause a condition known as ischemic colitis, and a history of radiation to the large intestine has been known to cause colitis. Symptoms of colitis include abdominal pain, diarrhea, dehydration, abdominal bloating, intestinal gas, and bloody feces.

Appendicitis

Appendicitis is inflammation of the appendix, which is a small, wormlike structure attached to the cecum on the lower right side of the abdomen. If untreated, an inflamed appendix can burst, causing a potentially fatal infection of the abdomen known as peritonitis. Appendicitis is most common in people ages 10 to 30, and although the cause is unknown, it may occur after a viral infection or when the opening connecting the large intestine and appendix becomes occluded. Appendicitis is considered an emergency, due to the risk of rupture.

The characteristics of appendicitis are:

- Pain in the right side of the abdomen
- Nausea
- Vomiting
- Constipation
- Diarrhea
- Low fever
- Abdominal swelling
- Loss of appetite

Appendicitis is treated by an appendectomy, which is surgery to remove the appendix. Laparoscopic surgery for appendectomies is now common. Laparoscopic surgery reduces the presence of a large scar on the abdomen because it only involves making tiny cuts and inserting a camera and surgical instruments to remove the appendix, rather than making a large incision, as was once common.

Hemorrhoids

About half of the American population will develop hemorrhoids by the age of 50. Figure 10-4 illustrates hemorrhoids, which are inflamed veins around the anus or lower rectum that often result from straining to defecate. They may also be associated with pregnancy, aging, chronic constipation or diarrhea, and anal intercourse. Hemorrhoids are common during pregnancy because the pressure of the fetus and hormonal changes cause the hemorrhoidal vessels to enlarge, although hemorrhoids are temporary for most pregnant women.

Hemorrhoids are usually not dangerous or life threatening, with symptoms subsiding in a few days. The most common characteristics of internal hemorrhoids are bright red rectal bleeding and painful swelling around the anus. Hemorrhoids may result from excessive straining, rubbing, or cleaning around the anus, which may all cause further inflammation and the development of more hemorrhoids.

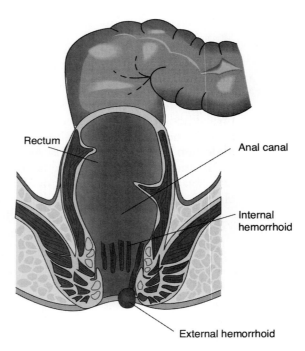

Rectum

Anal canal

Internal hemorrhoid

External hemorrhoid

Figure 10-4 Internal and external hemorrhoids.

Exercise and increased fiber in the diet helps reduce constipation and straining by producing feces that is softer and easier to pass. Good sources of fiber are fruits, vegetables, and whole grains. Drinking six to eight glasses of water daily also reduces constipation and strain during defecation.

Hepatitis

This section presents a general overview of hepatitis; viral forms of hepatitis are discussed in greater detail in Part Two. Hepatitis is inflammation of the liver, and it can be caused by infections from parasites, bacteria, or viruses. Hepatitis may also be caused by illicit drugs or poisonous mushrooms (Hart 2003a). An overdose of acetaminophen (such as Tylenol) in combination with excessive alcohol can also cause a fatal form of hepatitis. The body's immune system can also attack the liver causing autoimmune hepatitis. Table 10-2 identifies certain medications that can contribute to hepatitis. Additionally, hepatitis may be associated with inherited diseases like cystic fibrosis, or it may be due to excess levels of copper in the body.

Acute hepatitis has a sudden onset and short duration, while chronic hepatitis may be a long-term disease. Hepatitis can cause progressive liver damage, liver failure, or liver cancer. Certain risk factors increase the chance of contracting hepatitis, including eating contaminated foods, unprotected sex with multiple partners, IV drug abuse, living in a nursing home, excessive alcohol consumption, organ transplant, AIDS, receiving a tattoo, and working in a healthcare setting or funeral home.

Although there are numerous types of hepatitis, some of the most common include hepatitis A, hepatitis B, hepatitis C, autoimmune hepatitis, drug-induced hepatitis, and alcoholic hepatitis. Symptoms of hepatitis may include dark urine, clay-colored feces, loss of appetite, fatigue, abdominal pain, abdominal distention, general itching, jaundice, nausea, vomiting, weight loss, and gynecomastia, which is the development of breasts in males.

There are two vaccines available for hepatitis. The hepatitis A vaccine is available for people such as day-care and nursing home workers, laboratory workers, and those traveling to areas of the world where hepatitis A is endemic, like Africa and Asia. The hepatitis B vaccine is given to all infants in the United States, as well as to unvaccinated children. Information about the hepatitis B vaccine concerning funeral home employees is provided in Part Two of this text.

Table 10-2 Medications Contributing to Hepatitis

Methyldopa	Used to treat hypertension
Isoniazide	Used to treat tuberculosis
Valproate or phenytoin	Used to treat seizures
Chlorpromazine or amiodarone	Used to treat irregular heart beat
Trimethoprim-sulfamethoxazole or erythromycin	Antibiotics used to treat infections
Methotrexate	Used to treat cancer and, in smaller doses, arthritis

Jaundice. Jaundice, which is also known as **icterus**, is not a disease, it is a symptom of disease. Jaundice is a yellow discoloring of the skin, mucous membranes, and eyes caused by an excess of bilirubin in the blood (see Color Plate 23). Bilirubin is a breakdown product of hemoglobin. Normally it is processed in the liver and then deposited in the intestine so that it can be excreted in the feces. Places to look for jaundice include the palms, soles, sclera of the eyes, mucous membranes, and fingernail beds. Jaundice ranges from mild to severe, and its presence should always alert the embalmer to the potential of a variety of microbial infections.

Cirrhosis

Cirrhosis is a chronic, degenerative disorder of the liver, and Figure 10-5 identifies some of the most common characteristics of cirrhosis of the liver. In the United States, cirrhosis of the liver is mainly caused by long-term alcoholism,

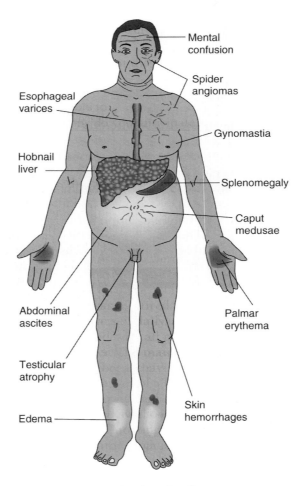

Figure 10–5 Clinical features of cirrhosis of the liver.

poisoning, or hepatitis. Cirrhosis of the liver is characterized by fatty and cellular infiltration and degeneration of liver cells, causing hardening of the liver. As a result of loss of liver function, increased blood pressure in the hepatic portal system may develop, leading to ammonia toxicity in the body. Liver disorders are characterized by any or all of the following:

- Ascites (abdominal edema)
- Mental dysfunction (dementia)
- Jaundice
- Blood clotting disorders

Cholelithiasis and Cholecystitis

Cholelithiasis is the formation of gallstones, and it is an inflammatory disorder of the gallbladder. There are three types of gallstones, the most common of which is composed of cholesterol. The other types include pigment gallstones and mixed gallstones. Each type is formed when bile becomes crystallized within the gallbladder or the bile duct, as shown in Figure 10-6.

When the gallstones block the flow of bile, the gallbladder and the bile duct can become inflamed. Gallstones are more common in women because they have more estrogen. The estrogen causes increased cholesterol secretion, while progesterone inhibits the flow of bile. Gallstones can cause inflammation of both the bile duct and the gallbladder. Inflammation of the bile duct is referred to as cholangitis, and inflammation of the gallbladder is known as cholecystitis.

Most gallstones cause no significant signs or symptoms because they do not block the flow of bile. However, when the flow of bile is blocked a common

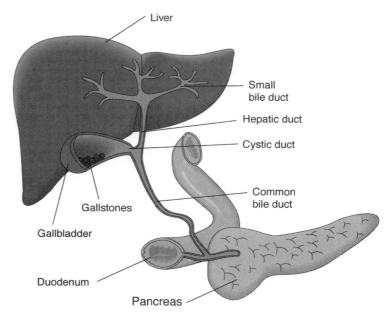

Figure 10-6 Cholelithiasis.

symptom is pain that radiates from the upper right quadrant of the abdomen to the shoulder. Other symptoms include indigestion, belching, bloating, and intolerance for fatty foods. The ingestion of fatty foods stimulates the release of bile for proper digestion, which causes pain because the bile duct is occluded.

Cholangitis

Cholangitis is an acute infection of the bile duct caused by blockage of the bile duct. The blockage of the flow of bile provides a breeding ground for the bacteria that cause the infection. Gallstones are the most common cause of obstruction, although strictures, stenosis, or tumors may also cause cholangitis. All of these causes slow the passage of bile, resulting in bacterial infection. Bacteria are not normally present in bile, but they are common in gallstones.

Mortality from cholangitis is high due to the common presence of other underlying diseases, and the spread of the infection throughout the blood. Historically, mortality was 100 percent, although currently it ranges from 7 percent to 40 percent (Santen 2001a).

Following are typical signs of advanced cholangitis:

- Pain in the upper right quadrant of the abdomen
- Fever
- Jaundice
- Mental status changes
- Blood poisoning

Pancreatitis

Pancreatitis is an inflammatory process in which the pancreas is digested by its own enzymes. The self-digestion of tissues by cellular enzymes is known as **autolysis**. Although the pancreas can heal without any anatomical or physiological impairment, permanent damage may also occur. The location of the pancreas in the retroperitoneal space, combined with its lack of an outer capsule, results in the easy spread of both infection and inflammation.

The primary causes of pancreatitis are a history of binge alcohol consumption and gallstones. If the gallstones become lodged in the pancreatic duct or the papilla of Vater, the flow of pancreatic juices becomes blocked and pancreatitis ensues. The autolytic enzymes in the pancreatic juices then begin to digest the pancreas.

Pancreatitis may be characterized by any or all of the following:

- Upper abdominal pain that radiates to the back
- Nausea
- Vomiting
- Mild jaundice
- Fever
- Bruising discolorations on the abdominal flanks

Pancreatitis is characterized by the presence of edema in the retroperitoneum and necrosis of the fat that surrounds the pancreas, which is known as peripancreatic fat. It can progress into a more severe form known as hemorrhagic or necrotizing pancreatitis. In this form of pancreatitis, the necrosis extends from the peripancreatic fat into the pancreas itself, and it is accompanied by hemorrhage and pancreas dysfunction. Pancreatic abscesses and cysts then form as a result of pancreatic juices being walled off by necrotic and bleeding tissue. Necrotizing pancreatitis can cause systemic effects such as vasodilatation, increased vascular permeability, pain, and accumulation of white blood cells in the walls of blood vessels.

Inflammatory exudates may spread from the pancreas to the left lung causing breathing difficulties, and muscular spasm may occur in the extremities due to calcium insufficiencies. Persons with severe pancreatitis may have a bluish discoloration on the flanks of their abdomen and their umbilical region. These discolorations are due to the leakage of blood from the pancreas in hemorrhagic pancreatitis.

Peritonitis

Peritonitis is an inflammation of the peritoneum, which is the membrane that lines the wall of the abdomen and covers the abdominal organs. Primary peritonitis occurs when an infection is present in the abdomen without obvious organ rupture. Primary peritonitis is the result of cirrhosis and fluid in the abdomen, especially in the cases of tuberculosis related to AIDS and in dialysis patients. Secondary peritonitis occurs when an organ is ruptured by the infection. Secondary peritonitis is usually the result of a ruptured appendix, perforated ulcer, abdominal trauma, or Crohn's disease. The air, acid, fecal material, and bacteria in the ruptured organ spill into the abdomen, resulting in infection. Peritonitis is characterized by abdominal pain, abdominal distention, fever, low urine output, thirst, fluid in the abdomen, inability to pass feces or gas, nausea, vomiting, shaking chills, and signs of shock. The cause of peritonitis must be identified and treated promptly. Typically, treatment involves surgery and antibiotics. The outcome for peritonitis is often good, but sometimes the outcome is poor, even with prompt and adequate treatment.

Diverticulosis

Diverticulosis is characterized by the development of small sacs in the wall of the colon, without inflammation or symptoms. These saculations are asymptomatic unless they become inflamed. Inflammation of diverticula occurs when feces is trapped inside these abnormal sacs, which can then stagnate in the colon and turn gangrenous with the possibility of perforation of the bowel. The inflammation of the diverticula is known as diverticulitis, and its symptoms are chronic constipation, mucus in the stool, and a gripping abdominal pain.

Bronze Diabetes

Bronze diabetes is a rare form of diabetes that affects the liver's ability to metabolize iron, causing enlargement of the liver and a bronze discoloration of the skin. Bronze diabetes should not be confused with Addison's disease, which also causes a bronze discoloration of the skin, but is due to a deficiency in the secretion of adrenocortical hormones from the suprarenal glands. Bronze diabetes is more common in men than women, and it generally occurs after the age of 40 as a symptom of diabetes mellitus. Bronze diabetes may lead to cardiac failure.

Hernia

Hernias are protrusions of an organ through the wall of the cavity containing the organ, as illustrated in Figure 10-7. Abdominal hernias are associated with pregnancy, heavy lifting, obesity, tumors, weakness from debilitating illness, and coughing. Hernias are more common in men because the abdominopelvic cavity is weak at the level at which the testicles descend. Coughing during a physical examination increases the intra-abdominal pressure exerted against the lower abdominal wall, allowing healthcare providers to feel a hernia. Hiatal hernias occur when digestive system organs protrude through the diaphragm (see Figure 10-8).

Stomach Cancer

Stomach cancer, which is also known as gastric cancer, can develop in any part of the stomach and can spread throughout the stomach and other organs. Initially, it spreads through the stomach wall to nearby lymph nodes and organs such as the liver, pancreas, and colon. Eventually, it can spread to distant organs, such as the lungs, the lymph nodes above the collar bone, and the ovaries. When stomach cancer metastasizes, the new tumor has the same kind of abnormal cells and the same name as the primary tumor.

Stomach cancer can be hard to diagnose because there are commonly no symptoms in its early stages. Often, stomach cancer has spread to other areas of the body before it causes symptoms significant enough to seek medical treatment and appropriate diagnosis. This lack of early symptoms explains the high

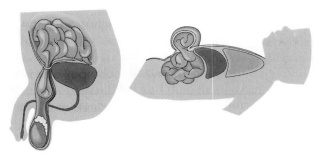

Inguinal   **Umbilical**

Figure 10-7 Inguinal and umbilical hernias.

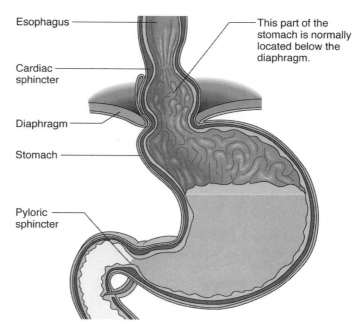

Figure 10-8 Hiatal hernia.

mortality rate associated with stomach cancer. The characteristics of stomach cancer are:

- Indigestion
- Abdominal pain
- Nausea
- Vomiting
- Diarrhea or constipation
- Bloating
- Loss of appetite
- Bloody vomit or feces

Liver Cancer

The liver is the largest internal organ in the body, and it is located under the right ribs just inferior to the lung and diaphragm. Several types of tumors can develop in the liver because it comprises several types of cells. The most common type of benign liver tumor is known as a hemangioma, and it starts in blood vessels within the liver. The most common form of liver cancer in adults is hepatocellular carcinoma. It begins in the hepatocytes, which are the most abundant cells in the liver.

Hepatocellular carcinoma sometimes begins as a single tumor that grows by expanding, and only metastasizes to the rest of the liver late in the disease. Another form of hepatocellular carcinoma begins as many tumors that spread tentacle-like growths throughout the liver, almost from the beginning of their formation. This form of liver cancer is most common among individuals with liver cirrhosis. Another form of liver cancer is cholangiocarcinoma, which starts in the bile ducts within the liver. The risk of developing cholangiocarcinoma is higher in the presence of gallstones, gallbladder inflammation, or chronic ulcerative colitis.

Most liver cancers do not originate in the liver; they spread from cancers in other places in the body. These tumors are named after their primary site. The liver is a common site of secondary metastasis of cancer because the blood is filtered by the liver. When the liver filters out the spreading malignant cells, the cells grow within the liver and cause the formation of secondary malignant tumors.

Colorectal Cancer

Cancer that begins in the colon is called colon cancer, and cancer that begins in the rectum is called rectal cancer. When cancer affects either of these portions of the large intestine, it may be called colorectal cancer. It is characterized by changes in bowel habits, diarrhea, constipation, bloody feces, gas, bloating, abdominal cramps, unexplained weight loss, and vomiting. Most colorectal cancer develops gradually from benign polyps. So, the early detection and removal of polyps may help prevent colorectal cancer.

Polyps

Polyps are benign tumors of vascular organs that contain a stem attaching the tumor to its surrounding tissue. Polyps are surgically removed if they are malignant or if they occlude the organ. They are typically found in vascular organs such as the nose, uterus, and rectum.

Obstructions

The small intestine and the large intestine are referred to as the *bowel*. When either becomes blocked, it is referred to as a bowel obstruction, which is depicted in Figure 10-9. The leading causes of bowel obstruction is postoperative adhesions. An **adhesion** occurs as part of the healing process after injury. If the intestine is cut during surgery, the two sides may grow together, effectively closing the lumen of the intestine. Other causes of bowel obstruction include cancer, Crohn's disease, bacterial infections, parasites, hernias, and paralysis of intestinal muscles. **Paralysis** is the loss of movement of muscles, and, in this case, paralysis of the peristaltic muscles in the bowel prevents the movement of materials within the bowel, leading to bowel obstruction. In children, bowel obstructions commonly result from congenital defects such as pyloric stenosis, volvulus, and intussusception of the intestines.

Figure 10-10 illustrates both intussusception and a volvulus. **Intussusception**, or invagination, of the intestine is characterized by one part of the intestine slipping into a previous segment of the intestine. Intussusception is more common in children than in adults, and it commonly occurs at the ileocecal juncture.

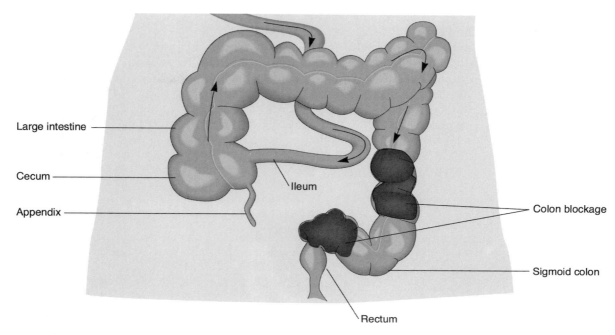

Figure 10-9 Colon blockage.

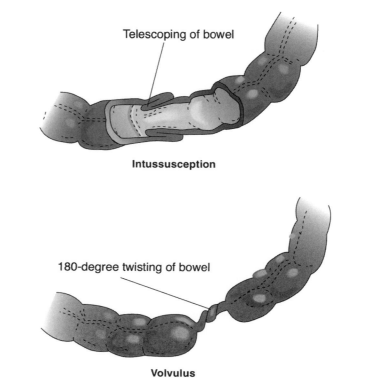

Figure 10-10 Intussusception and volvulus.

A **volvulus** occurs when the intestine twists on itself, causing obstruction of the movement of fecal material through the bowel. If the mesentery stretches out of shape, it frequently causes a volvulus in the intestine.

Bowel obstructions are serious because the blood vessels may also become compressed within the occlusion, leading to a lack of blood flow to the bowel and resulting in necrosis. Vomiting causes distention of the small intestine leading to increased pressure within the lumen of the intestines. The increased pressure compresses the lymphatic vessels in the mucosal layer of the intestines. The compression of the lymphatic vessels prevents them from removing excess fluid, and lymphedma appears within the lumen of the intestine. The fluid loss and dehydration that ensue are often a fatal combination.

POSTMORTEM CONDITIONS ASSOCIATED WITH DIGESTIVE DISORDERS

Embalming the remains of someone who dies as a result of a digestive system disorder can pose unique challenges to the embalmer. There are ten postmortem conditions associated with digestive system disorders with which the embalmer should be familiar:

1. Ascites
2. Edema
3. Dehydration
4. Emaciation
5. Rapid decomposition
6. Rapid coagulation of blood
7. Jaundice
8. Hemorrhage
9. Purge
10. Abdominal distention

The pathological changes that the body undergoes before death impact the embalming process. The most significant changes associated with digestive disorders are changes in the fluid levels within the tissues. Ascites, edema, dehydration, and emaciation are all related to either an excess or a reduction in the level of fluids in the tissues. Disorders such as cancers, Crohn's disease, and the inflammatory diseases of the digestive system can each alter the level of fluids within the body's tissues.

These changes in the level of fluids in the tissues persist after death. The presence of excess fluids in the tissues of the deceased is related to increased rates of tissue decomposition due to hydrolysis and the promotion of microbial growth. The high temperature within the abdomen also provides optimum temperature levels for microbial growth after death. In addition, the combination of excess fluids in some tissues and reduced levels of tissue fluids in dehydrated tissues can result in stasis of blood flow, leading to rapid coagulation of the blood.

Liver damage may also contribute to blood clotting abnormalities due to altered function of the liver, which produces several of the components found in blood. These components affect both blood clotting and blood volume. Hemorrhaging may also occur within the abdomen, causing discolorations in connection with digestive disorders such as hemorrhagic pancreatitis. Jaundice is also a discoloration commonly found in the remains of someone who dies from a liver disorder.

The combination of the accumulation of fluids within the abdomen, the presence of microbes, and the growth of malignant tumors may result in distention of the abdomen and purge. During the arterial embalming of the deceased, the arterial embalming fluid does not enter the lumen of the digestive system. Excess fluids and microbes within the lumen will not be directly affected by the arterial embalming fluid. It is, therefore, necessary to thoroughly aspirate and treat the abdominal and thoracic cavities with cavity fluid to remove edematous fluids, which may later purge from the nose and mouth, and to control the growth of microorganisms. Packing the anus with cotton treated with a mortuary-grade disinfectant is also advised.

Before embalming the remains of someone who has died as a result of digestive system pathologies, the embalmer must conduct a thorough case analysis. The proper volume, strength, and type of embalming chemical to employ depends on the condition of the remains. For example, the presence of edematous fluids in the abdomen also increases dilution of cavity embalming fluids, requiring the use of more astringent embalming chemicals. Nonetheless, the embalmer must be judicious in the use of high concentrations and large volumes of embalming fluids when presented with jaundiced or dehydrated tissues, which require larger volumes of lower-strength embalming fluids. The use of astringent embalming fluids can result in formaldehyde burn and discoloration of the tissues.

The combination of differing fluid levels within the tissues and the pressure exerted on the large blood vessels within the abdomen can require the use of multiple injection and drainage sites, as well as the use of different strengths, quantities, and types of embalming fluids.

Finally, treatments for digestive system disorders may include the use of devices such as colostomy bags or feeding tubes. A feeding tube, which is technically referred to as a gastronomy tube, is pictured in Figure 10-11. All external

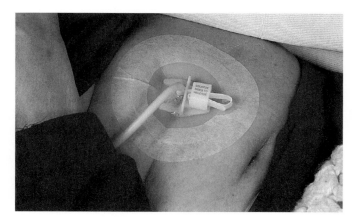

Figure 10–11 Gastronomy tube.

medical devices should be removed, disinfected, and properly discarded in the biohazardous waste. Any open wounds associated with these devices should be disinfected, preserved, dried, sutured, sealed, and covered with absorbent material and plastic.

REVIEW QUESTIONS

Matching

1. _____ volvulus
2. _____ peritonitis
3. _____ jaundice
4. _____ cholangitis
5. _____ intussusception

a. also known as icterus
b. inflammation of the membrane surrounding the abdominal cavity
c. inflammation of the gallbladder
d. disorder in which one part of the intestine slips into a previous segment of the intestine
e. disorder in which the intestine twists on itself

Multiple Choice

1. Which of the following is an inflammation of the stomach lining that can be caused by chronic, excessive alcohol consumption?
   a. esophagitis
   b. gastritis
   c. gingivitis
   d. stomach cancer

2. Which of the following does not describe Crohn's disease?
   a. an inflammatory bowel disease
   b. ileitis
   c. enteritis
   d. ulcerative colitis

3. Which of the following disorders is characterized by an intolerance for fatty foods?
   a. esophagitis
   b. Crohn's disease
   c. cholelithiasis
   d. pancreatitis

4. Which of the following disorders of the pancreas can cause a bluish discoloration on the flanks of the abdomen and the umbilical region?
   a. pancreatic cancer
   b. hemorrhagic pancreatitis
   c. necrotizing pancreatitis
   d. diabetes mellitus

5. Which of the following is caused by the liver's inability to metabolize iron?

    a. bronze diabetes

    b. liver cancer

    c. cirrhosis of the liver

    d. hepatitis

Putting Learning to Work!

The purpose of the following case analysis is to allow you to apply the information you have learned in a real-world situation. Read the case carefully and try to answer the following questions:

    What disorder do you suspect the person had at the time of death?

    What potential embalming complications do you anticipate?

    What precautions should you take as the embalmer to limit the effects of these complications?

Case Analysis

A 17-year-old student died on an airplane while flying between Hong Kong and New York City. The man spent one year as an exchange student and was returning home to New York City. He complained of indigestion for the week prior to his return. The day before his flight, he vomited and complained of abdominal pain. His host mother told him that he was probably just nervous about returning home.

    During the first leg of his flight between Hong Kong and Anchorage, Alaska, he experienced fever, nausea, abdominal pain in his lower right quadrant, which radiated toward his groin, and vomiting. He went into a coma somewhere over Ohio, after approximately 19 hours of travel. He had placed a blanket over his head to get some rest, and the flight attendant assumed he had fallen asleep.

Bibliography

Appendicitis. (2002). Retrieved June 7, 2003, from the National Digestive Diseases Information Clearinghouse, National Institutes of Health at http://www.niddk.nih.gov/health/digest/summary/append/.

Cirrhosis of the liver. (2002). Retrieved June 7, 2003, from the National Digestive Diseases Information Clearinghouse, National Institutes of Health at http://www.niddk.nih.gov/health/digest/pubs/cirrhosi/cirrhosi.htm.

Crohn's disease. (2000). Retrieved June 7, 2003, from the National Digestive Diseases Information Clearinghouse, National Institutes of Health at http://www.niddk.nih.gov/health/digest/pubs/crohns/crohns.htm.

Gastritis. (2002). Retrieved June 7, 2003, from the National Digestive Diseases Information Clearinghouse, National Institutes of Health at http://www.niddk.nih.gov/health/digest/summary/gastritis/gastritis.htm.

Hart, Jacqueline A. (2003a). Hepatitis. In *Medical Encyclopedia*. Retrieved March 15, 2004, from MedlinePlus, the U.S. National Library of Medicine and the National Institutes of Health at http://www.nlm.nih.gov/medlineplus/ency/article/001154.htm.

Hart, Jacqueline A. (2003b). Peptic ulcers. In *Medical Encyclopedia*. Retrieved March 15, 2004, from MedlinePlus, the U.S. National Library of Medicine and the National Institutes of Health at http://www.nlm.nih.gov/medlineplus/ency/article/000206.htm.

Hemorrhoids. (2002). Retrieved June 7, 2003, from the National Digestive Diseases Information Clearinghouse, National Institutes of Health at http://www.niddk.nih.gov/health/digest/pubs/hems/hemords.htm.

Hurtado, Rocio. (2003). Pharyngitis. In *Medical Encyclopedia*. Retrieved March 15, 2004, from MedlinePlus, the U.S. National Library of Medicine and the National Institutes of Health at http://www.nlm.nih.gov/medlineplus/ency/article/000655.htm.

Khoury, G., & Deeba, S. (2001). *Pancreatitis*. Retrieved June 7, 2003, from eMedicine at http://www.emedicine.com/EMERG/topic354.htm.

Kumar, V., Cotran, R., & Robbins, S. (2003). *Robbins basic pathology* (7th ed.). Philadelphia: Saunders.

Mayer, R. (2000). *Embalming: History, theory, & practice* (3rd ed.). New York: McGraw-Hill.

Muir, Andrew J. (2002). Colitis. In *Medical Encyclopedia*. Retrieved March 15, 2004, from MedlinePlus, the U.S. National Library of Medicine and the National Institutes of Health at http://www.nlm.nih.gov/medlineplus/ency/article/001125.htm.

Neighbors, M., & Tannehill-Jones, R. (2000). *Human diseases*. Clifton Park, NY: Thomson Delmar Learning.

Nobie, B., & Kahlsa, S. (2001). *Bowel obstruction, small*. Retrieved June 7, 2003, from eMedicine at http://www.emedicine.com/EMERG/topic66.htm.

Pathology for funeral service. (1999). Dallas, TX: Professional Training Schools.

Santen, S. (2001a). *Cholangitis*. Retrieved June 7, 2003, from eMedicine at http://www.emedicine.com/EMERG/topic96.htm.

Santen, S. (2001b). *Cholecystitis and biliary colic*. Retrieved June 7, 2003, from eMedicine at http://www.emedicine.com/EMERG/topic98.htm.

Santen, S. (2001c). *Cholelithiasis*. Retrieved June 7, 2003, from eMedicine at http://www.emedicine.com/EMERG/topic97.htm.

Shelton, H. (1992). *Boyd's introduction to the study of disease*. (11th ed.). Philadelphia: Lea & Febiger.

Stone, Christian. (2003). Enteritis. In *Medical Encyclopedia*. Retrieved March 15, 2004, from MedlinePlus, the U.S. National Library of Medicine and the National Institutes of Health at http://www.nlm.nih.gov/medlineplus/ency/article/001149.htm.

Tsoi, L. (2002). *Esophagitis*. Retrieved June 7, 2003, from eMedicine at http://www.emedicine.com/EMERG/topic175.htm.

Ulcerative colitis. (2003). Retrieved June 7, 2003, from the National Digestive Diseases Information Clearinghouse, National Institutes of Health at http://www.niddk.nih.gov/health/digest/pubs/colitis/colitis.htm.

Van Wynseberghe, D., Noback, C., & Carola, R. (1995). *Human anatomy & physiology* (3rd ed.). New York: McGraw-Hill.

Venes, D. (Ed.). (2001). *Taber's cyclopedic medical dictionary* (19th ed.). Philadelphia: F. A. Davis.

Viral hepatitis A. (2003). Retrieved July 22, 2003, from the National Center for Infectious Diseases, Division of Hepatitis, Centers for Disease Control and Prevention at http://www.cdc.gov/ncidod/diseases/hepatitis/a/index.htm.

Viral hepatitis B. (2003). Retrieved July 22, 2003, from the National Center for Infectious Diseases, Division of Hepatitis, Centers for Disease Control and Prevention at http://www.cdc.gov/ncidod/diseases/hepatitis/b/index.htm.

Viral hepatitis C. (2003). Retrieved July 22, 2003, from the National Center for Infectious Diseases, Division of Hepatitis, Centers for Disease Control and Prevention at http://www.cdc.gov/ncidod/diseases/hepatitis/c/index.htm.

What is liver cancer? (n.d.). Retrieved June 7, 2003, from the American Cancer Society at http://www.cancer.org/docroot/cri/content/cri_2_2_1x_what_is_liver_cancer_25.asp.

What you need to know about cancer of the colon and rectum. (2002). Retrieved June 7, 2003, from the National Cancer Institute, National Institutes of Health at http://www.cancer.gov/cancerinfo/wyntk/colon-and-rectum.

What you need to know about cancer of the pancreas. (2002). Retrieved June 7, 2003, from the National Cancer Institute, National Institutes of Health at http://www.cancer.gov/cancerinfo/wyntk/pancreas.

CHAPTER 11

Diseases of the Respiratory System

Learning Objectives

Upon completion of the chapter, review questions, and case analysis, the reader should be able to:

- Compare and contrast emphysema, bronchitis, and asthma.
- Describe the disease complications of the common cold, pneumonia, fungal diseases of the respiratory system, and tuberculosis.
- Explain the etiology and pathogenesis of pneumoconiosis, including the affects of coal dust, silicon, asbestos, and beryllium on the respiratory system.
- Compare and contrast the causes of lung abscess and respiratory polyps.
- Explain the effects of airway obstructions, including COPD, drowning, and strangulation.
- Differentiate between rhinitis and sinusitis.
- Compare and contrast pharyngitis, laryngitis, and tracheitis.
- Explain the difference between pleurisy and atelectasis.
- Describe cystic fibrosis.
- Discuss the effects of carbon monoxide on the body.
- Explain how respiratory diseases impact the condition of the deceased.

Key Terms

asphyxia	cyanosis
asthma	emphysema
atelectasis	empyema
bronchitis	laryngitis
cavitation	pleurisy

DISORDERS OF THE RESPIRATORY SYSTEM

Disorders of the respiratory system are typically classified as either upper respiratory diseases or lower respiratory diseases. Upper respiratory disorders tend to be confined to the nose, throat, and trachea, while lower respiratory diseases involve the bronchi and lungs. However, this method of classification is deceptive because disorders significant enough to cause death are likely to involve the entire respiratory system, as well as several other systems of the body. Table 11-1 lists and describes some of the inflammatory disorders of the respiratory tract that may be present in diseases of the respiratory system.

Instead of following the traditional method of classifying diseases of the respiratory system by location, this text categorizes them as either pathological or microbiological. Pathological disorders of the respiratory system are described in more detail in this chapter, and infectious diseases of the respiratory system are described in greater detail in Part Two, where they are classified according to the type of microorganism causing the disease. While reading this chapter, the reader may review the anatomy of the respiratory system by referring to Appendix F.

Rhinitis and Sinusitis

According to the American College of Allergies, Asthma, and Immunology (*Advice* 2000), *rhinitis* is a term describing the symptoms produced by nasal irritation or inflammation, while *sinusitis* is inflammation of any or all of the four sinus cavities of the skull that open into the nasal passage. Both conditions are typified by runny nose, itching, sneezing, and stuffy nose due to blockage or congestion. Itching of the eyes is also commonly associated with both rhinitis and sinusitis. Either infections or chemical irritants can cause both rhinitis or sinusitis; however, chronic rhinitis is usually due to an allergy commonly referred to as hay fever.

The normal process of trapping small particles such as dust, pollen, and microorganisms in the mucus of the nose results in mucus flowing from the nose or draining into the throat. This drainage causes runny nose and coughing in many people. Infections of the sinus cavities associated with sinusitis can also cause pressure and pain in the face, as well as dark circles under the eyes.

Table 11-1 Inflammations of the Respiratory Tract

Rhinitis	Inflammation of the nasal passages
Sinusitis	Inflammation of a sinus in a bone
Pharyngitis	Inflammation of the pharynx
Tracheitis	Inflammation of the trachea
Bronchitis	Inflammation of the bronchi
Laryngitis	Inflammation of the larynx

Pharyngitis and Laryngitis

Pharyngitis is inflammation of the pharynx (throat), while **laryngitis** is inflammation of the larynx (voice box). A combination of pharyngitis and laryngitis results in a sore throat and the loss of one's voice. Both of these conditions are commonly found as symptoms of many respiratory infections such as the common cold or strep throat.

Common Cold

According to the National Institute of Allergy and Diseases (The common cold 2001), over 1 billion colds occur in the United States each year. The signs and symptoms of the common cold are some of the most common of any illness known, since almost everyone has experienced them at some point in time. The common cold begins with sneezing, scratchy throat, and a runny nose. These symptoms and signs generally last only one to two weeks, but the common cold is one of the leading causes of healthcare visits and school or job absences. In 1996, colds caused 45 million days of restricted activity and 22 million days lost from school in the United States.

There are more than 200 different viruses known to cause the symptoms of the common cold. Rhinoviruses and coronaviruses are two of the most common causes of colds. The common cold is age dependent, with children having between six and ten colds per year due to their relative lack of resistance to infection, while people over 60 having one or fewer colds per year. Children in school or day care, and adults who work with children are more likely to get a cold.

Symptoms of the common cold usually begin about two or three days after infection and often include nasal discharge, obstructed nasal breathing, swelling of the sinuses, sneezing, sore throat, cough, and headache. Occasionally, colds lead to secondary bacterial infections of the middle ear or sinuses. Since colds are spread through both direct and indirect contact, handwashing is one of the best ways to reduce the spread of the common cold.

Tracheitis

Tracheitis is any inflammation of the trachea; however, the term normally refers to a bacterial infection of the trachea resulting in blockage of the wind pipe. It is most often caused by *Staphylococcus aureus,* and tracheitis frequently follows viral upper respiratory infections (Newman 2003). Typically, young children are affected, possibly because their trachea is easily blocked by swelling. Due to the blockage of the airway, tracheitis almost always requires hospitalization and the insertion of a breathing tube known as an endotracheal tube. Some of the signs of tracheitis include a deep, barking cough, crowing sounds during inhalation, high fever, difficulty breathing, and intercostal retractions. Intercostal retractions occur when the muscles between the ribs pull in as the person attempts to breathe.

Bronchitis

Bronchitis is an inflammation of the bronchi, which are the main air passages to the lungs. The two forms of bronchitis are acute and chronic. To be classified as chronic bronchitis, there must be the presence of a cough with mucus most days of the month for at least three months per year (Hart 2003).

Acute bronchitis usually follows a viral respiratory infection that generally begins in the nose, sinuses, and throat and then spreads to the bronchi and lungs. In addition to the viral infection of the bronchi, a secondary bacterial infection of the bronchi is not uncommon. Thus, acute bronchitis is frequently both viral and bacterial.

Chronic bronchitis is a long-term disorder of the bronchi accompanied by excessive mucus production and a productive cough, which means that mucus is being coughed up to clear the respiratory tract. Chronic bronchitis is almost always due to inflammation of the bronchi and not an infection. It is a component of chronic obstructive pulmonary disease, which is described later in this chapter.

Asthma

Asthma is a condition, which is sometimes chronic, in which the bronchi are hypersensitive to stimuli. Not unlike an allergic reaction, the mucous lining of the bronchi become irritated, and the bronchi proceed to swell shut, causing a reduction in airflow. This condition often causes the individual to hunch forward in an attempt to inhale. Individuals with asthma also have a characteristic wheezing sound accompanied by shortness of breath. Asthma tends to occur more frequently in children than adults.

Asthma attacks may be caused by allergens such as pollen, dust, mold spores, or animal dander. Respiratory tract infections may also cause asthma attacks. Certain foods such as eggs, shellfish, and chocolate may bring about an asthma attack. The individual's emotional state plays a role in asthma attacks as well—increased fatigue adds to the likelihood of an attack.

Pneumonia

Pneumonia is an inflammation of the lungs, although the term is clinically used to refer to an infection of the lungs. The majority of cases of pneumonia are due to a bacterial infection, but viruses also cause pneumonia. Pneumonias are categorized by the site of the infection and by the causative agent. Lobar pneumonia affects a single lobe of the lung, while bronchial pneumonia affects smaller lung areas in several lobes.

Pleurisy

Pleurisy is an inflammatory condition of the pleurae that surround the lungs. When the pleural space is invaded by microbes, the ensuing infection causes a variety of possible complications. The exudate that develops between the pleura may contain pus, causing a condition known as **empyema**. Pleurisy may also involve the development of fibrous materials, causing the pleura to adhere to the diaphragm or the chest wall. A condition known as hemorrhagic pleurisy also exists, wherein blood is found in the pleural space. Pleurisy may by characterized by any or all of the following:

- Stabbing pain in the affected area
- Worsening pain during deep breathing
- Chills
- Coughing
- Fever
- Pale and anxious face
- Guarding the affected side or lying on the affected side

Tuberculosis

According to the World Health Organization (*Tuberculosis* 2002), tuberculosis (TB) causes the death of over 2 million people each year. WHO has declared tuberculosis a global emergency due to what it calls the global breakdown in health services, the spread of HIV/AIDS, and the emergence of multidrug–resistant forms of TB.

Tuberculosis is a highly contagious disease that is spread through the air. When infected persons sneeze or cough, the bacterium that causes TB, *Mycobacterium tuberculosis* (described in Part Two) is spread.

One of the primary concerns about TB is that it has become multidrug–resistant, meaning that there are strains of TB that are resistant to all major anti-TB drugs. Multidrug–resistant TB has several contributing causes:

- Inconsistent or partial treatment
- Patients who do not take all of their drugs regularly for the required period because they start to feel better
- Healthcare providers who prescribe the wrong treatment or prescribe drugs that are unreliable

The bacterium that causes tuberculosis has a waxy coat that allows it to withstand extreme changes in its environment. It can survive for long periods of time in dried sputum or blood. TB affects the lungs, but it may spread to other parts of the body. TB gets its name from the formation of lesions known as tubercles that occur when the immune system walls off the TB bacterium, which then ruptures and spreads. The surrounding tissue becomes necrotic and forms a cheeselike substance known as caseation. TB is often accompanied by hemorrhaging resulting in hemoptysis, which is spitting up of blood. Persons with TB are often emaciated and dehydrated due to the chronic nature of the disease process. Tuberculosis also causes **cavitation** in the lungs, which is the formation of cavities within the lung tissue or other organs affected by tuberculosis.

Pneumoconiosis

Pneumoconiosis is an inflammatory disorder of the respiratory system caused by the inhalation of mineral dusts. Although some experts include the inhalation of certain organic compounds and chemical fumes and vapors as causes of pneumoconiosis, this text restricts the term to mineral dusts. The four most common pneumoconioses result from the inhalation of coal dust, silica, asbestos, and beryllium. Although pneumoconioses were once thought to be strictly occupational disorders among individuals who worked with these minerals, the increased frequency of cancers in family members extends the potential of these irritants to cause disease outside the workplace.

The reaction of the lung to mineral dusts depends on the size, shape, solubility, and reactivity of the dust particles. Large particles do not reach the distal airway, while extremely small pieces could potentially enter the alveoli and the blood. Coal dust is relatively inert and usually requires a fairly large amount of dust to accumulate before a disease reaction occurs in the body; however, silica, asbestos, and beryllium are more reactive than coal and cause disease at lower concentrations.

Most mineral dust is trapped by the mucus in the respiratory system and removed by the ciliated epithelial lining of the respiratory tract. Some dust, however, can become trapped in the respiratory system, causing macrophages to accumulate locally. These phagocytic cells release chemicals that are hazardous to the lungs, as they attempt to remove and destroy the inhaled dust particles. The combination of the presence of the mineral particles and the immune system response causes the formation of fibrous masses in the lungs.

The damage caused to the respiratory system can spread throughout the lymphatic system of the body. Smoking tobacco worsens the effects of all inhaled mineral dusts, but it is especially harmful in the case of asbestos exposure. Pneumoconiosis is typically associated with other respiratory disorders, heart failure, cancer, and death.

Coal Worker's Pneumoconiosis. Coal worker's pneumoconiosis is also known as black lung disease or anthracosis. At one time, coal miners spent a lifetime underground with picks and shovels, breathing the contaminants of coal mining. Although coal mostly consists of carbon, coal dust contains all of the minerals in the rock that surrounds the coal, including crystalline silica. As the miners swung picks into the face of the rock, they created tremendous amounts of dust that had nowhere to go. Proper ventilation and the use of respirators was not a priority in the early days of mining. Modern mining operations are much safer than those 50 years ago and earlier. Figure 11-1 depicts the lungs of a coal worker with pneumoconiosis. Note the excessive amount of coal dust lodged in the fine tissues of the lung, which causes them to harden, making breathing difficult.

Silicosis. Silicosis is the inhalation of crystalline silica, which primarily occurs as a result of occupational exposure. Some of the occupations that are at high risk of silica exposure include sandblasting, quarry mining, drilling, tunneling, and stone cutting. Crystalline forms of silica include quartz, cristobalite, and

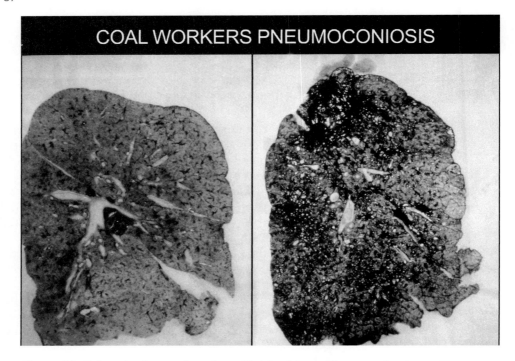

Figure 11-1 Lungs of a coal worker with black lung disease. (Courtesy of the Centers for Disease Control and Prevention, Atlanta, GA.)

tridymite. These crystals are used in artwork, watches, lenses, ceramics, plastics, and products such as bricks, chalk, and gypsum board.

Asbestosis. Asbestosis is a pneumoconiosis resulting from the inhalation of asbestos, which is a crystalline form of silica that has a fibrous structure. The extremely fine strands of asbestos are capable of reaching far down the respiratory tract, where they interact with macrophages to cause fibrous lesions, which can develop into cancer. Asbestos was once used in flame-retardant materials, in insulation, roofing shingles, floor tiles, siding, and joint compounds. Remember that all pneumoconioses result from the inhalation of mineral dust. Asbestos must be inhaled to cause asbestosis.

Berylliosis. Beryllium is the second lightest of all metals, and is, therefore, a useful component in nuclear, aerospace, and manufacturing industries. Beryllium is found in coal, oil, soil, volcanic ash, and in many rocks. Berylliosis is a pneumoconiosis caused by inhalation of beryllium dust. Beryllium is used in the manufacture of golf clubs, dental applications, nonsparking tools, wheelchairs, and a variety of electronic instruments.

Atelectasis

Atelectasis is commonly referred to as a collapsed lung, and it literally means "incomplete expansion." **Atelectasis** is the loss of lung volume due to inadequate expansion of airspaces, which results in inadequate oxygen and carbon dioxide exchange within the lungs. The result is that blood is not able to eliminate carbon dioxide and refresh itself with the oxygen it needs.

There are two categories of collapsed lung, obstructed and nonobstructed. Obstructive atelectasis is the most common type of collapsed lung, and it results when the trachea or bronchi becomes blocked. Causes of obstructive atelectasis include choking on a foreign body, tumors in the airway, fungal respiratory infections, or the presence of excessive amounts of mucus that plug the airway. Examples of diseases associated with mucus blockage include bronchial asthma, chronic bronchitis, cystic fibrosis, paralysis, and amyotrophic lateral sclerosis. Depending on the level of obstruction, the entire lung, a single lobe, or a segment of the lung may collapse.

Nonobstructive atelectasis can be caused by loss of contact between the parietal and visceral pleurae, compression, loss of surfactant, and replacement of lung tissue by scarring. Congestive heart failure can cause the accumulation of fluids resulting in nonobstructive lung collapse, or it may be caused by blood or air within the pleural cavity. Penetrating trauma, such as gunshot wounds or stab wounds, can allow air to leak from inside the lung into the pleural space. The trapped air between the outside and inside of the lung prevents the lung from fully expanding and causes it to collapse; this condition is referred to as a pneumothorax. If blood becomes trapped in the same space, the condition is referred to hemothorax.

Emphysema

Emphysema is a chronic inflammatory disease of the respiratory system, characterized by the presence of air pockets at the terminal ends of the bronchioles. The walls of the alveolar sacs become desiccated and tear. Because the individual is able to inhale, but is unable to properly exhale, a characteristic barrel chest develops, as illustrated in Figure 11-2. Individuals with emphysema may also purse their lips when exhaling in an effort to expel trapped air from the alveoli. Emphysema is often a secondary disease brought on by infections, long-term smoking, or pneumoconiosis.

Lung Abscess

A lung abscess is an area of inflamed, pus-filled tissue in the lung caused by infection. It is usually caused by bacteria that have been inhaled from the nose and mouth, resulting in an infection. Periodontal gum diseases are frequently the cause of a lung abscess (Beers 2004). A lung abscess may also be associated with a tumor in the lung, or it may associated with pneumonia. Although most people only develop one lung abscess, multiple lung abscesses have been noted in IV

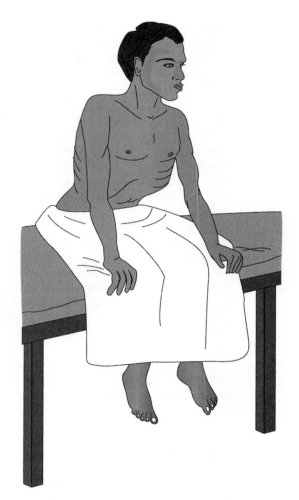

Figure 11-2 Pursed lips and barrel chest of emphysema.

drug users who use contaminated needles. In these cases, the infection begins at the site of injection and spreads to the lungs through the blood.

A lung abscess will eventually rupture, causing the formation of a cavity filled with fluid and air in the lung. The rupture of an abscess produces a large quantity of pus, fluid, and blood that is coughed up and expectorated. If the lung abscess ruptures into the pleural space, pus may fill the space causing empyema.

Fungal Diseases

There are a variety of fungal diseases that affect the respiratory system. Many fungal diseases of the respiratory system are complications of AIDS. Some of the most common fungal diseases of the respiratory system include histoplasmosis, aspergillosis, and coccidioidomycosis. Chapter 28 describes each of these fungal diseases in detail.

Cystic Fibrosis

Cystic fibrosis is the most common fatal genetic disease in the United States. It is a terminal disease in most cases at an average age of 20. According to the National Human Genome Research Institute (*Learning about cystic fibrosis* 2003), about 30,000 people in the United States have the disease. It is caused by mutations in the cystic fibrosis transmembrane regulator gene. The protein associated with this gene should allow cells to release chloride and other ions, but in CF, the cells are defective and do not release the chloride. The lack of chloride results in a salt imbalance in the cells. The defective cells produce a thick, sticky mucus that clogs the lungs, leads to infection, and blocks the pancreas. In addition, the presence of this thick mucus stops digestive enzymes from reaching the intestine, where they are required for proper digestion. Diabetes mellitus is frequently found in cases of CF. Researchers are focusing on ways to cure CF by correcting the defective gene, or correcting the defective protein.

Respiratory Polyps

Although polyps can occur anywhere along the respiratory tract, they are most common in the nose and throat of people with chronic allergic rhinitis or sinusitis. A polyp is a tumor with a pedicle, which is a stem that attaches it to surrounding tissue and supplies it with blood. Polyps bleed easily, and they may become malignant. Large respiratory polyps may interfere with breathing and are often removed surgically to ease breathing and reduce chronic inflammation and symptoms of allergy.

Carbon Monoxide Poisoning

Carbon monoxide (CO) is a colorless, tasteless, odorless gas produced by burning material containing carbon. Carbon monoxide poisoning is sometimes referred to as a silent killer because carbon monoxide is nonirritating, unlike other gases like formaldehyde, which has an irritating effect on the respiratory system causing watery eyes, runny nose, and a burning sensation in the throat.

The most common sources of CO are:

- Gas water heaters
- Kerosene space heaters
- Charcoal grills
- Propane stoves and heaters
- Propane-fueled forklifts
- Gas-powered concrete saws
- Indoor tractor pulls
- Swimming behind a motorboat
- Inhaling spray paint, solvents, or degreasers

- Riding in the back of an enclosed pickup truck
- Working indoors with combustion engines
- Steel foundries
- Home fires
- Fireplaces and woodstoves

Carbon monoxide poisoning is often associated with malfunctioning or obstructed exhaust systems and with suicide attempts. In a small, closed garage, the average car exhaust can induce a lethal coma within five minutes.

In the red blood cell, it is hemoglobin that transports carbon dioxide and oxygen. Hemoglobin has an affinity 200 times stronger for carbon monoxide than it does for oxygen, meaning that once carbon monoxide bonds with hemoglobin, the mere introduction of oxygen is not sufficient to restore proper levels of oxygen in the blood. Carbon monoxide kills by inducing central nervous system impairment, which prevents the person being poisoned from recognizing its effects and seeking help. Some of the most common characteristics of carbon monoxide poisoning are:

- Headache
- Dizziness
- Nausea
- Drowsiness
- Shortness of breath
- Chest pain
- Impaired judgment
- Confusion
- Hallucination
- Agitation
- Vomiting
- Abdominal pain
- Visual impairment
- Seizure

Among individuals who die from carbon monoxide poisoning, a characteristic cherry-red discoloration of the skin and mucous membranes is present due to carboxyhemoglobin in the blood. If the time between initial poisoning and death is long, swelling and hemorrhaging of the brain can also occur.

Flail Chest

The arched design of the rib cage allows it to absorb some blunt force due to its flexibility, and the intercostal muscles and fascia offer further strength and stability. Crushing injuries associated with heavy objects or sudden deceleration injuries may break a rib in one position, but only a significant impact breaks a rib in two or more positions.

A flail chest is the paradoxical movement of a segment of chest wall caused by three or more ribs broken in two or more places. Paradoxical movement means that as someone with a flail chest inhales, the portion of the rib cage that is fractured does not move with the expanding chest wall. The opposite is also the case: When the person exhales, and the chest wall moves inward, the fractured portion bulges out slightly, as indicated in Figure 11-3.

However, it is not the flail chest itself that is most significant; it is the amount of injury to the respiratory system and heart that typically causes fatality. A flail chest can be caused by such trauma as motor vehicle accidents, falls, and physical assault, although it may also result from minor trauma in persons with an underlying disease such as osteoporosis, which weakens the ribs.

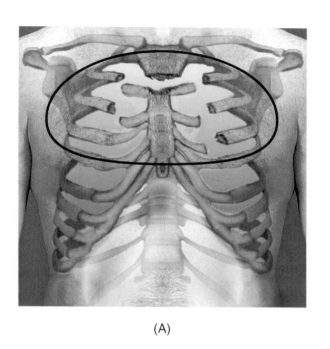

(A)

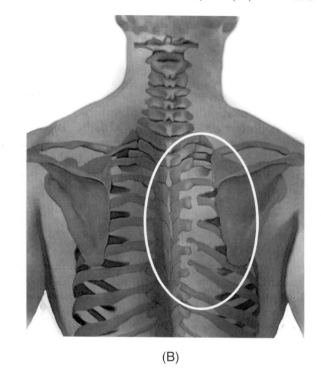

(B)

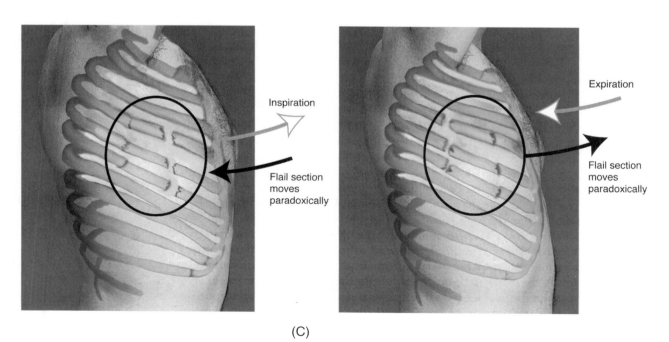

(C)

Figure 11-3 Flail chest: (A) anterior, (B) posterior, (C) lateral.

Flail chest may also occur during the embalming of the deceased as a result of aspiration of the thorax. In individuals with a compromised rib cage due to disorders such as bone cancer, osteoporosis, or blunt force trauma, the aspirator may exert enough pressure to fracture the sternum or ribs, collapsing a portion of the chest wall. Although this event may be disconcerting to the embalmer, it is simply the result of physical forces and does not represent an error on the part of the embalmer. The embalmer should continue to thoroughly aspirate the thorax and abdomen.

After thorough aspiration, and before the injection of cavity fluid, the embalmer should disconnect the trocar from the aspirator and reinsert the trocar into the abdomen. Angle the trocar tip toward the flail portion of the chest, and use the tip of the trocar to elevate the chest to its normal position. The embalmer should avoid exerting pressure on the surface of the chest wall during the injection of cavity fluid and the subsequent performance of cosmeticizing, dressing, and casketing the deceased.

Lung Cancer

Lung cancer is a leading cause of cancer deaths in both men and women in the United States. According to the Physicians Desk Reference Series (*Lung cancer* 2003), it is estimated that, in 2000, approximately 164,000 new cases of lung cancer were diagnosed and about 157,000 people died of the disease. Although smoking accounts for the vast majority of cases, there are other risk factors. Exposure to high levels of certain compounds encountered in mining and manufacturing can raise the risk of lung cancer. Such compounds include asbestos, a group of fibrous minerals that can lodge in the lungs when inhaled; bischloromethyl ether and chloromethyl ether, used to produce other chemicals; chromium, used in the manufacture of chrome plating; beryllium, used in aircraft, telecommunications, and high-technology industries; and arsenic, a byproduct of copper.

The characteristics of lung cancer—which often go undiagnosed until the cancer is advanced because they are common to many disorders—can include any or all of the following:

- Chest pain
- Shortness of breath
- Hoarseness
- Coughing
- Coughing up blood
- Pneumonia
- Bronchitis
- Wheezing
- Swelling of the neck and face
- Chest, shoulder, or arm pain
- Headache
- Unexplained fever

Lung cancers are divided into two categories: small cell lung cancer and nonsmall cell lung cancer. Small cell carcinomas, which are also known as oat cell carcinomas because they look like oats under the microscope, are normally associated with a history of cigarette smoking. These tumors grow very rapidly and quickly spread to other organs.

Nonsmall cell cancers account for the majority of lung cancers. The three types of nonsmall cell cancers are squamous cell carcinoma, adenocarcinoma, and large cell carcinoma. Squamous cell carcinoma usually begins in the bronchi and is closely associated with a history of smoking. Adenocarcinoma often develops along the outer edges of the lungs and under the membranes lining the bronchi. Large cell carcinomas are a group of cancers with large, abnormal-looking cells called "giant" or "clear" cells. They can appear in any part of the lung and tend to spread to other parts of the body.

By the time lung cancer is diagnosed, it usually has spread beyond the primary tumor. Lung cancer is rarely found in its early development because early-stage disease generally produces few, if any, symptoms, and those that do occur tend to be ignored. Lung cancer also has a tendency to spread quickly. The lungs are especially well supplied by the blood and lymph systems, which serve to carry cells to other parts of the body.

Chronic Obstructive Pulmonary Disease

Chronic obstructive pulmonary disease (COPD) is commonly listed by physicians as a cause of death on death certificates. It is a respiratory disorder in which the bronchioles become occluded, and the alveolar sacs become dehydrated. COPD complicates chronic bronchitis when bronchioles become plugged with mucus. The plugged bronchioles develop a bacterial infection that makes breathing difficult. Emphysema is typically found in association with chronic bronchitis under the umbrella of COPD. The individual is unable to draw a normal breath due to the bacterial obstruction and is unable to exhale normally due to the pockets of air that develop in the lungs.

Hanging and Strangulation

Deaths due to either hanging or strangulation are classified as asphyxias. The term **asphyxia** is defined as the inability to take in necessary amounts of oxygen. The physical constriction and squeezing of the soft tissues not only prevents breathing, it affects the cardiovascular system, the central nervous system, and body metabolism as well. The most common signs of asphyxia:

- Congestion of the veins of the face
- Facial edema
- Cyanosis
- Petechial hemorrhages of the face and eyes
- Ligature marks on the neck

Compression of the jugular veins with or without concurrent compression of the carotid arteries leads to a reduction in the amount of oxygen reaching the brain, the loss of consciousness, and eventually death. If both carotid arteries are compressed, it takes approximately ten seconds to lose consciousness. If only the jugular veins are compressed, it takes approximately one minute to lose consciousness. Given continued compression, the time frame from the loss of consciousness to death is only a matter of minutes.

Airway obstruction occurs when the hyoid bone and tongue are pushed in a superior and posterior direction forcing the laryngopharynx closed. It is also believed that pressure exerted on the carotid arteries over the carotid sinus provokes a reflex that slows the heart and produces a fatal arrhythmia.

Classic signs of hanging or strangulation begin with congestion of the face due to blood pooling in the veins. In cases of strangulation, bruising of the neck is common (see Color Plate 24). The veins become congested with blood because compression of the jugular veins prevents the return of blood to the heart. Another classic sign is facial edema due to the increased venous blood pressure. The head develops a bluish discoloration referred to as **cyanosis** that results from the presence of deoxyhemoglobin in the blood. Another characteristic sign of asphyxia is petechial hemorrhage in the skin and eyes, particularly in the eyelids, conjunctiva, sclera, face, lips, and behind the ears. The person pictured in Figure 11-4 exhibits the characteristic signs of traumatic asphyxia as a result of being pinned under an overturned vehicle.

Petechia is a pinpoint bleeding in the capillary beds due to increased venous pressure in the case of hanging and strangulation. Color Plate 25 depicts petechiae in the feet due to increased blood pressure. The final sign of hanging or strangulation is ligature marks on the neck. Thin ligature lacerates the tissue, while wide ligature results in characteristic bruising patterns that match the design of the ligature. Hanging usually results in marks high on the neck due to the weight of the body as it hangs, while strangulation marks are typically lower on the neck.

Drowning

According to the National Center for Health Statistics (2000), there were 4,406 drownings in 1998, including 1,003 children under the age of 15. The United States Coast Guard (*U.S. Coast Guard boating statistic* 1992) also received 6,000 reports of crashes involving recreational boats that resulted in 3,700 injuries and 816 deaths in 1992. Of all injury deaths for children, drowning was the second leading cause in 1998, and in that same year, over 80 percent of drownings were men. Most striking is the disparity between African American children and Caucasian children in their rates of drowning. In 1998, African American children ages 5 to 19 drowned at a rate 2.5 times higher than Caucasian children. Among adult drownings in 1992, about half were alcohol related. The majority of all child drownings occur in home swimming pools. According to the Consumer Product Safety Commission (*Large buckets* 1989), mop buckets, especially plastic five-gallon buckets, pose a drowning hazard to young children.

Drowning is defined as death secondary to asphyxia while immersed in a liquid, usually water, or within 24 hours of submersion (Shepherd and Martin 2002). The popular image of a drowning victim thrashing about and gasping for

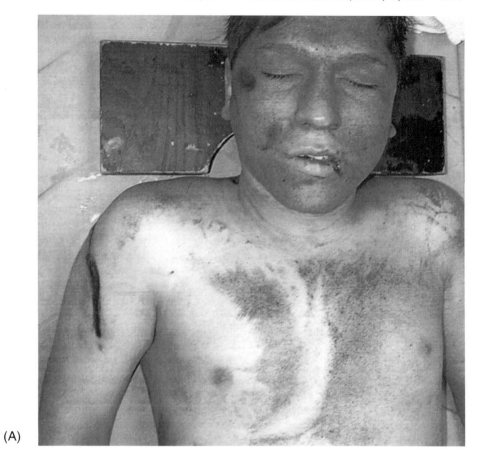

(A)

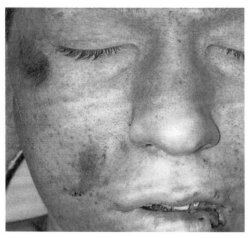

(B)

Figure 11-4 (A) Death due to traumatic asphyxia while pinned under a vehicle. (B) Note petechiae and congestion of the face. (Reprinted with permission from Vincent J. DiMaio and Dominick DiMaio, 2001, *Forensic pathology*, 2nd ed. Copyright CRC Press, Boca Raton, FL.)

air is rarely reported. In actuality, most drowning victims are motionless individuals who float in the water or quietly disappear beneath the surface of the water. After a brief period of initial gasping, and possibly inhaling water, remaining under water stimulates hyperventilation, followed by a period of holding one's breath until spasms of the larynx occur. As the oxygen level decreases in the body causing hypoxemia, anaerobic respiration occurs in the cells increasing the level of lactic acid in the body's tissues and causing a condition known as lactic acidosis. The combination of these factors eventually leads to cardiac arrest or brain death. Thereafter, the airway relaxes, and the lungs fill with water, although in about 10 percent to 20 percent of the cases the airway remains closed and the lungs do not fill with water. In short, drowning victims do not die from water filling their lungs, they die from a lack of air. The lungs only fill with water after death in most drowning cases.

POSTMORTEM CONDITIONS ASSOCIATED WITH RESPIRATORY DISORDERS

Respiratory illnesses can cause a variety of effects on the body that may complicate the embalming process. The embalmer should recognize five postmortem conditions in the deceased that potentially signal death resulting from respiratory illnesses.

1. Cyanosis
2. Emaciation
3. Hydrothorax
4. Hemorrhage
5. Cavitation

Because respiratory illnesses are associated with a lack of appropriate oxygenation of tissues, a characteristic blue discoloration of the skin and mucous membranes known as cyanosis is typically present. The blue discoloration is the result of the presence of deoxyhemoglobin in the blood. Cyanosis is an antemortem, intravascular discoloration that is removed during the process of arterial injection of embalming fluids. The adequate removal of cyanosis depends on proper distribution and profusion of arterial embalming fluid in the tissues of the deceased. Gentle massage and copious amounts of nonastringent arterial fluids may be required depending on the length of time between death and embalming, which is referred to as the *postmortem interval*.

Many respiratory disorders are chronic, and death may occur only after a long period of disease. The lack of proper respiration frequently results in debilitation that is characterized by emaciation. Abnormal respiratory function also affects circulation resulting in hydrothorax and hemorrhage. Thorough aspiration of the deceased is a critical component in the inhibition of the formation of purge.

Purge from the respiratory system is typically reddish-pink and frothy due to the combination of blood, edematous fluids, and air. It is also essential that proper cavity treatment occur to retard the spread of microbial agents in cases of respiratory infection such as tuberculosis, which causes cavitation of the lung tissue. The embalmer must follow universal precautions and utilize personal protective equipment because respiratory infections can potentially spread from the deceased to the embalmer and the public.

Injuries to the trachea or larynx may necessitate either a tracheotomy or a laryngectomy, in which a stoma is created in the neck. Figure 11-5 pictures a man with stoma of the neck along with a prosthesis. Scar tissue associated with stomas in the neck may complicate the arterial injection of the common carotid arteries. Some embalmers prefer to utilize the femoral artery and femoral vein for the arterial injection of persons with a stoma in the neck.

The stoma should be disinfected and cauterized. Drying powder and absorbent material should be inserted in the stoma, and the stoma should be sutured and sealed. It may be necessary to apply mortuary wax to the sutures used to close the stoma to attain an aesthetically pleasing restoration of the neck.

The postmortem conditions associated with drowning victims are unique to each case. Among young children who drown in cold water, a diving reflex may occur that constricts nonessential blood vessels to shunt blood to the heart and brain. The location of the drowning is also important. Depending on location, the victim may have vomit, sand, silt, or sewage anywhere in the respiratory system. Individuals who survive for a period of time between the drowning and death may also experience pulmonary edema following the spasms of the larynx. Edema of the central nervous system may also occur.

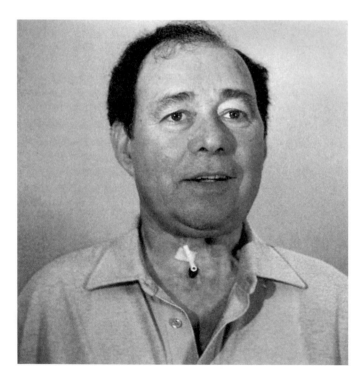

Figure 11-5 Laryngeal stoma.

Embalming a drowning victim, like any other case, must begin with a thorough case analysis. Although the embalmer may anticipate the need to aspirate water from the thorax, it may be possible that there will be no excess water due to contraction of the larynx. Pulmonary and cerebral edema may also need to be treated. The distribution of arterial embalming fluids may be inhibited by vasoconstriction in peripheral tissues. It is also important to examine the deceased thoroughly for masked injuries. Drownings may be caused by seizure disorders, heart attacks, neuromuscular diseases, diabetes, drug or alcohol abuse, shark bite, jelly fish stings, or trauma to the spine or head associated with surfing, water skiing, or falling from a boat. Identifying the cause of the drowning may help the embalmer more effectively embalm the deceased.

REVIEW QUESTIONS

Matching

1. _____ rhinitis
2. _____ emphysema
3. _____ carbon monoxide poisoning
4. _____ pleurisy
5. _____ sinusitis

a. inflammation of the sinuses
b. characterized by a barrel chest
c. pus between the pleura
d. inflammation of the nasal passage
e. characterized by a cherry-red discoloration

Multiple Choice

1. Which of the following is a condition in which the mucous lining of the bronchi become irritated, and the bronchi proceed to swell shut causing a reduction in air flow?
   a. emphysema
   b. COPD
   c. asthma
   d. pneumoconiosis

2. Which of the following conditions is characterized by a loss of lung volume due to inadequate expansion of airspaces?
   a. asthma
   b. atelectasis
   c. COPD
   d. emphysema

3. Which of the following occurs after death in most drownings?
   a. water enters the lungs
   b. hypoxemia
   c. lactic acidosis
   d. heart or brain failure

4. Which of the following conditions is a respiratory disorder involving both asthma and emphysema?

   a. anthracosis

   b. berylliosis

   c. pleurisy

   d. COPD

5. Which of the following is a condition characterized by blood in the pleural space?

   a. silicosis

   b. hemorrhagic pleurisy

   c. flail chest

   d. cyanosis

Putting Learning to Work!

The purpose of the following case analysis is to allow you to apply the information you have learned in a real-world situation. Read the case carefully and try to answer the following questions:

     What disorder do you suspect the person had at the time of death?

     What potential embalming complications do you anticipate?

     What precautions should you take as the embalmer to limit the effects of these complications?

Case Analysis

A 25-year-old male died as a result of a motor vehicle accident. The man was driving a five-speed pickup truck. The gearshift was missing its knob. When the man was struck from the passenger side in a T-bone collision, he was thrown to the right. The man was not wearing a seatbelt, and the force of the impact impaled the gearshift into his right abdominal flank just below his rib cage. The angle of the gearshift was such that the tip punctured his right lung. On aspiration, you discover a large quantity of blood in the right side of his thorax, and a whistling sound is present through the puncture wound in the man's chest.

Bibliography

Advice from your allergist: Rhinitis. (2000). Retrieved March 16, 2004, from the American College of Allergy, Asthma, and Immunology at http://allergy.mcg.edu/advice/rhin.html.

Beers, Mark H. (Ed.). (2004). Lung abscess. In *The Merck Manual: 2nd Home Edition.* Retrieved March 16, 2004, from http://www.merck.com/mrkshared/mmanual_home2/sec04/ch043/ch043a.jsp.

Cole, C. (2002). *Carbon monoxide poisoning.* Retrieved June 9, 2003, from eMedicine http://www.emedicine.com/aaem/topic92.htm.

The common cold. (2001). In *Health matters.* Retrieved March 16, 2004, from the National Institute of Allergy and Infectious Diseases, National Institutes of Health, U.S. Department of Health and Human Services at http://www.niaid.nih.gov/factsheets/cold.htm.

Cystic fibrosis research directions. (1997). Retrieved May 30, 2003, from the National Institutes of Health, National Institute of Diabetes and Digestive and Kidney Disorders at http://www.niddk.nih.gov/health/endo/pubs/cystic/cystic.htm.

Fretz, P., & Hughes, J. (2003). *Adenocarcinoma: Lung tumors.* Retrieved May 29, 2003, from the Virtual Hospital, University of Iowa Health Care at http://www.vh.org/adult/provider/radiology/LungTumors/PathologicTypes/Text/Adenocarcinoma.html.

Hart, Jacqueline. (2003). Bronchitis. In *Medical Encyclopedia.* Retrieved March 16, 2004, from MedlinePlus, the U.S. National Library of Medicine and the National Institutes of Health at http://www.nlm.nih.gov/medlineplus/ency/article/001087.htm.

Kumar, V., Cotran, R., & Robbins, S. (2003). *Robbins basic pathology* (7th ed.). Philadelphia: Saunders.

Large buckets are drowning hazards for young children. (1989). Retrieved April 10, 2004, from News from CPSC, U.S. Consumer Product Safety Commission at http://www.cpsc.gov/cpscpub/prerel/prhtml89/89065.html.

Learning about cystic fibrosis. (n/d). Retrieved May 30, 2003, from the National Institutes of Health. National Human Genome Research Institute at http://www.genome.gov/page.cfm?pageID=10001213.

Lung cancer: Hard to cure; easy to prevent. (2003). Retrieved July 23, 2003, from Thomson Learning at http://www.gettingwell.com/content/lifelong_health/chapters/fgac30.shtml.

Mayer, R. (2000). *Embalming: History, theory, & practice* (3rd ed.). New York: McGraw-Hill.

National Center for Health Statistics (NCHS). (2000). *National Mortality Data*, 1998. Hyattsville, MD: NCHS.

Neighbors, M., & Tannehill-Jones, R. (2000). *Human diseases.* Clifton Park, NY: Thomson Delmar Learning.

Newman, Jason. (2003). Tracheitis. In *Medical Encyclopedia.* Retrieved March 16, 2004, from MedlinePlus, the U.S. National Library of Medicine and the National Institutes of Health at http://www.nlm.nih.gov/medlineplus/ency/article/000988.htm.

Pathology for funeral service. (1999). Dallas, TX: Professional Training Schools.

Sharma, S. (2003). *Atelectasis.* Retrieved June 9, 2003, from eMedicine at http://www.emedicine.com/med/topic180.htm.

Shelton, H. (1992). *Boyd's introduction to the study of disease* (11th ed.). Philadelphia: Lea & Febiger.

Shepherd, S., & Martin, J. (2002). *Submersion injury, near drowning.* Retrieved May 27, 2003, from eMedicine at http://www.emedicine.com/emerg/topic744.htm.

Tuberculosis. (2003). Retrieved July 26, 2003, from MedlinePlus, the U.S. National Library of Medicine and the National Institutes of Health at http://www.nlm.nih.gov/medlineplus/tuberculosis.html.

Tuberculosis. (2003). Retrieved July 26, 2003, from the National Center for HIV, STDs, and TB Prevention, Division of Tuberculosis Elimination, Centers for Disease Control and Prevention at http://www.cdc.gov/nchstp/tb/faqs/qa.htm.

Tuberculosis. (2002). Retrieved March 16, 2004, from the World Health Organization at http://www.who.int/mediacentre/factsheets/fs104/en/.

Tuberculosis resources. (n/d). Retrieved July 26, 2003, from the Department of Biomedical Informatics at Columbia University at http://www.cpmc.columbia.edu/tbcpp/.

U.S. Coast Guard boating statistic. (1992). Washington, DC: U.S. Department of Transportation.

Venes, D. (Ed.). (2001). *Taber's cyclopedic medical dictionary* (19th ed.). Philadelphia: F. A. Davis.

CHAPTER 12

Diseases of the Urinary System

Learning Objectives

Upon completion of the chapter, review questions, and case analysis, the reader should be able to:

- Describe the lesions and disease conditions associated with uremia, focusing on the significance of uremia on the embalming process.
- Compare and contrast pyelitis, pyelonephritis, ureteritis, cystitis, and urethritis.
- Differentiate between nephrolithiasis and polycystic kidney.
- Compare and contrast renal cell carcinoma and carcinoma of the urinary bladder.
- Explain the relationship between renal failure and dialysis.
- Compare and contrast glomerulonephritis and hydronephrosis.
- Explain the impact of urinary system diseases on the condition of the deceased.

Key Terms

dialysis
dysplasia
nitrogen

uremia
urotropin

DISORDERS OF THE URINARY SYSTEM

Disorders of the urinary system are extremely important to the embalmer due to the associated accumulation of nitrogen in the tissues of the body. **Nitrogen** as a gas is colorless and odorless, and is generally considered an inert element. Nitrogen compounds, however, are found in foods, organic materials, fertilizers, poisons, and explosives. As a liquid, nitrogen is also colorless and odorless, and is similar in appearance to water. The more nitrogen present in the tissues of the deceased, the higher the formaldehyde demand during the embalming process. Not only is nitrogen released in the tissues during decomposition of human remains, it is also present in the form of several nitrogenous waste products when the urinary system fails to function properly. Urinary disorders can also result in edematous tissues that may be laden with microbial agents. The combination of the nitrogenous compounds, excess fluids, and microbial agents may all yield increased rates of decomposition and retardation of the effective distribution and diffusion of embalming fluids.

Table 12-1 lists some significant inflammatory disorders of the urinary system. While reading this chapter, the reader may review the anatomy of the urinary system by referring to Appendix G.

Uremia

Uremia is a disorder of the urinary system caused by retention in the blood of nitrogenous waste products normally excreted in the urine. Uremia is noticeable to the embalmer by its strong odor and possible yellow discoloration of the tissues. Because of the high nitrogenous waste levels in the remains, the formaldehyde demand is greatly increased and dehydration and edema are commonly present, as observed in Color Plate 26. If any yellow discoloration is present, the embalmer should err on the side of caution and utilize a jaundice fluid rather than a high index embalming fluid.

Some of the most common characteristics of uremia are:

- Nausea
- Vomiting
- Headache
- Dizziness
- Reduced vision
- Coma or convulsions

Table 12-1 Inflammatory Disorders of the Urinary System

Glomerulonephritis	Microbial inflammation of the glomerulus and the nephron
Pyelonephritis	Inflammation of the kidney and the nephron
Pyelitis	Inflammation of the renal pelvis of the kidney
Nephrolithiasis	Kidney stones (renal calculi)
Ureteritis	Inflammation of the ureter
Cystitis	Inflammation of the urinary bladder
Urethritis	Inflammation of the urethra

- Urinous odor of the breath and perspiration
- Stupor
- Lack of pupil reaction
- Dry skin
- Hard, rapid pulse
- High blood pressure

Bright's Disease

Bright's disease is an antiquated name for kidney disease in general. Richard Bright, an English physician, performed groundbreaking work in describing renal insufficiency between 1827 and 1836. Since the 1960s, renal diseases have been classified in more specific terms.

Glomerulonephritis

Bright initially described acute glomerulonephritis in 1827, and acute nephritic syndrome remains the most serious and potentially devastating form of renal disorders. Acute glomerulonephritis is characterized by the sudden onset of blood and protein in the urine accompanied by salt and water retention. There are both structural and functional changes associated with acute glomerulonephritis.

At the cellular level, there is an increase in the number of epithelial and endothelial cells in the glomerulus. Immune system cells known as neutrophils and monocytes are also present in large numbers in the glomerulus. The capillary walls within the glomerulus also thicken. As a result of these anatomical changes, the glomerulus undergoes physiological changes such as the excess secretion of proteins in the urine, blood in the urine, edema, and high blood pressure. Acute glomerulonephritis can be caused by streptococcal throat infection, skin infection, hepatitis, diabetes, or intravenous drug use. Depending on etiology, glomerulonephritis is treated with antibiotics. Acute glomerulonephritis can be accompanied by any or all of the following:

- Loss of appetite
- Generalized itching
- Nausea
- Easy bruising
- Nose bleeds
- Facial swelling
- Leg edema
- Shortness of breath
- Ascites
- Skin rash
- Pale skin
- Joint swelling

Acute glomerulonephritis may progress into chronic glomerulonephritis. In cases of chronic glomerulonephritis, the glomerulus becomes fibrous. Symptoms of chronic glomerulonephritis include weakness, loss of appetite, weight loss, pus in the urine, early morning nausea and vomiting, change in taste sensation, sleeping during the day and wakefulness at night, seizures, and tremors. The excess amount of fluid in the body may also result in distention of the internal jugular veins. When introducing a drain tube into the internal jugular vein during arterial embalming, the embalmer may notice the odor of urine in the blood and tissue fluids.

Urinary Tract Infections

There are a variety of microorganisms that can cause urinary tract infections. These infections are typically categorized by the portion of the urinary tract that is affected, as illustrated in Figure 12-1. Some of the most common microorganisms that cause urinary tract infections include *Neisseria gonorrhea*, *Chlamydia trachomatis*, *Escherichia coli*, *Proteus* species, and *Pseudomonas* species.

Pyelitis and Pyelonephritis. Pyelitis is any inflammation of the renal pelvis and the calyces of the kidneys, while pyelonephritis is an inflammatory disorder of the nephrons of the kidney caused by renal infections. Pyelonephritis is commonly known as a kidney infection, and it is an infection of both the renal pelvis and the remainder of the kidney. Many microorganisms, especially bacteria, can invade the body by traveling through the urethra to the bladder and then up the ureters to the kidneys, and both pyelitis and pyelonephritis may migrate from the bladder. Chronic pyelonephritis occurs almost exclusively in persons with major anatomic anomalies such as urinary tract obstructions, kidney stones, or structural birth defects of the kidneys. The characteristics of pyelonephritis are:

- Fever
- Nausea
- Vomiting
- Pain in the flanks of the abdomen
- High blood pressure
- Lack of sufficient urine production

Ureteritis. Ureteritis is an inflammation of one or both of the ureters, which are the tubes that connect the kidneys to the urinary bladder. Typically, ureteritis occurs when an infection spreads from the kidneys to the urinary bladder. Alternatively, it may occur if the nerves that cause the ureters to function become defective. Damage to the nervous supply to the ureter can cause the muscular layers of the ureters to malfunction, which slows the flow of urine and results in ureteritis (Beer 2004a).

Cystitis. Cystitis is any inflammation of the urinary bladder, and interstitial cystitis is a recurring condition characterized by discomfort and pain in the bladder and the surrounding pelvic region. Symptoms of interstitial cystitis include an

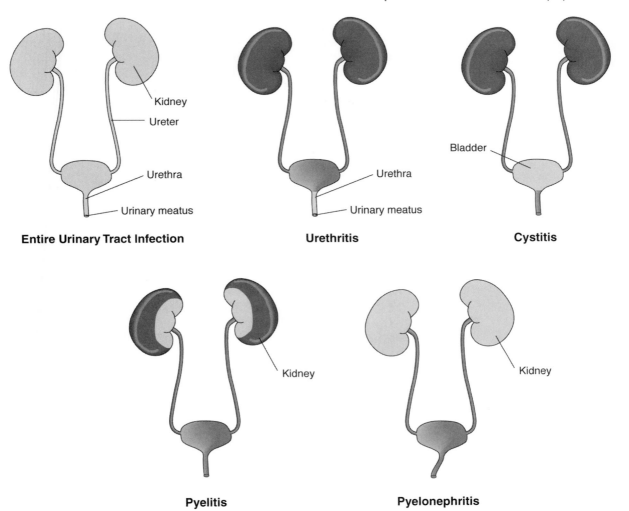

Entire Urinary Tract Infection

Kidney
Ureter
Urethra
Urinary meatus

Urethritis

Urethra
Urinary meatus

Cystitis

Bladder

Pyelitis

Kidney

Pyelonephritis

Kidney

Figure 12-1 Inflammatory disorders of the urinary tract.

urgent need to urinate, a need to urinate as many as 60 times a day, and increasing pain as the bladder fills with urine or as it empties. Women's symptoms worsen during menstruation. Through time, the bladder wall may become irritated or scarred, and pinpoint bleeding caused by recurrent irritation may appear on the bladder wall. Interstitial cystitis is idiopathic, and antibiotics are not effective in its treatment. Currently there is no cure for interstitial cystitis.

Urethritis.   Urethritis is an inflammatory condition of the urethra, which is the tube that carries urine out of the body from the urinary bladder. A variety of microorganisms can cause urethritis. Urethritis is commonly referred to as a urinary tract infection, and women are far more likely than men to develop this type of infection. In women, the infectious microorganisms travel from the vagina and the anus to the urethra where they can cause urethritis. *Neisseria gonorrhea, Chlamydia,* and the herpes simplex virus are all causative agents of sexually transmitted diseases that can cause urethritis. In men, trichomonas, which is type of microscopic parasite, is more likely to cause urethritis than in women (Beer 2004b). The symptoms of urethritis related to sexually transmitted diseases includes painful urination and a yellow-green discharge of pus from the urethra.

Hydronephrosis

Hydronephrosis is a condition that occurs as part of a disease; it is not a disease itself. Hydronephrosis occurs when a kidney becomes distended due to a backup of urine, as illustrated in Figure 12-2. When both kidneys are involved, the condition is called bilateral hydronephrosis, while the involvement of a single kidney is referred to as unilateral hydronephrosis. Hydronephrosis may accompany pregnancy, or it may be caused by obstruction of the renal system, backflow of urine from the bladder into the ureter and kidney, and kidney stones. Occasionally, unilateral hydronephrosis may not present any signs or symptoms.

Hydronephrosis can be treated by inserting a stint that allows urination; however, this remedy only allows the removal of excess urine. The original cause of the hydronephrosis must still be treated, as prolonged hydronephrosis eventually results in renal failure. The following may indicate the presence of hydronephrosis:

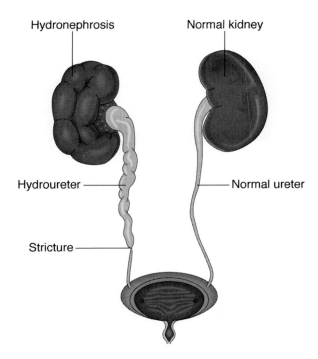

Figure 12-2 Hydronephrosis.

- Abdominal flank pain
- Abdominal mass
- Nausea
- Vomiting
- Urinary tract infections
- Fever
- Disruption of urinary output
- Frequency of urination
- Urgency to urinate

Nephrolithiasis

Nephrolithiasis is a condition in which one or more kidney stones are present in the urinary system. The technical name for kidney stones is *renal calculi*. Kidney stones may form when the urine becomes overconcentrated with substances such as calcium, oxalates, phosphates, and carbonate. Stones are often asymptomatic until they begin to move down the ureter, causing pain that starts in the abdominal flank and leads to the groin. Kidney stones are common, and recurrence is common, especially if a person has had more than two episodes of kidney stones. Premature infants are more likely to develop kidney stones, and some types of stones tend to run in families.

The following are common signals of kidney stones:

- Nausea
- Vomiting
- Urinary frequency
- Hematuria (blood in the urine)
- Severe pelvic and abdominal pain
- Fever
- Chills
- Discoloration of the urine

Most kidney stones are passed spontaneously through the urine; however, surgical removal of stones may be required. An alternative to surgery may be lithotripsy, which is illustrated in Figure 12-3. Ultrasonic waves are used to break up stones, so that they may be expelled in the urine or removed with an endoscope, which is inserted into the kidney through a small incision.

Polycystic Kidney

Polycystic kidney disease is an inherited disorder characterized by bilateral, grapelike clusters of cysts that replace normal renal tissue. Figure 12-4 illustrates how the presence of these cysts can greatly enlarge the size of the kidneys externally, thereby compressing the nephrons inside. This compression eventually disrupts the filtration of the blood as well as the production of urine.

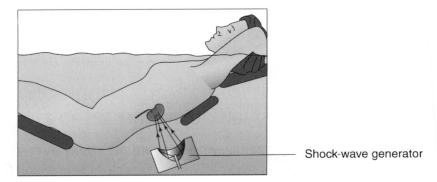

Figure 12-3 Lithotripsy.

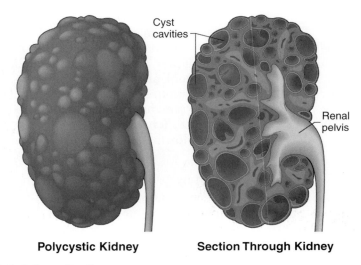

Polycystic Kidney   **Section Through Kidney**

Figure 12-4 Polycystic disease.

Kidney Malformations

According to the American Urological Association, one in 4,000 infants are born with only one kidney, which is a condition known as *renal agenesis*. The absence of a kidney typically goes undetected until an image is taken as an adult for some unrelated reason, for example during pregnancy screening in women. In cases of renal **dysplasia**, an abnormal tissue development occurs in the kidney that is arranged in a specific pattern within one kidney, or it may be randomly present throughout both kidneys. Some people have smaller than normal kidneys, which is known as renal hypoplasia. A small kidney may be otherwise normal; however, by the time a child reaches adulthood, the smaller kidney may not be able to function due to the increase in body size. Any developmental malformation of the kidneys may result in malfunction of the urinary system.

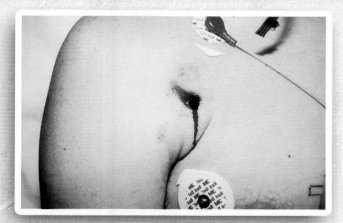

Color Plate 1 An entrance wound typically has a round or oval shape accompanied by a narrow area of abrasion and burns from the weapon. (Courtesy of Dr. Deborah Funk, Albany Medical Center, Albany, NY.)

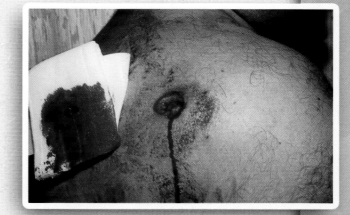

Color Plate 2 Exit wounds are typically irregular in shape or slitlike. (Courtesy of Dr. Deborah Funk, Albany Medical Center, Albany, NY.)

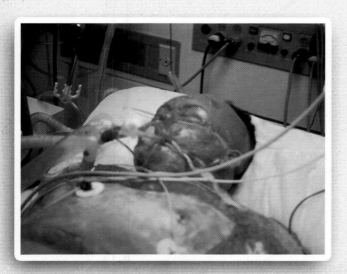

Color Plate 3 Burn wound edema. Note the facial swelling. (Courtesy of Ernest Grant, North Carolina Jaycee Burn Center.)

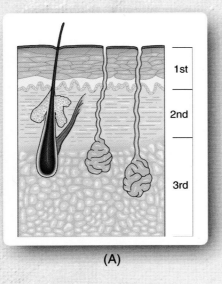

(A)

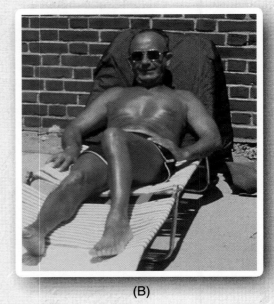

(B)

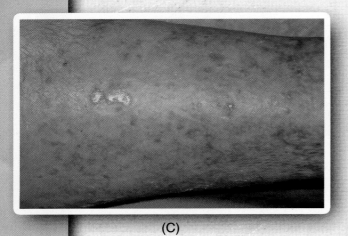

(C)

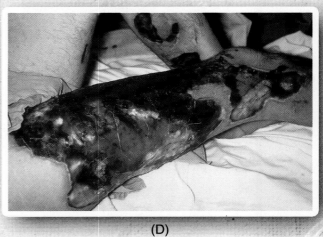

(D)

Color Plate 4 (A) Layers of skin in relation to degree of burn. (B) First-degree burns. (C) Second-degree burns. (D) Third degree burns. (B, C, and D Courtesy of the Phoenix Society of Burns Survivors, Inc.)

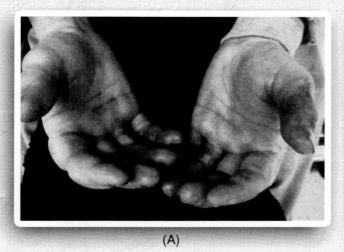
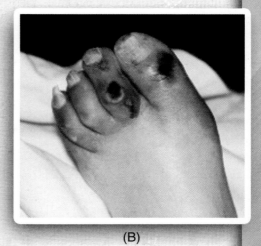

(A)   (B)

Color Plate 5 (A) Edema and blister formation 24 hours after frostbite injury. (Courtesy of Kevin Reilly, Albany Medical Center, Albany, NY.) (B) Deep frostbite results in permanent damage to tissue. (Courtesy of Dr. Deborah Funk, Albany Medical Center, Albany, NY.)

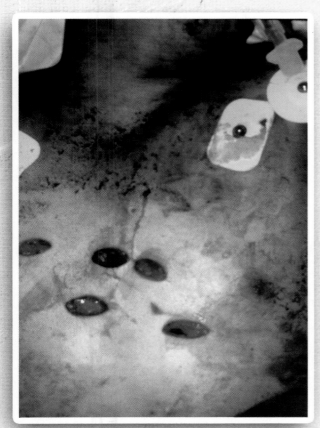

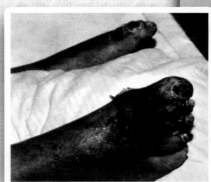

Color Plate 7 Gas gangrene.

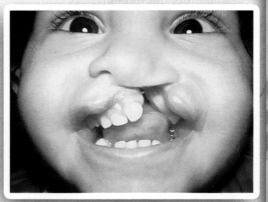

Color Plate 6 Appearance of stab wound. (Courtesy of Dr. Deborah Funk, Albany Medical Center, Albany, NY.)

Color Plate 8 Cleft Lip. (Courtesy of Dr. Joseph Konzelman, School of Dentistry, Medical College of Georgia.)

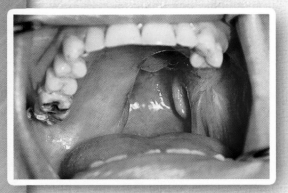

Color Plate 9 Cleft Palate. (Courtesy of Dr. Joseph Konzelman, School of Dentistry, Medical College of Georgia.)

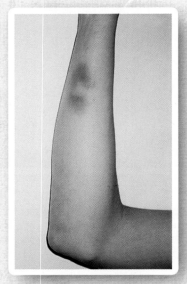

Color Plate 12 Ecchymosis.

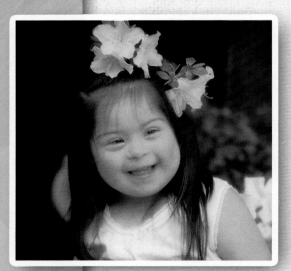

Color Plate 10 Down Syndrome. (© Marijane Scott, Marijane's Designer Portraits, Down Right Beautiful 1996 Calendar.)

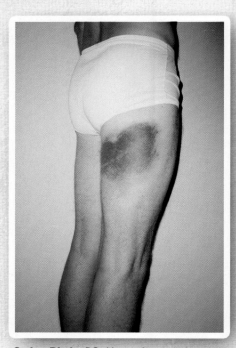

Color Plate 13 Hematoma.

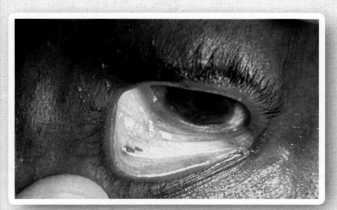

Color Plate 11 Petechia on the lower right eyelid. (Courtesy of the CDC, Dr. Thomas F. Sellers, Emory University.)

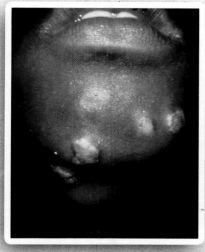

Color Plate 14 Papilloma on the chin. (Courtesy of the CDC, Dr. Peter Perine.)

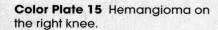

Color Plate 15 Hemangioma on the right knee.

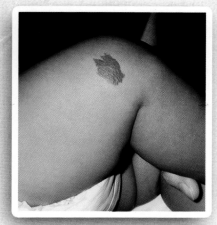

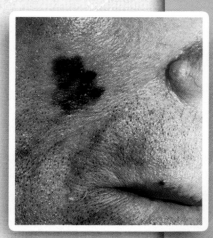

Color Plate 16 Malignant melanoma. (Courtesy of Robert A. Silverman, MD, Pediatric Dermatology, Georgetown University.)

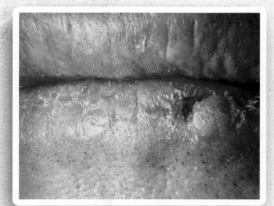

Color Plate 17 Squamous cell carcinoma on the lower lip. (Courtesy of Dr. Joseph Konzelman, School of Dentistry, Medical College of Georgia.)

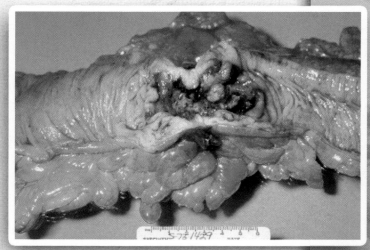

Color Plate 18 Adenocarcinoma of the colon. (Courtesy of the CDC, Dr. Edwin P. Ewing, Jr.)

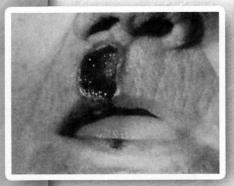

Color Plate 19 Basal cell carcinoma.
(Courtesy of Robert A. Silverman, MD, Pediatric
Dermatology, Georgetown University.)

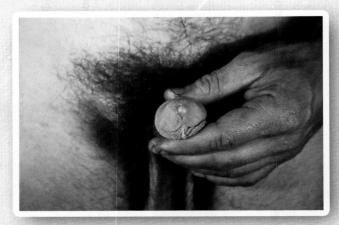

Color Plate 20 Epidermoid cyst occluding the
urethra. (Courtesy of the CDC, William R. Smart, San Rafael,
California/ Susan Lindsley.)

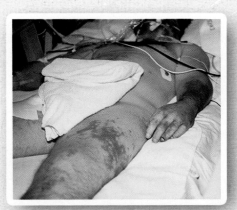

Color Plate 21 Purpura. (Courtesy of
Dr. Mark Dougherty, Lexington, KY.)

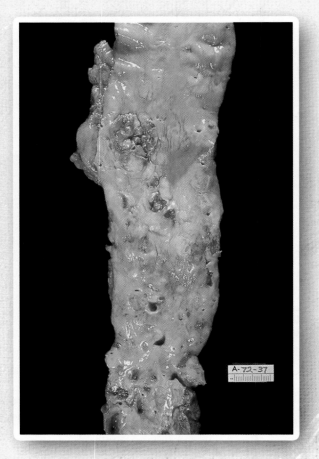

Color Plate 22 Atherosclerosis of
the aorta. (Courtesy of the CDC, Dr.
Edwin P. Ewing, Jr.)

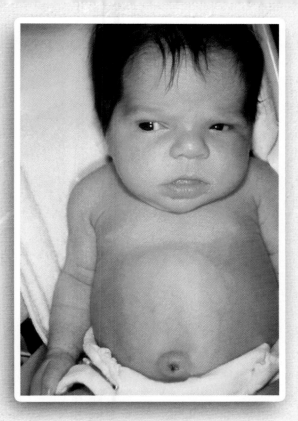

Color Plate 23 Jaundice.
(Courtesy of the CDC, Dr. Hudson.)

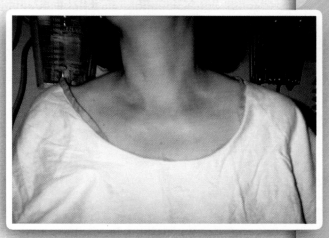

Color Plate 24 Bruising of the neck due to strangulation.

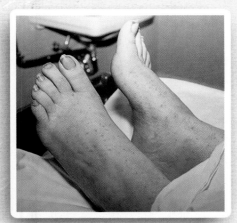

Color Plate 25 Petechiae on the feet. (Courtesy of Dr. Mark Dougherty, Lexington, KY.)

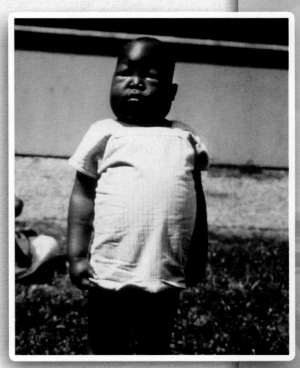

Color Plate 26 Edema due to nephrosis. (Courtesy of the CDC, Dr. Myron Schultz.)

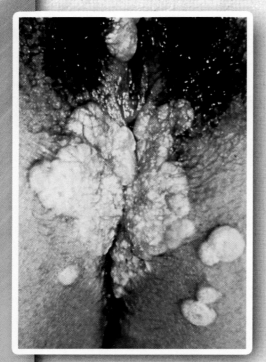

Color Plate 27 Genital warts. (Courtesy of the CDC.)

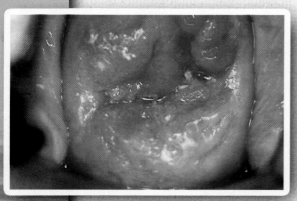

Color Plate 28 Cervical cancer. (Courtesy of the CDC.)

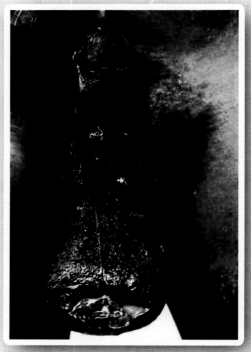

Color Plate 29 Cancer of the scrotum. (Courtesy of the CDC, Robert S. Craig.)

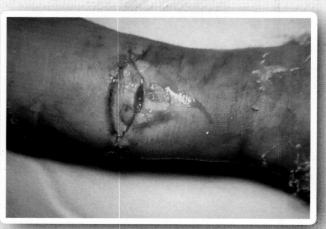

Color Plate 30 Wound botulism involvement of a compound fracture of the right ulna. (Courtesy of the CDC.)

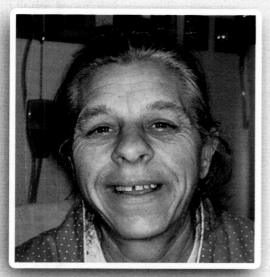

Color Plate 31 Note the wide nose, spaced teeth, and enlarged lips of this person with acromegaly. (Courtesy of Matthew C. Leinung, MD, Acting Head, Division of Endocrinology, Albany Medical College, Albany, NY.)

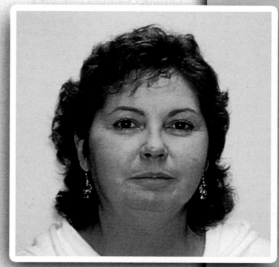

Color Plate 32 Cushing's syndrome. (Courtesy of Matthew C. Leinung, M.D., Acting Head, Division of Endocrinology, Albany Medical College, Albany, NY.)

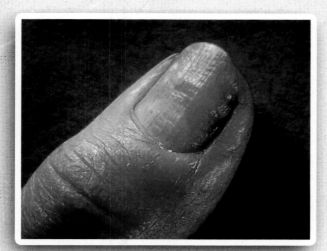

Color Plate 33 Fungal infection of the fingernail. (Courtesy of the CDC, Sherry Brinkman.)

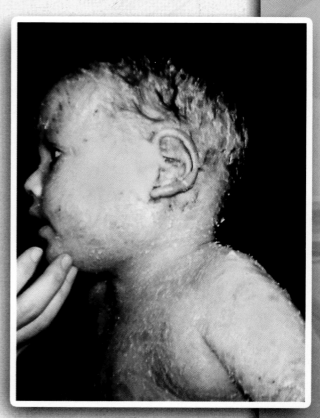

Color Plate 34 Seborrheic dermatitis. (Courtesy of the CDC, Susan Lindsley.)

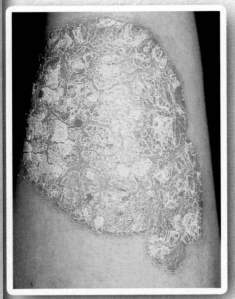

Color Plate 35 Psoriasis. (Courtesy of Robert A. Silverman, MD, Pediatric Dermatology, Georgetown University.)

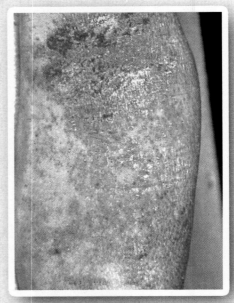

Color Plate 36 Eczema. (Courtesy of the CDC.)

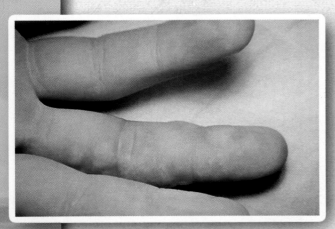

Color Plate 37 Lesions due to secondary herpes simplex infection in a patient with a primary meningococcal infection. (Courtesy of the CDC, Dr. Thomas F. Sellers, Emory University.)

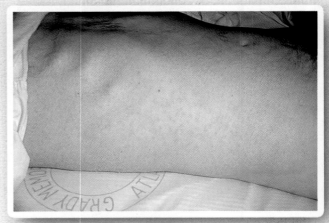

Color Plate 38 Rash due to septicemia. (Courtesy of the CDC, Dr. Thomas F. Sellers, Emory University.)

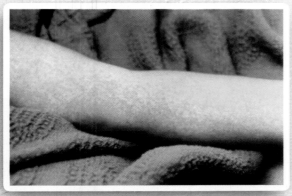

Color Plate 39 Rash on the arm 3 to 5 days after onset of toxic shock syndrome. (Courtesy of the CDC.)

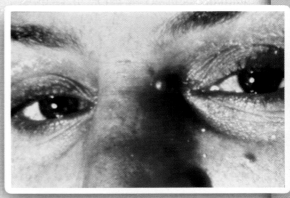

Color Plate 40 Involvement of the eyes in toxic shock syndrome infection. (Courtesy of the CDC.)

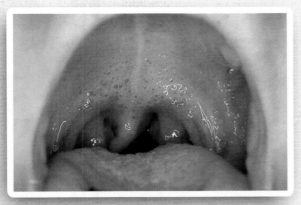

Color Plate 41 Petechiae and inflammation caused by strep throat. (Courtesy of the CDC, Dr. Heinz F. Eichenwald.)

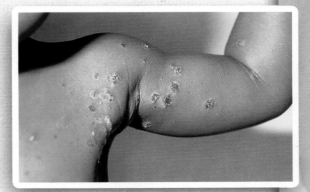

Color Plate 42 Impetigo. (Courtesy of Robert A. Silverman, MD, Pediatric Dermatology, Georgetown University.)

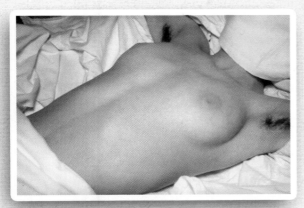

Color Plate 43 Rash due to scarlet fever. (Courtesy of the CDC.)

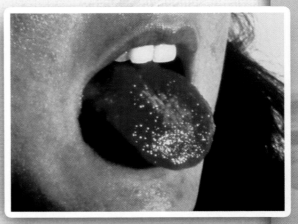

Color Plate 44 Strawberry tongue. (Courtesy of the CDC.)

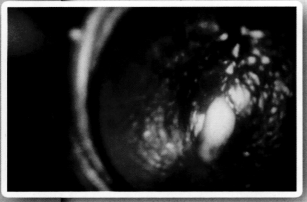

Color Plate 45 Discharge from penis due to gonorrhea. (Courtesy of the CDC, Susan Lindsley.)

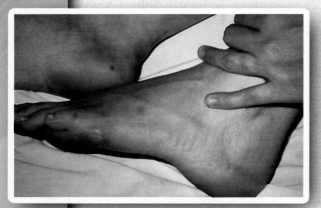

Color Plate 47 Foot lesions due to gonorrhea infection. (Courtesy of the CDC, J. Pledger, Dr. S. E. Thompson, VDCD.)

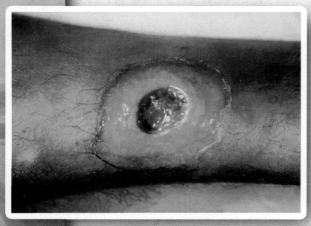

Color Plate 49 Diphtheria skin lesion on the leg. (Courtesy of the CDC.)

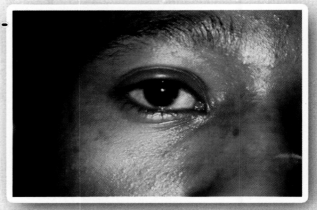

Color Plate 46 Gonorrheal infection of the eye. (Courtesy of the CDC, Joe Miller.

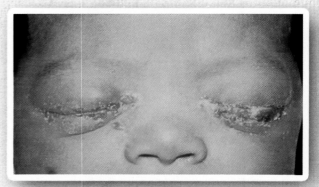

Color Plate 48 Ophthalmia neonatorum due to gonorrhea infection. (Courtesy of the CDC, J. Pledger.)

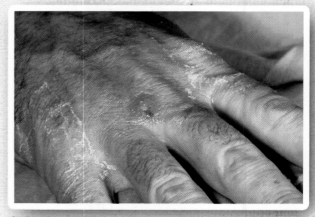

Color Plate 50 Tularemia lesion on the dorsal skin of the right hand caused by Francisella tularensis. (Courtesy of the CDC, Dr. Brachman.)

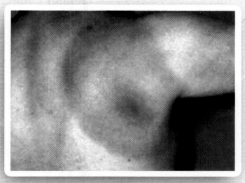

Color Plate 51 Bull's-eye rash caused by Borrelia burgdorferi in a case of Lyme disease. (Courtesy of the CDC.)

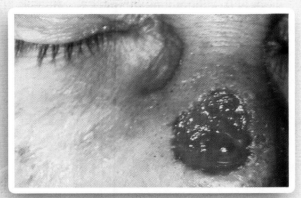

Color Plate 53 Gumma on the nose of a person in tertiary stage of syphilis. (Courtesy of the CDC, J. Pledger.)

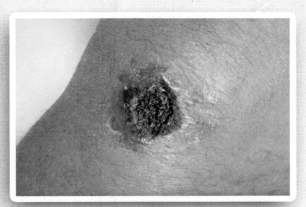

Color Plate 55 Anthrax lesion on the skin of the forearm. (Courtesy of the CDC, James H. Steele.)

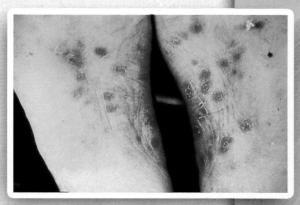

Color Plate 52 Rash on the feet during secondary stage of syphilis. (Courtesy of the CDC, Dr. Gavin Hart.)

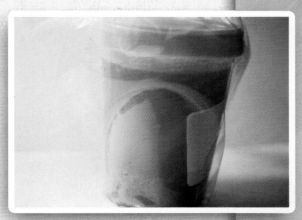

Color Plate 54 A cup of "rice-water" stool from a cholera patient. (Courtesy of the CDC.)

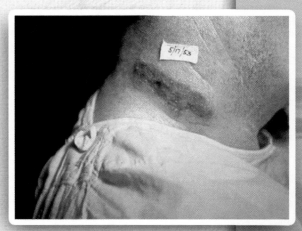

Color Plate 56 Anthrax lesion on the skin of the neck. (Courtesy of the CDC.)

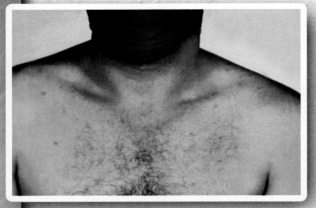

Color Plate 57 Rose spots on the chest of a man with typhoid fever. (Courtesy of the CDC, Armed Forces Institute of Pathology, Charles N. Farmer.)

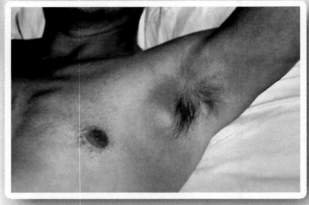

Color Plate 58 An axillary bubo in a person with plague. (Courtesy of the CDC, Margaret Parsons, Dr. Karl F. Meyer.)

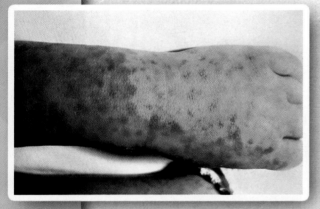

Color Plate 59 Rash on the foot associated with Rocky Mountain spotted fever. (Courtesy of the CDC.)

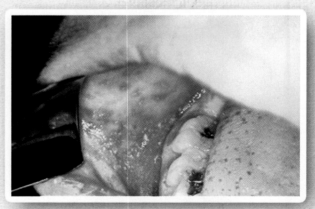

Color Plate 60 Koplik's spots in rubeola. (Courtesy of the CDC.)

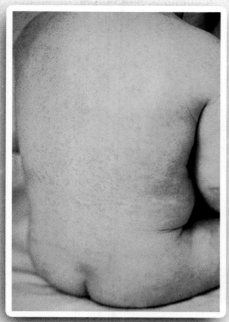

Color Plate 61 Rubella rash. (Courtesy of the CDC.)

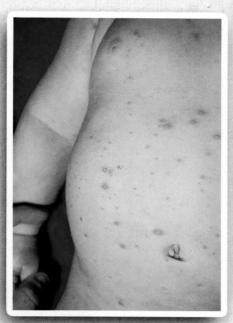

Color Plate 62 Varicella rash. (Courtesy of Robert A. Silverman, MD, Pediatric Dermatology, Georgetown University.)

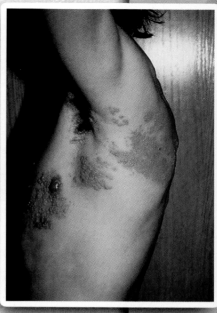

Color Plate 63 Shingles. (Courtesy of Robert A. Silverman, MD, Pediatric Dermatology, Georgetown University.)

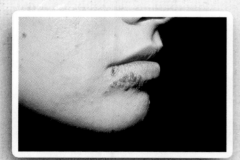

Color Plate 64 Cold sores caused by herpes simplex 1 virus. (Courtesy of Robert A. Silverman, MD, Pediatric Dermatology, Georgetown University.)

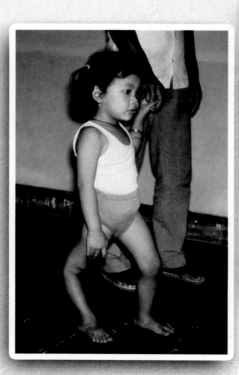

Color Plate 65 This child displays a deformity of her right lower extremity due to poliovirus infection. (Courtesy of the CDC.)

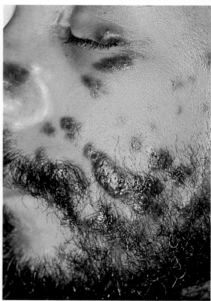

Color Plate 66 Kaposi's sarcoma. (Courtesy of Robert A. Silverman, MD, Pediatric Dermatology, Georgetown University.)

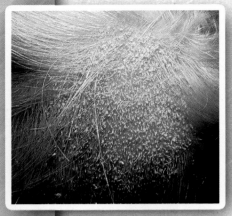

Color Plate 67 *Tinea capitis.* (Courtesy of Robert A. Silverman, MD, Pediatric Dermatology, Georgetown University.)

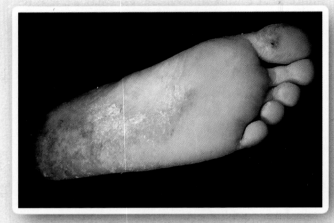

Color Plate 68 *Tinea pedis.* (Courtesy of the CDC.)

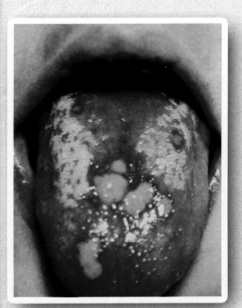

Color Plate 69 White patches on the tongue in a case of thrush.

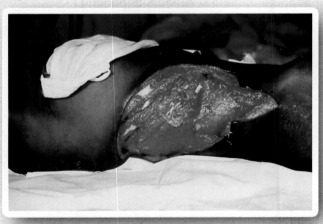

Color Plate 70 Extraintestinal amebiasis involving the right flank. (Courtesy of the CDC.)

Renal Cell Carcinoma

One form of kidney cancer is renal cell carcinoma, which is characterized by a lack of early warning signs, diverse clinical manifestations, and resistance to both radiation and chemotherapy. Originally, it was believed that renal cell carcinoma was derived from the adrenal glands, hence the alternate name of hypernephroma. Renal cell carcinoma typically originates in the epithelium of the proximal renal tubule. Renal cell carcinoma is the sixth leading cause of cancer death in the United States, and it is more common among persons of European descent than Asian or African descent. Renal cell carcinoma is also twice as prevalent in men as it is in women. It frequently metastasizes to the lung, soft tissues, bone, liver, and brain. The combination of its rapid metastasis and its resistance to conventional treatments explains its high mortality.

The following can indicate the presence of renal cell carcinoma:

- Hematuria (blood in the urine)
- Abdominal flank pain
- Abdominal mass
- Weight loss
- Fever
- Hypertension
- Night sweats

Carcinoma of the Urinary Bladder

Bladder cancer is typically caused by transitional cell carcinomas, which may appear in any part of the urinary tract including the renal pelvis, ureter, bladder, or urethra. Bladder cancer is categorized as low grade or high grade and as superficial or muscle invasive. Primary bladder tumors are rare but may include small cell carcinoma, lymphoma, or sarcoma. Urinary bladder cancers may also include adenocarcinomas, squamous cell carcinomas, leiomyosarcomas, or rhabdomyosarcomas. One of the only initial signs of bladder cancer is painless hematuria, which is blood in the urine. It is believed that bladder cancer may be due to the carcinogenic agents in cigarette smoke (i.e., nitrosamine, 2-naphthylamine, and 4-aminobiphenyl) and industrial exposure to aromatic amines in dyes, paints, solvents, leather dust, inks, combustion products, rubber, and textiles.

Renal Failure

The loss of function of the kidneys is known as renal failure. There are two forms of renal failure: acute and chronic. The kidneys filter wastes and excrete fluid by using the bloodstream's natural pressure, so there are numerous potential causes of kidney failure. Acute renal failure results from a sudden drop in blood pressure brought on by trauma, complications in surgery, septic shock, hemorrhage, burns, or dehydration. Acute renal failure can also occur as a result of blockage or narrowing of the renal artery, which inhibits blood flow and proper oxygenation of renal tissues. Infections such as acute pyelonephritis or septicemia may also cause acute renal failure. Acute renal failure can be accompanied by any or all of the following:

- Decreased urine output
- Decreased urine volume (oliguria)
- Lack of urine output (anuria)
- Coma
- Edema of the ankles, feet, or legs
- Bruising easily
- Hallucinations
- Nosebleeds
- Vomiting blood
- Seizures

Unlike acute renal failure with its sudden reversible failure of kidney function, chronic renal failure is slowly progressive and rarely reversible. It may progress to a fatal stage. Chronic renal failure typically results from other major diseases such as glomerulonephritis, polycystic kidney disease, kidney stones, and chronic infections.

Chronic renal failure results in the accumulation of fluid and waste products in the body, causing uremia. Uremia is the buildup of nitrogenous waste products in the blood, which may occur without symptoms. Most body systems are affected by uremia. Some of the diseases that can result in chronic renal failure include congestive heart failure, diabetes, hypertension, urinary tract infections, kidney stones, obstructions of the urinary tract, and glomerulonephritis. Kidney transplant may eventually be required in cases of chronic renal failure, which is characterized by the following:

- Weight loss
- Nausea
- Vomiting
- Headache
- Frequent hiccups
- Generalized itching (pruritus)
- Changes in urine output
- Easy bruising
- Easy bleeding
- Hematuria
- Melena
- Delirium
- Coma
- Muscle twitching or cramps
- Seizures
- Deposits of white crystals in and on the skin

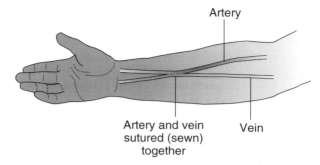

Figure 12-5 Fistula used for dialysis.

Dialysis. **Dialysis** is a processes of diffusing blood across a semipermeable membrane to remove toxic materials and to maintain fluid, electrolyte, and acid–base balance in cases of impaired kidney function or absence of the kidneys. It is a method of removing toxic substances from the blood when the kidneys are unable to do so. Dialysis is most frequently used for patients who have kidney failure, but may also be used to quickly remove drugs or poisons in emergency situations.

One type of dialysis is hemodialysis, which works by circulating the blood through special filters in a hemodialysis machine. The blood flows across a semipermeable membrane, along with solutions that help facilitate removal of toxins. During hemodialysis, an artificial kidney is used to clear urea, metabolic waste products, toxins, and excess fluid from the blood. Hemodialysis is used to treat end-stage renal failure, transient renal failure, and some cases of poisonings. In the United States, more than 200,000 patients undergo hemodialysis regularly for end-stage renal diseases.

Before hemodialysis can be performed, there needs to be adequate access to the vascular system. Access is usually established through either an arteriovenous fistula or arteriovenous graft. An arteriovenous fistula involves the surgical joining of an artery and vein, which increases blood volume and stretches the vein to allow a larger volume of blood flow (see Figure 12-5). When a person's veins are not suitable for an arteriovenous fistula, a portion of the person's saphenous vein, a carotid artery from a cow, or a synthetic graft is surgically implanted and is known as an arteriovenous graft. Once the two sites are accessible, a hemodialysis machine is connected. Blood is taken from the artery, filtered in the machine, and returned through the vein.

POSTMORTEM CONDITIONS ASSOCIATED WITH URINARY DISORDERS

There are four significant postmortem conditions with which the embalmer should be familiar when embalming the remains of persons who have died as a result of urinary diseases.

1. Edema
2. Uremia
3. Dehydration
4. Odor

Although each case is unique, and a thorough case analysis should always be conducted prior to embalming any human remains, urinary disorders typically require astringent embalming chemicals and copious amounts of arterial embalming fluid. The presence of nitrogenous compounds in the tissues due to uremia has two significant effects on the embalming process.

First, nitrogenous waste products increase formaldehyde demand due to their neutralizing effects on formaldehyde. Ammonia and formaldehyde react to form urotropin. **Urotropin** is formed due to the affinity of formaldehyde for nitrogen. As nitrogenous waste products accumulate in the tissues due to renal dysfunction, more formaldehyde is needed to overcome the neutralizing effects of the nitrogen present in the tissues.

Second, nitrogenous tissues have altered protein structures that inhibit formaldehyde's ability to cross-link proteins. In addition, both edema and odor can be significantly reduced through aggressive arterial embalming techniques. Nonetheless, the presence of dehydrated tissues and the possible presence of jaundice related to liver failure are contraindications for the use of strong embalming chemicals. Instead, specially designed jaundice embalming fluids should be utilized for their cosmetic effects, as well as their inclusion of buffers, which counter the pH-altering effects of nitrogenous waste products in the tissues. Embalming fluids require specific pH levels to function properly in the tissues and are disrupted by the acidic tissues of human remains exhibiting uremic poisoning.

REVIEW QUESTIONS

Matching

1. _____ uremia
2. _____ hematuria
3. _____ cystitis
4. _____ urethritis
5. _____ oliguria

a. inflammation of the urethra
b. decreased urine output
c. the build-up of nitrogenous waste products in the blood
d. blood in the urine
e. inflammation of the urinary bladder

Multiple Choice

1. Which of the following is characterized by the sudden onset of blood and protein in the urine accompanied by salt and water retention?
   a. pyelitis
   b. cystitis
   c. hydronephrosis
   d. acute glomerulonephritis

2. Which of the following is a disease condition of the kidney brought on by excess buildup of urine?

a. renal failure
b. Bright's disease
c. hydronephrosis
d. nephrolithiasis

3. What effect does excess nitrogenous waste in the tissues have on the embalming process?

i. It increases formaldehyde demand.
ii. It causes cavitation of the lung tissue.
iii. It causes an odor.
iv. It can spread to the public causing an infectious disease.

a. i and ii
b. ii and iii
c. iii and iv
d. i and iii

4. Transitional cell carcinoma is most likely to occur in which of the following organs?

a. urinary bladder
b. trachea
c. kidney
d. lung

5. Which of the following is commonly referred to as a kidney infection?

a. pyelitis
b. pyelonephritis
c. cystitis
d. glomeruloneprhosis

Putting Learning to Work!

The purpose of the following case analysis is to allow you to apply the information you have learned in a real-world situation. Read the case carefully and try to answer the following questions:

What disorder do you suspect the person had at the time of death?

What potential embalming complications do you anticipate?

What precautions should you take as the embalmer to limit the effects of these complications?

Case Analysis

A 57-year-old man died in the intensive care unit of a local hospital. The deceased is approximately 5'10" and weighs 240 pounds. He has edema of all his tissues, and he has a strong odor of urine. You notice a recent surgical scar on his forearm, and he has ulcers on his feet and legs. During the injection of arterial embalming solution, you are able to establish adequate distribution, but the embalming fluid diffuses poorly.

Bibliography

Angelo, S. (2002). Acute renal failure. In *Medical Encyclopedia*. Retrieved June 9, 2003, from MedlinePlus, the U.S. National Library of Medicine and the National Institutes of Health at http://www.nlm.nih.gov/medlineplus/ency/article/000501.htm.

American Urological Association page. (n/d). Retrieved March 16, 2004, from http://www.urologyhealth.org/adult/index.cfm?cat=02&topic=119.

Beer, Mark H. (Ed.). (2004a). Ureteritis. In *The Merck Manual: 2nd Home Edition*. Retrieved March 16, 2004, from http://www.merck.com/mrkshared/mmanual_home2/sec11/ch149/ch149d.jsp.

Beer, Mark H. (Ed.). (2004b). Urethritis. In *The Merck Manual: 2nd Home Edition*. Retrieved March 16, 2004, from http://www.merck.com/mrkshared/mmanual_home2/sec11/ch149/ch149b.jsp.

Dorn, J. M., & Hopkins, B. M. (1998). *Thanatochemistry: A survey of general, organic, and biochemistry for funeral service professionals* (2nd ed.). Upper Saddle River, NJ: Prentice Hall.

Frasseto, L., & Sant, G. (2002). *Cystitis, nonbacterial*. Retrieved June 9, 2003, from eMedicine at http://www.emedicine.com/med/topic2850.htm.

Gowda, A., & Nzerue, C. (2003). *Pyelonephritis, chronic*. Retrieved June 9, 2003, from eMedicine at http://www.emedicine.com/med/topic2841.htm.

Interstitial cystitis. (2002). Retrieved June 9, 2003, from the National Kidney and Urologic Diseases Information Clearinghouse, National Institutes of Health at http://www.niddk.nih.gov/health/urolog/pubs/cystitis/cystitis.htm.

Konety, B., & Pirtskhalaishvili, G. (2002). *Transitional cell carcinoma, renal*. Retrieved May 29, 2003, from eMedicine at http://www.emedicine.com/med/topic2003.htm.

Koren, A. (2001). Chronic renal failure. In *Medical Encyclopedia*. Retrieved June 9, 2003, from MedlinePlus, the U.S. National Library of Medicine and the National Institutes of Health at http://www.nlm.nih.gov/medlineplus/ency/article/000471.htm.

Koren, A. (2001). Nephrolithiasis. In *Medical Encyclopedia*. Retrieved June 9, 2003, from MedlinePlus, the U.S. National Library of Medicine and the National Institutes of Health at http://www.nlm.nih.gov/medlineplus/ency/article/000458.htm.

Kumar, V., Cotran, R., & Robbins, S. (2003). *Robbins basic pathology* (7th ed.). Philadelphia: Saunders.

Mayer, R. (2000). *Embalming: History, theory, & practice* (3rd ed.). New York: McGraw-Hill.

Neighbors, M., & Tannehill-Jones, R. (2000). *Human diseases*. Clifton Park, NY: Thomson Delmar Learning.

Parmar, M. (2002). *Glomerlulonephritis, acute*. Retrieved June 9, 2003, from eMedicine at http://www.emedicine.com/med/topic879.htm.

Pathology for funeral service. (1999). Dallas, TX: Professional Training Schools.

Sachdeva, K., & Makhoul, I. (2002). *Renal cell carcinoma*. Retrieved June 9, 2003, from eMedicine at http://www.emedicine.com/MED/topic2002.htm.

Salifu, M., & Delano, D. (2002). *Glomerulonephritis, chronic*. Retrieved June 9, 2003, from eMedicine at http://www.emedicine.com/emerg/topic219.htm.

Sant, G. (Ed.). (1997). *Interstitial cystitis*. Philadelphia: Lippincott-Raven.

Shelton, H. (1992). *Boyd's introduction to the study of disease* (11th ed.). Philadelphia: Lea & Febiger.

Steinberg, G., & Kim, H. (2002). *Bladder cancer*. Retrieved June 9, 2003, from eMedicine at http://www.emedicine.com/med/topic2344.htm.

Venes, D. (Ed.). (2001). *Taber's cyclopedic medical dictionary* (19th ed.). Philadelphia: F. A. Davis.

Young, K. (2002). Unilateral hydronephrosis. In *Medical Encyclopedia*. Retrieved June 9, 2003, from MedlinePlus, the U.S. National Library of Medicine and the National Institutes of Health at http://www.nlm.nih.gov/medlineplus/ency/article/000506.htm.

CHAPTER 13

Diseases of the Nervous System

Learning Objectives

Upon completion of the chapter, review questions, and case analysis, the reader should be able to:

- Differentiate between meningitis, encephalitis, myelitis, and neuritis.
- Explain both why hydroncephalus can cause skull deformation and the role of a shunt in the treatment of this disease.
- Compare and contrast multiple sclerosis, Parkinson's disease, Alzheimer's disease, and amyotrophic lateral sclerosis.
- Describe the hazards related to embalming persons who die from Creutzfeldt-Jakob disease.
- Compare and contrast concussions and contusions.
- Differentiate epilepsy, glioma, and cerebral palsy.
- Compare and contrast strokes and hematoma.
- Explain the impact of nervous system disease on the condition of the deceased.

Key Terms

concussion
contusion
convulsions
dementia
encephalitis

epilepsy
meningitis
seizures
sundowning

DISORDERS OF THE NERVOUS SYSTEM

This chapter focuses on pathological conditions associated with the nervous system. Several infectious diseases are described in this chapter as they relate to functional pathological changes in the body. In addition, many of the infectious diseases described in this chapter may have several different microbiological causes, each of which is described in greater detail in Part Two. While reading this chapter, the reader may review the anatomy of the nervous system by referring to Appendix H.

Meningitis

According to the Division of Bacterial and Mycotic Diseases of the Centers for Disease Control and Prevention (*Meningococcal diseases* 2003), **meningitis** is an infection of the cerebrospinal fluid, which is the fluid surrounding the spinal cord and brain. It is sometimes referred to as spinal meningitis, and it is usually caused by a virus or bacterium. Viral meningitis is usually less severe than bacterial meningitis. Before the 1990s, *Haemophilus influenzae* was the leading cause of bacterial meningitis, but today *Streptococcus pneumoniae* and *Neisseria meningitidis* are the leading causes. A less common, but severe form of meningitis is fungal meningitis, which is also known as cryptococcal meningitis.

Meningitis is characterized by stiff neck, headache, and high fever. In addition, symptoms of nausea, vomiting, discomfort under bright lights, confusion, and sleepiness may also signal meningitis. As meningitis progresses, seizures are common. Depending on the cause, meningitis is contagious, and may be treated with antibiotics.

Hydrocephalus

Hydrocephalus is a degenerative disorder of the nervous system. It is a condition in which the cerebrospinal fluid fails to be properly drained or absorbed, causing the ventricles of the brain to fill with cerebrospinal fluid. The condition can be caused by developmental anomalies, infection, injury, or brain tumors. The cerebrospinal fluid can be surgically shunted away from the scull via an implant, as illustrated in Figure 13-1. Among infants, hydrocephalus may cause extreme distention and disfigurement of the head because the cranial sutures have not yet formed.

Encephalitis

Encephalitis is inflammation of the brain. When used clinically, the term refers to an infection of the brain caused by a virus (Edwards 2003). Although rare, encephalitis can be a severe and potentially fatal disease. The two forms of encephalitis are primary encephalitis and secondary encephalitis. Primary encephalitis occurs when a virus directly invades the brain and spinal cord. In cases of secondary encephalitis, which is also known as postinfectious encephalitis, the virus first infects another part of the body and then spreads to the brain.

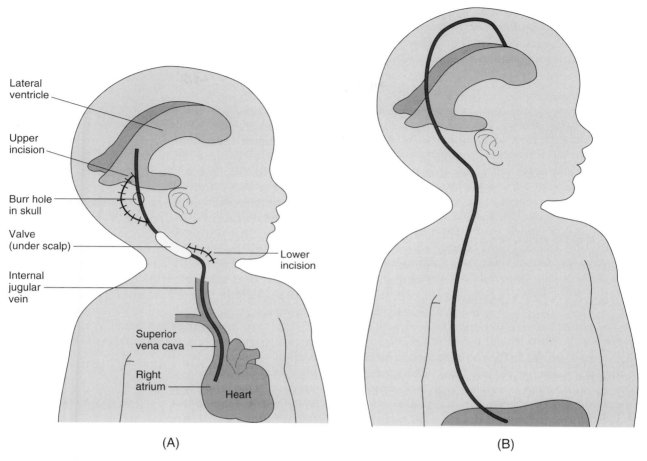

Lateral ventricle

Upper incision

Burr hole in skull

Valve (under scalp)

Internal jugular vein

Superior vena cava

Right atrium

Heart

Lower incision

(A)

(B)

Figure 13-1 (A) A ventriculoatrial shunt drains spinal fluid into the circulation of the heart. (B) A ventriculo-peritoneal shunt drains spinal fluid into the peritoneum.

Although most people with encephalitis have few or no symptoms, more se-vere cases can include drowsiness, confusion, seizures, fever, headache, nausea, vomiting, convulsions, or tremors. **Convulsions** are an abnormal, violent, and involuntary contraction or series of contractions of the muscles, while **seizures** are sudden, uncontrolled discharges of electrical activity in the brain. Seizures may cause convulsions, although convulsions can have other causes. Addition-ally, seizures may not manifest in convulsions, and may result in immediate un-consciousness or immobility.

Encephalitis is caused by three broad categories of viruses, including herpes virus, childhood infections, and arboviruses. Both herpes simplex virus types 1 and 2 are the most common causes of encephalitis, with herpes sim-plex virus 1 causing more cases than herpes simplex virus 2. If untreated, en-cephalitis caused by the herpes simplex viruses is fatal between 60 percent and 80 percent of the time. If treated, it is fatal at the rate of between 15 percent and 20 percent. Another potential cause of encephalitis is the Varicella-Zoster virus, which causes chickenpox and shingles. Finally, the Epstein-Barr virus, which causes infectious mononucleosis, can cause a form of encephalitis that results in death about 8 percent of the time.

Myelitis

Myelitis is an inflammation of the spinal cord, resulting from an infection in the spinal cord, noninfectious necrosing of the spinal cord, or demyelization of the spinal cord. Myelitis is characterized by flaccid limb paralysis, incontinence, and weakness or numbness of the limbs. One form of myelitis is transverse myelitis.

Transverse myelitis is an inflammatory disorder of the spinal cord. It occurs as a result of a process known as demyelization, which is the loss of the fatty tissue that surrounds the nerves. Transverse myelitis can have an acute onset, characterized by low back pain, spinal cord dysfunction, muscle spasms, headache, loss of appetite, and numbness or tingling in the legs. It can be caused by viral infections, spinal cord injuries, immune reactions, or insufficient blood flow to the spinal cord. It may also occur as a complication of disorders such as multiple sclerosis, smallpox, measles, or chickenpox. There is no treatment for transverse myelitis, except to treat the symptoms of the disorder. The prognosis for complete recovery from transverse myelitis is poor, with most individuals encountering considerable disability.

Neuritis

Neuritis is inflammation of a nerve or nerves. Some causes of neuritis include trauma, infection, and poisons. Trauma to the nerve causes it to become inflamed. Neuritis caused by infections can be either directly caused by an infection of the nerve, or it can be the result of complications due to infections such as tuberculosis, tetanus, or measles. Neuritis caused by poisons and other toxins are rare.

Epilepsy

Epilepsy is a recurrent degenerative disorder of the nervous system marked by repetitive abnormal electrical discharges within the brain known as seizures. Epilepsy is characterized by sudden convulsions and seizures or altered consciousness, depending on the type of attack. There are two basic types of seizures associated with epilepsy: grand mal and petite mal.

Grand mal seizures are characterized by fecal and urinary incontinence, uncontrolled contraction of the muscles of the extremities, loss of consciousness, and a cry caused by contraction of the respiratory muscles forcing exhalation. Petite mal seizures differ from grand mal seizures in that the individual ceases activity for a few seconds. Petite mal seizures are more common in children, who often outgrow the disorder. Epilepsy is controlled in most cases through medication.

Television epilepsy is a related disorder, in which the attacks occur while the individual is watching television. It is assumed that the horizontal and vertical lines of a television cause the seizures, rather than the flicker of the screen. There have also been cases of children who experienced seizures while playing video games.

Rabies

Rabies is an infection that affects the nervous system, and it is caused by the rabies virus, which is described in greater detail in Part Two of this book. If untreated, rabies can be fatal. Rabies may also be known as hydrophobia, which refers to a fear of water. Humans and nonhuman animals salivate during advanced rabies because of damage to the nervous system that prevents proper swallowing, and even the sound of running water has been known to cause convulsions in persons with rabies, which explains the name hydrophobia. Rabies is usually contracted by bite from the contaminated saliva of animals like raccoons, foxes, bats, skunks, and dogs. Figure 13-2 is a close-up of a dog's face during late-stage "dumb" paralytic rabies. Animals with "dumb" rabies appear

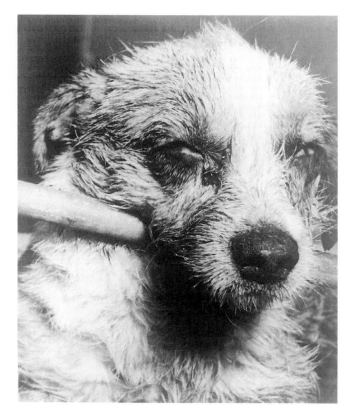

Figure 13–2 A dog during late-stage "dumb" rabies.

depressed and tired. Eventually, both nonhuman animals and humans with rabies become completely paralyzed.

Multiple Sclerosis

Multiple sclerosis (MS) is an inflammatory disease of the central nervous system in which infiltrating lymphocytes, predominantly T cells and macrophages, degrade the myelin sheath of nerves. It is assumed that this autoimmune disease is linked to a viral infection. There is no treatment for MS except the use of steroids and other symptom-related medications. Persons with MS typically experience periods of exacerbation and remission of the disease. The average person with MS lives over 30 years with the disease; however, some die within a few months of its onset.

Parkinson's Disease

Parkinson's disease was first formally described in "An Essay on the Shaking Palsy," published in 1817 by a London physician named James Parkinson, but the disease has existed for many thousands of years. Its symptoms and potential therapies were mentioned as early as 5000 BC in the system of medicine known as the Ayurveda in India; in addition, the Chinese described what has become known as Parkinson's disease over 2,500 years ago in Nei Jing, the first Chinese medical text (*Parkinson's disease backgrounder* 2001).

Parkinson's disease is a chronic nervous disease characterized by a fine, slowly spreading tremor, muscular weakness and rigidity, and a peculiar gait (see Figure 13-3). Persons with Parkinson's disease have diminished levels of dopamine, a neurotransmitter, in their brains, which causes them to exhibit signs of a fine tremor of the hands or feet that spreads to other parts of the body.

In advanced cases of Parkinson's, individuals have an expressionless face and a speech impairment. In addition, they have a bowed head, a forward bend to their body, and thumbs that are turned in towards their palms. Parkinson's causes flexed arms as the muscles become rigid. Recovery from Parkinson's disease rarely occurs.

Alzheimer's Disease

Dementia is a condition of deteriorated mental ability accompanied by emotional instability. It is a progressive, irreversible decline in mental function, marked by memory impairment and, often, deficits in reasoning, judgment, abstract thought, registration, comprehension, learning, task execution, and use of language. The most common form of dementia among older people in the United States is Alzheimer's disease. It involves the parts of the brain that control thought, memory, and language. Alzheimer's is an idiopathic disorder for which there is currently no cure. It usually begins after age 60, although it is possible for younger people to develop Alzheimer's disease. The disease is named after Dr. Alois Alzheimer, a German doctor, who, in 1906, noticed changes in the brain tissue of a woman who had died of an unusual mental illness. He found clumps

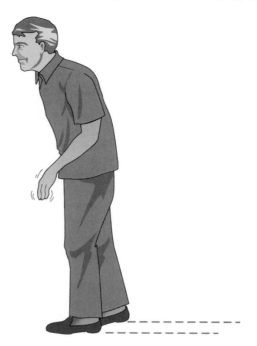

Figure 13-3 A person with Parkinson's disease exhibits tremor, a bowed head, forward bend to the body, and a peculiar gait.

of starchlike material known as amyloid plaques and bundles of fibers known as neurofibrillary tangles in her brain.

In addition to amyloid degeneration and neurofibrillary tangles in the brain tissue, Alzheimer's disease also causes the degeneration of nerve cells in the areas of the brain responsible for memory and mental capacity. There is also a reduction in the amount of necessary chemicals, referred to as neurotransmitters, in the brain that allow communication between cells.

At first, the only characteristic of Alzheimer's disease may be mild forgetfulness. People may only have trouble remembering recent events or the names of familiar people at this stage, although long-term memory is typically not affected. As the disease progresses, individuals may forget how to do simple tasks like brushing their teeth or combing their hair, and they may begin to have problems speaking, understanding, reading, or writing.

In the latter stages of Alzheimer's disease, people become anxious or aggressive and may wander away from home. Eventually, most people with Alzheimer's disease will require total care. The extreme demands of caregiving may result in mixed emotions for the care giver at the time of death. Although they experience grief as a result of the death, they may also experience guilt due to feelings of relief of their caregiving responsibilities.

Individuals with Alzheimer's disease may also experience sundowning, which is common to people suffering from dementia. **Sundowning** is confusion or disorientation that increases in the afternoon or evening. During sundowning, individuals may become more confused, restless, and insecure in the early evening, and the condition worsens after a move or change in routine. Persons experiencing sundowning become more demanding, restless, upset, suspicious, or disoriented, and they may hallucinate at night. It is believed that sundowning may be the result of a lack of stimulation by light and daily activity experienced in the dark. The lack of sensory inputs fails to stimulate certain areas of the brain exacerbating the manifestations of dementia. It is a common finding in patients with cognitive disorders and tends to improve when the patient is reassured and reoriented.

The only definitive diagnosis of Alzheimer's disease is the observation of plaques and tangles in brain tissue, which can only be done at autopsy. There is currently no way to definitively diagnose Alzheimer's disease while a person is living. Although there is no cure for Alzheimer's disease, some medicines may help control behavioral symptoms such as sleeplessness, agitation, wandering, anxiety, and depression.

Amyotrophic Lateral Sclerosis

Amyotrophic lateral sclerosis (ALS) is a progressive, fatal, neurological disease that belongs to a class of disorders known as motor neuron diseases. Although ALS was first reported in a woman in 1869, it received the name Lou Gehrig's disease for a baseball player who died of it in 1941.

Amyotrophic lateral sclerosis is the result of the degeneration of specific nerve cells in the central nervous system that control voluntary movement. The degeneration of these motor neuron cells results in the weakening and eventual atrophy of the muscles they control. The deterioration of the muscles leads to paralysis. The signs and symptoms of ALS, which depend on the affected muscles, are:

- Tripping and falling
- Loss of motor control in hands and arms
- Speech impairment
- Difficulty swallowing (dysphagia)
- Breathing impairment
- Persistent fatigue
- Severe muscle twitching and cramping

Amyotrophic lateral sclerosis typically affects middle-aged men, although women may also develop it. There is no cure and no proven therapy that will prevent its progression. It is usually fatal within five years after diagnosis.

Glioma

Gliomas are malignant tumors of glial cells, which provide supporting structure to the neurons of the brain. Malignancies of the glial cells tend not to metastasize outside of the skull. Gliomas are extremely difficult to remove from the brain surgically because they do not encapsulate; instead, they grow into the surrounding brain tissue, making it difficult to know the extent of brain tissue to remove. Gliomas are fast growing tumors resulting in high mortality.

Creutzfeldt-Jakob Disease

According to the National Institute of Neurological Disorders and Strokes (NINDS Creutzfeldt-Jakob disease 2001), Creutzfeldt-Jakob disease (CJD) is a rare, degenerative brain disorder with no known cure. It is fatal in 90 percent of the cases within one year, and there is currently no treatment to control its progress. There is no diagnostic test for CJD, which is categorized as either sporadic CJD, hereditary CJD, or acquired CJD. The only way to confirm a diagnosis of CJD is by biopsy of the brain during an autopsy. A confirmed diagnosis of CJD while the person is still alive does not help the patient, so a brain biopsy of a living patient is rarely performed, unless it is used to confirm a treatable nervous system disorder. In the early stages of CJD, symptoms include failing memory, behavioral changes, lack of coordination, and visual disturbances. As the disease progresses, the individual experiences mental deterioration, involuntary movements, blindness, and coma.

Cerebral Palsy

Cerebral palsy is a term used to describe a group of chronic disorders characterized by the impairment of control over movement. The impairment generally appears in the first few years of life and typically does not progress over time. It is believed that cerebral palsy is caused by developmental anomalies or damage to areas in the brain, disrupting its ability to control movement and posture.

Individuals with cerebral palsy have difficulty with their fine motor tasks, such as writing or using scissors. In addition, they struggle to maintain balance and walk. They may also lack full control of their voluntary movements. Symptoms may be as severe as having seizures or mental impairment, but symptoms differ between individuals and can change through time.

Signs of cerebral palsy are typically apparent by the age of three. Infants may develop normally, but exhibit difficulty learning to roll over, sit, crawl, smile, or walk. Some of the causes of cerebral palsy include head injury, jaundice, Rh incompatibility, and German measles. There is currently no cure for cerebral palsy, but it is usually neither progressive nor fatal.

Spina Bifida

Spina bifida is a congenital defect in which the spinal cord protrudes. As a result of this deficiency, the membranes of the spinal cord push through the opening. The opening is typically located in the lumbar vertebrae, forming a tumor in a condition known as spina bifida cystica.

Stroke

Strokes, which are also known as apoplexy, transient ischemic attacks (TIAs), or cerebrovascular accidents (CVAs), occur in the blood vessels of the brain. For a variety of reasons, a blood vessel bursts within the brain causing a loss of blood flow to the tissues of the brain, resulting in death of the brain tissue. Figure 13-4

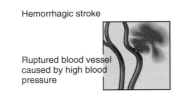

Hemorrhagic stroke

Ruptured blood vessel
caused by high blood
pressure

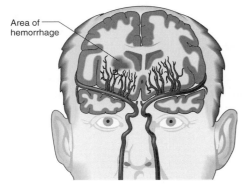

Area of
hemorrhage

Ischemic stroke

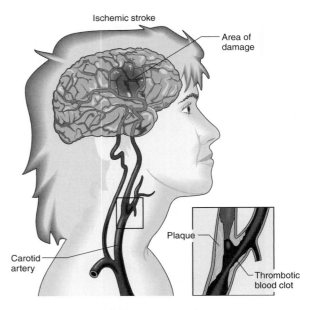

Area of
damage

Plaque

Carotid
artery

Thrombotic
blood clot

Figure 13–4 An ischemic stroke occurs when a cerebral vessel is occluded and the brain cells go without oxygenated blood for a time.

Figure 13–5 Rupture of cerebral blood vessels results in damage to surrounding brain tissue during a hemorrhagic stroke.

illustrates an ischemic stroke, in which a cerebral blood vessel becomes occluded. Figure 13-5 illustrates a hemorrhagic stroke, in which a cerebral blood vessel ruptures, causing internal bleeding.

The effects of a stroke are numerous and varied depending on the area of the brain in which the vessel ruptures. Loss of motor control, loss of sensory perception, and loss of speech are common effects of stroke. Since each hemisphere of the brain controls the opposite side of the body, if the symptoms are present on the right side of the body, the left side of the brain was the site of injury, and vice versa. Extensive therapy aids the stroke patient to recovery, if recovery is possible.

A TIA is a stroke that lasts only a few minutes. It occurs when the blood supply to the brain is briefly interrupted. The symptoms of a TIA are similar to a more severe stroke, but they do not last as long. Most symptoms of a TIA last only about an hour, but they may persist for as much as a day or so.

TRAUMA OF THE NERVOUS SYSTEM

Traumatic injuries to the nervous system are a leading cause of death and long-term disability in the United States. Most fatal or debilitating traumas result from head injuries caused by blunt force trauma associated with motor vehicle accidents, falls, gunshot wounds, or physical assaults, including child and spousal abuse. Severe trauma to the brain need not be fatal, however.

In 1848, Phineas Gage, a 25-year-old railroad construction foreman, accidentally caused an explosion that drove an iron bar through his head. The bar entered his left jaw and exited the top of his forehead. Amazingly, Gage survived and was declared recovered in a few weeks. Although he lived 13 more years, his personality changed completely. He became loud, profane, and irresponsible; he was unable to plan and think ahead. Gage's personality changed because of trauma to specific areas of the brain by the iron rod.

Concussion and Contusion

A **concussion** is a traumatic injury to the head resulting in temporary loss of consciousness, paralysis, vomiting, and seizures. Recovery occurs in hours or days, without permanent injury, with the exception of memory loss surrounding the traumatic event. Figure 13-6 illustrates damage to the brain resulting from concussion.

Contusions are more serious than concussions because contusions include hemorrhaging into the brain tissue (see Figure 13-7). A **contusion** is a head injury of sufficient force to bruise the brain, which often involves the surface of the brain and can cause an extravasation of blood without rupture of the meninges. Contusions can occur at any point at which the brain is in contact with the skull, but are most common in the frontal, temporal, and occipital lobes of the brain. Although the skull is often intact, it can contain fractures.

Interestingly, the site of contusion does not indicate the point of blunt force trauma. For example, if the head is struck with a hammer with sufficient force, contusions will develop at the site of impact. In contrast, trauma to the back of the head encountered in a falling accident may result in contusions in the frontal lobe as the brain is jarred against the frontal bone, with no contusion present in the occipital lobe.

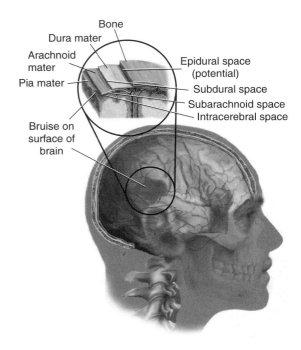

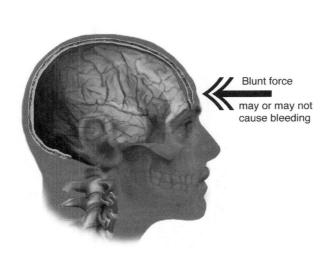

Figure 13-6 Concussion.

Figure 13-7 Contusion.

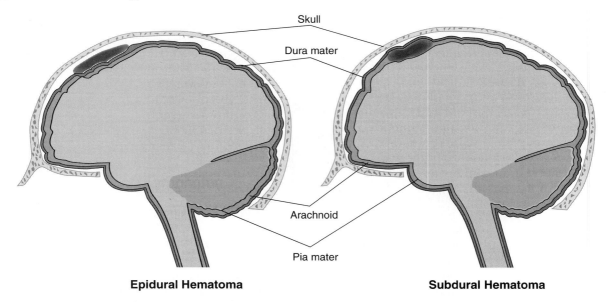

Skull

Dura mater

Arachnoid

Pia mater

Epidural Hematoma   **Subdural Hematoma**

Figure 13-8 Epidural and subdural hematomas.

 ## Hematoma

Figure 13-8 illustrates the area of bleeding associated with both epidural hematomas and subdural hematomas, while Table 13-1 lists and defines common sites of intracranial hemorrhage.

Epidural hematoma is a traumatic accumulation of blood between the skull and the dural membrane, which is most frequently due to rupture of a meningeal artery. The inciting event often is a focused blow to the head, such as that produced by a hammer, baseball bat, or windshield. The middle meningeal artery is firmly attached to the skull at the squamous portion of the temporal bone, so injury to the temple region of the head frequently results in its rupture. In most cases this trauma results in an overlying fracture. Because the underlying brain usually has been minimally injured, prognosis is excellent, if treated aggressively. Notice in Figure 13-9 how the brain tissue is compressed by the hematoma.

An acute subdural hematoma is a rapidly clotting blood collection below the inner layer of the dura, but external to the brain and arachnoid membrane. Acute subdural hematomas are almost always directly the result of blunt force

Table 13-1 Intracranial Hemorrhaging

Extradural (epidural)	Bleeding between the dura mater and the skull
Subdural	Bleeding between the dura mater and the arachnoid membrane
Subarachnoid	Bleeding between the pia mater and the arachnoid membrane

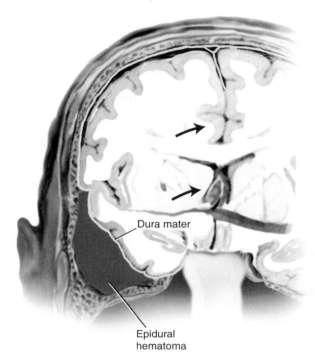

Figure 13-9 Note the shift of midline structures (small arrows) caused by epidural hematoma.

traumas to the head, such as whiplash or violently shaking an infant. Chronic subdural hematomas are less frequently the result of blunt force trauma than the result of brain atrophy in association with nervous disorders like Alzheimer's disease. Notice in Figure 13-10 that the brain and other cranial tissues are displaced and compressed by intracranial bleeding.

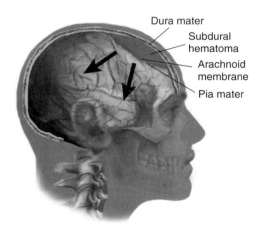

Figure 13-10 Note the shift of midline structures (small arrows) caused by subdural hematoma.

POSTMORTEM CONDITIONS ASSOCIATED WITH NERVOUS DISORDERS

Like pathologies of other systems of the body, pathologies of the nervous system result in unique complications during the embalming process. There are four common postmortem conditions associated with nervous disorders with which the embalmer should be familiar:

1. Brain purge
2. Hemorrhage
3. Atrophy
4. Diminished circulation

The effect of nervous system disorders is often paralysis or, at a minimum, severe restriction of movement. These restrictions result in atrophy of muscles and diminished circulation. In such cases, the deceased's blood vascular system may not be conducive to the proper distribution and diffusion of arterial embalming fluids. Sectional embalming techniques may be necessary in such cases, which call for the injection of copious amounts of lower than usual index arterial fluids, under low pressure, accompanied by gentle massage. This slow method of embalming the deceased is preferable to astringent techniques, which may result in only superficial results. Allowing the fluids to slowly build pressure within the blood vascular system, by alternating injection and drainage, will further add to the thorough distribution and diffusion of arterial fluids within the tissues of the deceased.

Injuries to the nervous system severe enough to result in death almost always result in cerebral edema in the deceased. Changes in the blood-brain barrier, which typically prevents fluids from leaking from the blood vessels and entering the brain tissues, allow the development of edema and hemorrhage. The absence of lymphatic drainage in the brain impairs the resorption of edematous fluids. Increased intracranial pressure, due to the presence of edematous fluid and internal bleeding, may result in severe distention and deformity of the deceased's head. In addition, a clear to pink fluid may also purge from the nose and ears.

The standard method of treating the cranial cavity after arterial embalming is to aspirate the excess fluid and then treat the tissues with cavity embalming fluids. Using an infant trocar, the embalmer inserts the tip into the nostril and penetrates the cribriform plate of the ethmoid bone. After thoroughly aspirating the cranial vault, a sufficient quantity of cavity fluid is introduced to attain preservation. Enough absorbent material is placed inside the nostril to prevent purge from the nose, which may result in chemical burns of the face. It is likely that the cranial cavity will need to be aspirated more than once, so no more absorbent material should be utilized than is necessary, as it must be removed for subsequent aspiration.

Just prior to cosmeticizing, dressing, and casketing, it may be advisable to place a desiccant powder in the nostril, and pack the nostril thoroughly with absorbent material. It is important not to alter the structure of the nose with excess packing materials, and the embalmer should be certain that no absorbent material is visible. If it is necessary to aspirate the cranial cavity after introducing desiccating powder into the nostril, the trocar should be inserted in the opposite nostril to prevent the trocar tip from becoming clogged with drying powder.

REVIEW QUESTIONS

Matching

1. _____ demyelization
2. _____ myelitis
3. _____ dementia
4. _____ sundowning
5. _____ contusions

a. increased confusion, restlessness, and insecurity in the early evening
b. the loss of the fatty tissue that surrounds the nerves
c. deteriorated mental ability accompanied by emotional instability
d. hemorrhages in the superficial brain tissue caused by blunt force trauma
e. inflammation of the myelin sheath that surrounds nerves

Multiple Choice

1. Alzheimer's disease is associated with which of the following tissue disorders?
   a. pigmentation
   b. amyloid degeneration
   c. necrosis
   d. inflammation
2. Which of the following is a type of brain cancer?
   a. glioma
   b. myelitis
   c. epilepsy
   d. spina bifida
3. Which of the following is a condition in which the cerebrospinal fluid fails to be properly drained or absorbed, causing the ventricles of the brain to fill with cerebrospinal fluid?
   a. Parkinson's disease
   b. Alzheimer's disease
   c. concussion
   d. hydrocephalus
4. Which type of hematoma typically results from degenerative disorders like Alzheimer's disease, rather than from blunt force trauma?
   a. chronic subdural
   b. epidural
   c. extradural
   d. subarachnoid

5. Which of the following disorders is characterized by flaccid limb paralysis, incontinence, and weakness or numbness of the limbs?

a. Parkinson's disease

b. Alzheimer's disease

c. myelitis

d. epilepsy

Putting Learning to Work!

The purpose of the following case analysis is to allow you to apply the information you have learned in a real-world situation. Read the case carefully and try to answer the following questions:

What disorder do you suspect the person had at the time of death?

What potential embalming complications do you anticipate?

What precautions should you take as the embalmer to limit the effects of these complications?

Case Analysis

A 73-year-old male died at his home. The man was a retired professor who spent the majority of his lifetime leading a healthy lifestyle. He exercised daily, ate a healthy diet, and avoided alcohol, medications, and tobacco. His children and wife all preceded him in death, and he had been cared for recently by his adult granddaughter. The man enjoyed dancing each week at the American Legion dances, but about a year ago, he began having difficulty coordinating his steps. He also noticed difficulty typing, and turning the pages of a book became difficult as well. Until last year, he spoke once a month as a guest lecturer at the local university, but he began having trouble speaking. About six months ago, he noticed swallowing complications, and his breathing became labored. In the last six weeks, he could no longer control his muscle twitching and cramping. As a result of being bedridden, he became emaciated.

Bibliography

Alzheimer's disease fact sheet. (2003). Retrieved June 10, 2003, from the National Institute on Aging, National Institutes of Health at http://www.alzheimers.org/pubs/adfact.html.

Cerebral palsy. (2003). Retrieved July 25, 2003, from MedlinePlus, the U.S. National Library of Medicine and the National Institutes of Health at http://www.nlm.nih.gov/medlineplus/cerebralpalsy.html.

Dementia and sundowning. (2002). Alzheimer's Australia Health Sheets. Retrieved June 10, 2003, from the Better Health Channel at http://www.betterhealth.vic.gov.au/bhcv2/bhcarticles.nsf/pages/Dementia_and_sundowning?OpenDocument.

Edwards, Brook F. (2003). *Encephalitis*. Retrieved March 16, 2004, from the Brain and Nervous Systems Center of the Mayo Clinic at http://www.mayoclinic.com/invoke.cfm?id=DS00226.

Hydrocephalus. (2003). Retrieved July 25, 2003, from MedlinePlus, the U.S. National Library of Medicine and the National Institutes of Health at http://www.nlm.nih.gov/medlineplus/hydrocephalus.html.

The Internet Stroke Center page. (2003). Retrieved July 25, 2003, from the University of Washington in St. Louis at http://www.strokecenter.org/prof/index.html.

Kumar, V., Cotran, R., & Robbins, S. (2003). *Robbins basic pathology* (7th ed.). Philadelphia: Saunders.

Macmillian, M. (2002). The Phineas Gage Information Page. Retrieved July 25, 2003, from the Department of Psychology, Deakin University, Victoria, Australia at http://www.deakin.edu.au/hbs/GAGEPAGE/.

Mayer, R. (2000). *Embalming: History, theory, & practice* (3rd ed.). New York: McGraw-Hill.

Meningococcal diseases. (2003). Retrieved March 16, 2004, from the Division of Bacterial and Mycotic Diseases, Centers for Disease Control and Prevention at http://www.cdc.gov/ncidod/dbmd/diseaseinfo/meningococcal_g.htm.

Mixed Giomas: The Cancer BACUP Factsheet. (2001). Retrieved May 29, 2003, from the British Association of Cancer United Patients at http://www.cancerbacup.org.uk/info/mixedglioma.htm.

Neighbors, M., & Tannehill-Jones, R. (2000). *Human diseases*. Clifton Park, NY: Delmar Thomson Learning.

New variant CJD. (2005). Retrieved January 8, 2005, at http://www.cdc.gov/ncidod/diseases/cid/cjd_fact_sheet.htm.

NINDS amyotrophic lateral sclerosis information page. (2001). Retrieved June 10, 2003, from the National Institute of Neurological Disorders and Stroke, National Institutes of Health at http://www.ninds.nih.gov/health_and_medical/disorders/amyotrophiclateralsclerosis_doc.htm.

NINDS cerebral palsy information page. (2001). Retrieved June 10, 2003, from the National Institute of Neurological Disorders and Stroke, National Institutes of Health at http://www.ninds.nih.gov/health_and_medical/disorders/cerebral_palsy.htm.

NINDS Creutzfeldt-Jakob disease information page. (2001). Retrieved March 16, 2004, from the National Institute of Neurological Disorders and Stroke, National Institutes of Health at http://www.ninds.nih.gov/health_and_medical/disorders/cjd.htm.

NINDS spina bifida information page. (2001). Retrieved May 30, 2003, from the National Institutes of Health, The National Institute of Neurological Disorders and Stroke at http://www.ninds.nih.gov/health_and_medical/disorders/spina_bifida.htm.

NINDS transverse myelitis information page. (2001). Retrieved June 10, 2003, from the National Institute of Neurological Disorders and Stroke, National Institutes of Health at http://www.ninds.nih.gov/health_and_medical/disorders/transversemyelitis_doc.htm.

Parkinson's disease backgrounder. (2001). Retrieved June 10, 2003, from the National Institute of Neurological Disorders and Stroke, National Institutes of Health at http://www.ninds.nih.gov/health_and_medical/pubs/parkinson's_disease_backgrounder.htm.

Pathology for funeral service. (1999). Dallas, TX: Professional Training Schools.

Poliomyelitis. (n.d.). Retrieved July 26, 2003, from the National Immunization Program, Centers for Disease Control and Prevention at http://www.cdc.gov/nip/publications/pink/polio.pdf.

Price, D., & Wilson, S. (2001). Epidural hematoma. Retrieved June 5, 2003, from eMedicine at http://www.emedicine.com/EMERG/topic167.htm.

Scaletta, T. (2002). *Subdural hematoma*. Retrieved June 5, 2003, from eMedicine at http://www.emedicine.com/EMERG/topic560.htm.

Shelton, H. (1992). *Boyd's introduction to the study of disease* (11th ed.). Philadelphia: Lea & Febiger.

Sowaka, J., Gurwood, A., & Kabat, K. (2001). Pituitary adenoma. In *Handbook of Ocular Disease Management*. Jobson Publishing. Retrieved May 29, 2003, from http://www.revoptom.com/handbook/SECT54a.HTM.

Types of seizures. (2003). Retrieved July 25, 2003, from the Epilepsy Foundation at http://www.epilepsyfoundation.org/answerplace/Medical/seizures/types/.

Update 2002: Bovine spongiform encephalopathy and variant Creutzfelt-Jacob disease. (2003). Retrieved July 26, 2003, from the National Center for Infectious Diseases, Division of Viral and Rickettsial Diseases, Centers for Disease Control and Prevention at http://www.cdc.gov/ncidod/diseases/cjd/bse_cjd.htm.

Van Wynseberghe, D., Noback, C., & Carola, R. (1995). *Human anatomy & physiology* (3rd ed.). New York: McGraw Hill.

Venes, D. (Ed.). (2001). *Taber's cyclopedic medical dictionary* (19th ed.). Philadelphia: F. A. Davis.

Walling, A. (1999). Amyotrophic lateral sclerosis: Lou Gehrig's disease. In *American Family Physician*. Retrieved June 10, 2003, from http://www.aafp.org/afp/990315ap/1489.html.

CHAPTER 14

Diseases of the Female Reproductive System

Learning Objectives

Upon completion of the chapter, review questions, and case analysis, the reader should be able to:

- Discuss the significant disease conditions associated with pelvic inflammatory disease.
- List the possible sites of ectopic pregnancies.
- Compare and contrast endometritis and endometriosis.
- Compare and contrast dermoid cysts and sebaceous cysts.
- Describe different forms of mastectomy based on the degree of breast removal.
- Differentiate between eclampsia and pre-eclampsia.
- Discuss the importance of regular examinations for cervical cancer.
- Explain the impact of diseases of the female reproductive system on the condition of the deceased.

Key Terms

ectopic pregnancy	lumpectomy
eclampsia	mastectomy
endometritis	oophoritis
endometriosis	salpingitis

DISORDERS OF THE FEMALE REPRODUCTIVE SYSTEM

This chapter describes some of the most significant pathological disorders of the female reproductive system. It also includes some infectious diseases of the female reproductive system, each of which is described in greater detail in Part Two. While reading this chapter, the reader may review the anatomy of the female reproductive system by referring to Appendix I.

Pelvic Inflammatory Disease

Salpingitis and pelvic inflammatory disease are synonymous terms used to describe infection and inflammation of the female upper genital tract, especially the fallopian tubes. Pelvic inflammatory disease is a condition that lacks a precise definition and may include infection of the endometrium (**endometritis**), the fallopian tubes (**salpingitis**), the ovaries (**oophoritis**), the uterine wall (myometritis), the uterine serosa and broad ligaments (parametritis), and the pelvic peritoneum. Most cases of pelvic inflammatory disease occur in two stages. During the first stage, a vaginal or cervical infection develops, and during the second stage, the infection spreads to the upper genital tract.

Table 14-1 lists some of the most common inflammatory conditions of the female reproductive system. Many cases of pelvic inflammatory disease are asymptomatic, and the only characteristic of symptomatic cases may be lower abdominal pain.

Sexually Transmitted Diseases

According to the National Institutes of Health (An introduction 1999), sexually transmitted diseases (STDs), which were once called venereal diseases (VD), are the most common infectious diseases in the United States, with over 20 identified STDs affecting more than 13 million people each year. The cost of STDs is estimated to exceed $10 billion dollars annually. Some of the significant STDs are AIDS, chlamydia, genital herpes, genital warts, gonorrhea, and syphilis. Part Two of this book describes each of these diseases and the microorganisms that cause them in detail. Although STDs often have recognizable lesions, in many cases, neither men nor women may have any external lesions indicating the presence of disease. The lack of obvious lesions is one of the factors that increases the rate of transmission of STDs.

Ectopic Pregnancy

Ectopic pregnancy is the implantation of the fertilized ovum in a site other than the normal one in the uterine cavity. In most cases, the egg implants within the

Table 14-1 Inflammatory Conditions of the Female Reproductive System

Endometritis	Inflammation of the lining of the uterus due to bacterial infection
Endocervicitis	Inflammation of the uterus and the cervix
Salpingitis	Inflammation of the fallopian (uterine) tube
Oophoritis	Inflammation of the ovary
Vaginitis	Inflammation of the vagina

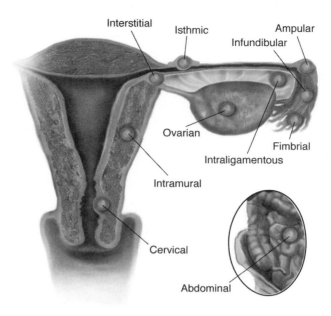

Figure 14-1 Possible sites of implantation in ectopic pregnancy.

fallopian tube, although it may implant in the ovary, abdomen, or cervix (see Figure 14-1). Ectopic pregnancies rarely progress to full term.

Ectopic pregnancies are usually caused by an obstruction of the passage of the fertilized egg through the fallopian tube to the uterus due to physical blockage in the tube or failure of the tubal epithelium to move the fertilized egg down the tube and into the uterus. Previous tubal infection or surgery might also have caused scarring of the lining of the tube, which can inhibit the passage of the fertilized egg toward the uterus. Many women who experience tubal pregnancies also have a history of salpingitis or pelvic inflammatory disease. Occasionally, ectopic pregnancies are due to unknown causes.

Pre-Eclampsia and Eclampsia

Pre-eclampsia is a serious condition that occurs during pregnancy. It is characterized by high blood pressure, weight gain, and protein in the urine. Pre-eclampsia may progress into **eclampsia**, which is the occurrence of seizures during pregnancy, which cannot be attributed to another cause, after the 20th week of gestation. The causes of both pre-eclampsia and eclamspia are unknown. There is an increased risk for pre-eclampsia with first pregnancies, teenage pregnancies, mothers older than 40, among African-American women, multiple pregnancies, and women with a history of diabetes, hypertension, or renal diseases.

Table 14-2 compares the characteristics of pre-eclampsia and eclampsia. The treatment for these disorders is to deliver as soon as it is safe for the fetus

Table 14-2 Characteristics of Pre-Eclampsia and Eclampsia

Pre-Eclampsia	Eclampsia
Swelling of hands and face on arising	Seizures
Sudden weight gain over one or two days	Severe agitation
Persistent headache	Periods of unconsciousness
Upper abdominal pain	Aches and pains after seizures

because prolonging such pregnancy usually results in fetal death and complications for the mother. Treatment includes medications to control elevated blood pressure and seizures and bed rest until delivery can safely occur.

Endometriosis

Endometriosis is a condition in which the tissue that normally lines the uterus, which is known as the endometrium, grows in other areas of the body, such as the pelvic area, the surface of the uterus, the ovaries, the intestines, the rectum, or the bladder (see Figure 14-2). Endometriosis is an idiopathic disorder, which can cause pain, irregular bleeding, and infertility as the disease progresses.

Each month the ovaries produce hormones that stimulate the cells of the uterine lining to multiply and prepare for a fertilized egg, at which point any endometrial cells outside of the uterus also respond to this signal. These misplaced cells, however, are incapable of separating themselves from the surrounding tissue and sloughing off during the next menstrual period. If this process continues, it can cause scarring and adhesions in the tubes and ovaries, which may inhibit the passage of a fertilized egg down the fallopian tube.

If the cells penetrate the ovary, they may collect large amounts of blood and form what is known as ovarian blood cysts or endometriomas. Ovarian blood cysts are also known as chocolate cysts, due to the darkening of the collected blood inside of them, and they can grow to the size of an orange.

Although some women are asymptomatic, the following are some of the most common characteristics of endometriosis:

- Increasingly painful periods
- Abdominopelvic pain and cramps lasting for a week surrounding menstruation
- Pain during or following sexual intercourse
- Painful bowel movements
- Premenstrual spotting of blood
- Infertility

Ovarian Cysts

Ovarian cysts are sacs filled with fluids that develop on or within the ovary, as illustrated in Figure 14-3. Typically, ovarian cysts are functional and disappear on their own. A functional disorder is one that is not caused by disease. A func-

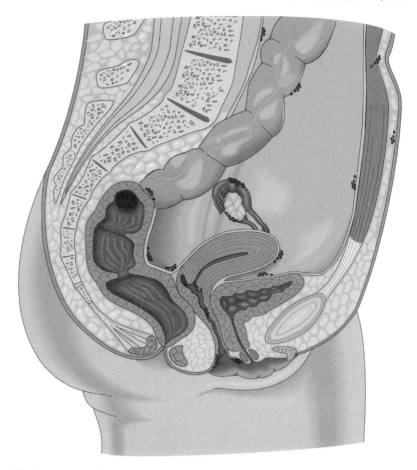

Figure 14-2 Endometriosis—common sites of endometrial implants.

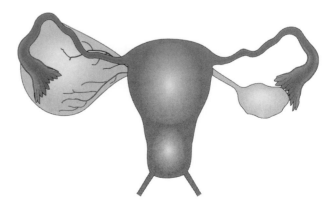

Figure 14-3 Ovarian cyst.

tional ovarian cyst forms during the days preceding ovulation, when a follicle grows, but fails to rupture and release an egg as it should. Instead of being re-absorbed, the fluid within the follicle forms a cyst that disappears within 60 days. Functional ovarian cysts differ from benign or malignant cysts, which must be treated to resolve. Some of the signs of a nonfunctional ovarian cyst include:

- Constant, dull, aching pelvic pain
- Pain during sexual intercourse or normal movement
- Pelvic pain shortly after beginning or ending of menses
- Changes in the normal pattern of menstrual bleeding
- Lengthened or shortened menstrual cycle
- Absence of menstruation
- Abdominal bloating or distention

A dermoid cyst is a tumor that is covered in dermislike tissue that contains sebaceous glands, hair, cartilage, bonelike structures, nails, or teeth (Ruszczak 2002). Although dermoid cysts can occur anywhere in both males and females, including the reproductive tract, specifically, a type of dermoid cyst tumor known as a cystic teratoma can occur in the ovary.

Cervical Cancer

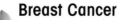

There are two primary categories of cervical cancer. The most common is squamous cell carcinoma, which develops from the flat cells covering the outer surface of the cervix at the top of the vagina. The other type is adenocarcinoma, which develops from the glandular cells lining the cervical canal. The best way to detect precancerous cells in the cervix is through regular cervical smears. Although the smear test is designed to detect precancerous cells, it may also detect an existing cancer. The most common symptoms of cervical cancer are abnormal bleeding between periods or after sexual intercourse, a malodorous vaginal discharge, and discomfort during intercourse. Color Plate 28 highlights the erosion of the cervix that accompanies cervical cancer.

Breast Cancer

The exact causes of breast cancer are not known, but the risk of developing breast cancer increases with age. Breast cancer is uncommon among women under the age of 35, and most cases occur in women over the age of 50. Caucasian women develop breast cancer more frequently than African-American or Asian-American women. In its early stages, breast cancer is painless and may present no signs or symptoms, but as the cancer grows, any or all of the following can be present:

- A lump or thickening in or near the breast or in the underarm area.
- A change in the size or shape of the breast.
- Nipple discharge or tenderness
- The nipple is pulled back (inverted) into the breast.

- Ridges or pitting of the breast which causes the breast to look like the rind of an orange.
- The breast, areola, or nipple may be warm, swollen, red, or scaly.

It may be necessary to examine tissue or fluids from the breast to determine if they are malignant. One of the most common ways to test tissues or fluids for malignancy is by taking a biopsy. The first way to obtain a biopsy is through fine-needle aspiration, in which a thin needle is used to remove fluid and cells from a breast lump. The second way to obtain a biopsy is to take a needle biopsy, which involves the use of a larger needle that can remove more tissue and fluid than a thin needle. The third way to obtain a biopsy is through a surgical procedure known as a **lumpectomy**, during which a surgeon removes the lump and an area of healthy tissue around its edges. A lumpectomy is preferable to the removal of the breast or a portion thereof, which is referred to as a **mastectomy**. Although breast reconstruction is sometimes possible, mastectomy has several noncosmetic disadvantages (e.g., psychological distress, invasiveness of the procedure, degree of anesthesia required, recovery time, necessity of physical therapy). Figure 14-4 illustrates a lumpectomy and three of the four types of mastectomy, while Figure 14-5 is a photograph of a woman whose breast cancer recurred after she underwent a radical mastectomy. There are four types of mastectomy:

1. Subcutaneous: removal of the entire breast leaving the nipple and areola.
2. Total (simple): removal of the entire breast, but not the axillary lymph nodes.
3. Modified radical: removal of the entire breast and most of the axillary lymph nodes.
4. Radical: removal of the pectoralis muscles and the breast and axillary lymph nodes. Although once considered the standard for breast cancer treatment, this procedure is mostly of historical interest because it is rarely used today.

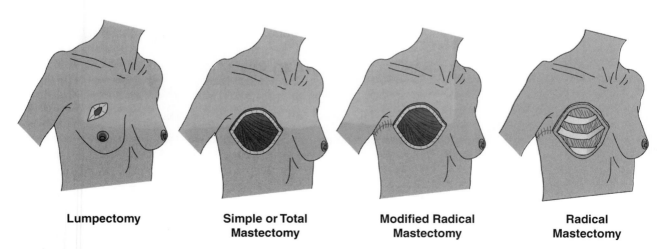

| **Lumpectomy** | **Simple or Total Mastectomy** | **Modified Radical Mastectomy** | **Radical Mastectomy** |

Figure 14-4 Types of mastectomy.

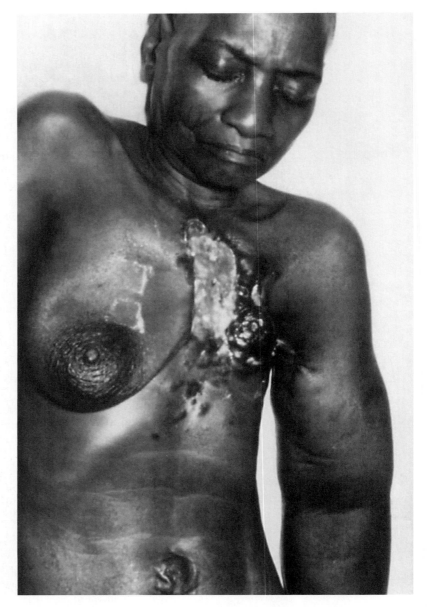

Figure 14-5 Breast cancer complications after a mastectomy. (Courtesy of the Centers for Disease Control and Prevention, Atlanta, GA, Robert S. Craig.)

POSTMORTEM CONDITIONS ASSOCIATED WITH REPRODUCTIVE SYSTEM DISORDERS

Many of the disorders associated with the reproductive system are both inflammatory and infectious. The immune system's response to these disorders results in postmortem conditions that can complicate the embalming processes. There are at least five postmortem conditions associated with reproductive system disorders that the embalmer should anticipate:

1. Rapid blood coagulation
2. Ascites
3. Edema
4. Infections
5. Discolorations

As with any infectious diseases, rapid blood coagulation can complicate the embalming processes. In addition, the lesions associated with infectious diseases may cause deformation and discoloration of tissues, necessitating restoration. Control of microbial agents associated with female reproductive system infections requires the thorough disinfection of the deceased during the embalming process. To this end, any surface lesions require the application of topical disinfectants and surface or hypodermic application of preservative chemicals.

REVIEW QUESTIONS

Matching

1. _____ oophoritis
2. _____ salpingitis
3. _____ endometritis
4. _____ endocervicitis
5. _____ vaginitis

a. inflammation of the ovary
b. inflammation of the vagina
c. inflammation of the fallopian tube
d. inflammation of the uterine wall
e. inflammation of the uterus and the cervix

Multiple Choice

1. Which of the following is a condition in which the fertilized egg fails to implant itself in the uterine wall and implants outside the uterus?
   a. endometritis
   b. endocervicitis
   c. ectopic pregnancy
   d. salpingitis
2. Which of the following disorders is related to seizures and sudden death of mothers after about the 20th week of pregnancy?
   a. ectopic pregnancy
   b. eclampsia
   c. epilepsy
   d. myalgia

3. Endometriomas are also known as which of the following?
   a. ovarian blood cysts
   b. tubal pregnancies
   c. orchitis
   d. endometriosis

4. Which type of mastectomy is most invasive?
   a. subcutaneous
   b. simple
   c. modified radical
   d. radical

5. Which of the following refers to sacs filled with fluids that develop on or within the ovary?
   a. cystitis
   b. ovarian cysts
   c. pre-eclampsia
   d. oophoritis

Putting Learning to Work!

The purpose of the following case analysis is to allow you to apply the information you have learned in a real-world situation. Read the case carefully and try to answer the following questions:

What disorder do you suspect the person had at the time of death?

What potential embalming complications do you anticipate?

What precautions should you take as the embalmer to limit the effects of these complications?

Case Analysis

A 63-year-old female died at her home. She weighs approximately 495 pounds, and she is 5'6" tall. Her son informs you that his mother has not left her home for the past six years due to her obesity. Before her death, she complained of constant abdominal pain, abdominal bloating and distention, and pain when she moved. She assumed the pain was due to her weight. She also experienced spotty bleeding from her vagina, although she was postmenopausal. During aspiration, you experience difficulty penetrating some of the viscera, and there is an excessive amount of fluid in the lower abdomen.

Bibliography

Bradley, C. (2002a). Endometrial biopsy. In *Medical Encyclopedia*. Retrieved July 25, 2003, from MedlinePlus, the U.S. National Library of Medicine and the National Institutes of Health at http://www.nlm.nih.gov/medlineplus/ency/article/003917.htm.

Bradley, C. (2002b). Endometriosis. In *Medical Encyclopedia*. Retrieved July 25, 2003, from MedlinePlus, the U.S. National Library of Medicine and the National Institutes of Health at http://www.nlm.nih.gov/medlineplus/ency/article/000915.htm.

Bradley, C. (2002c). Endometritis. In *Medical Encyclopedia*. Retrieved July 25, 2003, from MedlinePlus, the U.S. National Library of Medicine and the National Institutes of Health at http://www.nlm.nih.gov/medlineplus/ency/article/001484.htm.

Brooks, M. (2001). *Pregnancy, eclampsia*. Retrieved July 25, 2003, from eMedicine at http://www.emedicine.com/emerg/topic796.htm.

Chen, P. (2020). Pelvic inflammatory disease. In *Medical Encyclopedia*. Retrieved July 25, 2003, from MedlinePlus, the U.S. National Library of Medicine and the National Institutes of Health at http://www.nlm.nih.gov/medlineplus/ency/article/000888.htm.

Chlamydia in the United States. (2001). Retrieved July 20, 2003, from the Division of Sexually Transmitted Diseases Prevention, National Center for HIV, STD, and TB Prevention. Centers for Disease Control and Prevention at http://www.cdc.gov/nchstp/dstd/Fact_Sheets/chlamydia_facts.htm.

Chlamydia pneumoniae. (2002). Retrieved from the National Center for Infectious Diseases, Division of Bacterial and Mycotic Diseases, Centers for Disease Control and Prevention at http://www.cdc.gov/ncidod/dbmd/diseaseinfo/chlamydiapneumonia_t.htm.

Donegan, W., Spratt, J., & Orsini, J. (Eds.). (2002). *Cancer of the breast*. Philadelphia: W.B. Saunders.

Genital herpes. (2001). Retrieved July 26, 2003, from the National Center for HIV, STDs, and TB Prevention, Division of HIV/AIDS Prevention, Centers for Disease Control and Prevention at http://www.cdc.gov/nchstp/dstd/Fact_Sheets/facts_Genital_Herpes.htm.

Gonorrhea. (2001). Retrieved July 26, 2003, from the National Center for HIV, STD, and TB Prevention, Division of Sexually Transmitted Diseases, Centers for Disease Control and Prevention at http://www.cdc.gov/nchstp/dstd/Fact_Sheets/FactsGonorrhea.htm.

Human papilloma virus. (1997). Retrieved May 29, 2003, from the Department of Gynecology and Obstetrics, University of Iowa at http://obgyn.uihc.uiowa.edu/Patinfo/Adhealth/hpv.htm.

An introduction to sexually transmitted diseases. (1999). In *Health matters*. Retrieved March 16, 2004, from the National Institute of Allergy and Infectious Diseases, National Institutes of Health: http://www.niaid.nih.gov/factsheets/stdinfo.htm.

Kendrick, J., Atrash, H., Strauss, L., Gargiullo, P., & Ahn, Y. (1997). Vaginal douching and the risk of ectopic pregnancy among black women. *American Journal of Obstetrics and Gynecology, 176,* 991–997.

Knopf, K. (2002). Endometrial cancer. In *Medical Encyclopedia*. Retrieved July 25, 2003, from MedlinePlus, the U.S. National Library of Medicine and the National Institutes of Health at http://www.nlm.nih.gov/medlineplus/ency/article/000910.htm.

Knowles, D. (2002). Leydig cell tumors. In *Medical Encyclopedia*. Retrieved July 25, 2003, from MedlinePlus, the U.S. National Library of Medicine and the National Institutes of Health at http://www.nlm.nih.gov/medlineplus/ency/article/000409.htm.

Kumar, V., Cotran, R., & Robbins, S. (2003). *Robbins basic pathology* (7th ed.). Philadelphia: Saunders.

Mayer, R. (2000). *Embalming: History, theory, & practice* (3rd ed.). New York: McGraw-Hill.

Miethke, M., & Raugi, G. (2003). *Leiomyoma*. Retrieved May 29, 2003, from eMedicine at http://www.emedicine.com/DERM/topic217.htm.

Neighbors, M., & Tannehill-Jones, R. (2000). *Human diseases*. Clifton Park, NY: Thomson Delmar Learning.

Ovarian cyst. (2003). Retrieved July 25, 2003, from the American Academy of Family Physicians at http://familydoctor.org/handouts/279.html.

Pathology for funeral service. (1999). Dallas, TX: Professional Training Schools.

Pre-eclampsia. (n.d.). Retrieved July 25, 2003, from the Action on Pre-Eclampsia Promoting Safer Pregnancy at http://www.apec.org.uk/apec_what.html.

Ruszczak, Zbigniew. (2002). *Dermoid cyst*. Retrieved March 16, 2004, from eMedicine at http://www.emedicine.com/derm/topic686.htm.

Shelton, H. (1992). *Boyd's introduction to the study of disease* (11th ed.). Philadelphia: Lea & Febiger.

Vanni, R. (2002). Uterus: Leiomyoma. In *Atlas of Genetics and Cytogenetics in Oncology Haematology*. Retrieved May 29, 2003, from http://www.infobiogen.fr/services/chromcancer/Tumors/leiomyomID5031.html.

Venes, D. (Ed.). (2001). *Taber's cyclopedic medical dictionary* (19th ed.). Philadelphia: F. A. Davis.

What is leiomyosarcoma? (2001). Retrieved May 29, 2003, from the British Association of Cancer United Patients at http://www.cancerbacup.org.uk/questions/specific/sarcomas/sts/leiomyosarcoma.htm.

CHAPTER 15

Diseases of the Male Reproductive System

Learning Objectives

Upon completion of the chapter, review questions, and case analysis, the reader should be able to:

- Describe the etiology and pathogenesis of orchitis.
- Compare and contrast cryptorchism and inguinal hernia.
- Describe the etiology and pathogenesis of prostatitis.
- Differentiate between prostate cancer and testicular cancer.
- Discuss hydrocele in relation to its postmortem presence and its postmortem embalming treatment.
- Explain the impact of diseases of the male reproductive system on the condition of the deceased.

Key Terms

cryptorchism
hydrocele
inguinal hernia

orchitis
prostatitis

DISORDERS OF THE MALE REPRODUCTIVE SYSTEM

This chapter describes some of the most significant pathological disorders of the male reproductive system. It also includes some infectious diseases of the male reproductive system, each of which is described in greater detail in Part Two. While reading this chapter, the reader may review the anatomy of the male reproductive system by referring to Appendix J.

Orchitis

Orchitis is a disorder with a long history, first being reported by Hippocrates in the 5th century. **Orchitis** is an acute inflammatory reaction in the testicle, occurring in boys under the age of ten, as a result of the mumps virus. However, it can be caused by other microbial infections. Orchitis currently occurs in approximately 20 percent of boys who contract mumps, and it normally develops between four and seven days after mumps virus infection. Orchitis of one testicle rarely results in sterility or increased risk of tumors in later life. The onset of orchitis is typically acute, often causing initial symptoms within hours. Orchitis is characterized by the following:

- Severe pain in the testicle and groin
- Fatigue
- Pain and tenderness in the muscles (myalgia)
- Fever and chills
- Nausea
- Headache

Prostatitis

According to the NKUDIC (*Prostatitis* 2003), prostatitis may account for up to 25 percent of all office visits by young and middle-aged men for complaints involving the genital and urinary systems. **Prostatitis** is inflammation of the prostate gland, and it can refer to four categories of disease. Acute bacterial prostatitis is the least common form of prostatitis, with symptoms of chills, fever, frequent urination, urgency in urination, burning urination, and lower back or genital pain. *Acute bacterial prostatitis* is treated with antibiotics to counter the infection. *Chronic bacterial prostatitis* is also relatively rare, and is characterized by the same signs and symptoms as acute bacterial prostatitis. The difference in acute and chronic prostatitis is that in cases of chronic prostatitis, the infection settles into the prostate gland due to a defect in the prostate gland. Treatment typically requires removal of the defective tissue in the prostate gland, followed by antibiotic treatment for the bacterial infection.

Chronic prostatitis, which is also known as chronic pelvic pain syndrome, is the most common form of prostatitis. Chronic prostatitis may or may not be accompanied by inflammation of the prostate. This form of prostatitis is poorly understood, and its symptoms, which are similar to those of bacterial prostatitis, can come and go without warning. Chronic prostatitis is currently treated with a combination of warm baths and medications that relax the prostate gland.

Finally, *asymptomatic inflammatory prostatitis* is a condition that, as its name suggests, does not have noticeable symptoms. It is an inflammatory condition of the prostate that is typically diagnosed when healthcare professionals conduct tests for the cause of infertility or the presence of prostate cancer in the male. Asymptomatic inflammatory prostatitis is not accompanied by pain or discomfort; however, immune system cells that combat infections are found in the male's semen.

Hydrocele

According to Kazzi (2002), **hydrocele** is a collection of edematous fluid in the scrotum. Specifically, the serous fluid accumulates in the scrotum as a result of either a defect or an irritation of the tunica vaginalis or the spermatic cord within the scrotum. Most hydroceles are congenital, meaning that their cause is present at birth, and they are most common in children between the ages of one and two years old. In adult males, most cases of hydrocele are observed in those over the age of 40. In adults, hydrocele is most commonly the result of cancer, infections, trauma to the testicles, hernias, or damage to the circulatory system within the male reproductive system.

Only about 1 percent of all males experience hydroceles. Most hydroceles are asymptomatic; however, they may be accompanied by a sensation of heaviness or dragging. A painless enlargement of the scrotum is also a common sign of hydrocele. Hydroceles can also causes mild discomfort that radiates from the scrotum to the mid-lower back. Hydrocele only occurs on both sides of the scrotum in about 7 percent to 10 percent of the cases. As described later in this chapter, hydrocele can complicate the embalming processes.

Cryptorchism

Cryptorchism, which is also known as cryptorchidism, is defined as failure of the testis to descend from its intra-abdominal location into the scrotum (see Figure 15-1). A normal testicle descends at approximately 36 weeks of age, but

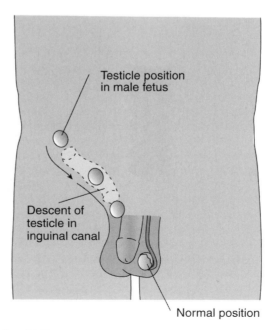

Figure 15-1 Cryptorchidism—pathway and common sites of hidden testis.

for unknown reasons, cryptorchism occurs in some male infants. It is treated by a procedure known as orchiopexy, in which the testicle is sutured into place in the scrotum.

Inguinal Hernia

An **inguinal hernia** is a condition in which part of the intestine bulges through a weakened area of the muscles in the inguinal canal, which is located in the groin. Hernias are more common in males, and they can be caused by obesity, heavy lifting, straining to defecate, or by any other activity that places increased pressure on the weakened muscles (*Inguinal hernia* 2002). Hernias can cause a lump in the groin, pain in the groin, and blockage of the intestine. If the intestine becomes twisted, or if the blood supply to the intestine is compromised in a condition known as a strangulated hernia, the affected portion of the intestine requires surgical removal. If the blood supply is cut off from the bowel for too long, it can lead to necrosis of the affected portion of the intestine.

Benign Prostatic Hyperplasia and Prostate Cancer

There is a difference in the benign enlargement of the prostate and prostate cancer. Benign prostatic hyperplasia is the abnormal growth of prostate cells, but the condition is not cancerous. In benign prostate growth, the prostate undergoes abnormal growth and presses against the urethra and bladder, interfering with the normal flow of urine (see Figure 15-2). As they age, most men will develop benign enlargement of the prostate, which can cause severe enough urinary dysfunction to warrant treatment.

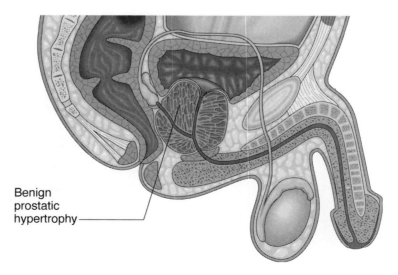

Benign
prostatic
hypertrophy

Figure 15–2 Enlarged prostate gland.

Prostate cancer is a much more serious disorder that affects African-American men more than Caucasians, Asian Americans, or Native Americans. Prostate cancer may be initially detected by a digital rectal exam, during which the healthcare professional inserts a lubricated, gloved finger into the rectum and feels the prostate through the rectal wall to check for lumps. There is also a blood test that measures prostate-specific antigen. Early prostate cancer often does not cause symptoms, but prostate cancer can cause any or all of the following:

- A need to urinate frequently, especially at night
- Difficulty starting urination or holding back urine
- Inability to urinate
- Weak or interrupted flow of urine
- Painful or burning urination
- Difficulty in having an erection
- Painful ejaculation
- Blood in urine or semen
- Frequent pain or stiffness in the lower back, hips, or upper thighs

If a pathologist determines that a tissue biopsy is malignant, the grade of the cancer will be reported to the oncologist. The grade tells how much the tumor tissue differs from normal prostate tissue and suggests how fast the tumor is likely to grow. The Gleason system uses scores between 2 and 10 to grade prostate cancer, and another system uses G1 through G4. The higher the grade, the more likely the tumor has grown and spread.

During stage I (stage A), the tumor cannot be felt during a rectal exam. During stage II (stage B), the tumor involves more tissue within the prostate, and it can be felt during a rectal exam. During stage III (stage C), the cancer has spread outside the prostate to nearby tissues. During stage IV (stage D), the cancer has spread to lymph nodes or to other parts of the body. If detected early, the survival rate of prostate cancer is higher than if it is detected in later stages.

Testicular Cancer

There are two broad categories of testicular cancer: seminoma and nonseminoma. The nonseminomas include choriocarcinoma, embryonal carcinoma, teratoma, and yolk sac tumors. Although the causes of testicular cancer are unknown, some of the risk factors include undescended testicles (cryptorchidism), abnormal testicular development, and Klinefelter's syndrome, which is a sex chromosome disorder characterized by low levels of male hormones, sterility, breast enlargement, and small testes. Most testicular cancers are found by men themselves, and any of the following should alert men to see their healthcare professional:

- A painless lump or swelling in either testicle
- Any enlargement of a testicle or change in the way it feels
- A feeling of heaviness in the scrotum
- A dull ache in the lower abdomen or the groin

- A sudden collection of fluid in the scrotum
- Pain or discomfort in a testicle or in the scrotum

Seminomas and nonseminomas grow and spread differently, necessitating different professionals for treatment, some of whom can include a surgeon, an oncologist, and a radiation oncologist. If necessary, surgery to remove the testicle, called a radical inguinal orchiectomy, is performed. Men with one remaining healthy testicle can still have normal erections and produce enough sperm to have children. There is also an artificial testicle that can be placed in the scrotum, which has the same weight and feel as a human testicle.

Sexually Transmitted Diseases

According to the National Institutes of Health (An introduction 1999), sexually transmitted diseases are the most common infectious diseases in the United States. Some of the most significant STDs are AIDS, chlamydia, genital herpes, genital warts, gonorrhea, and syphilis. Part Two of this book describes each of these diseases and the microorganisms that cause them in detail.

POSTMORTEM CONDITIONS ASSOCIATED WITH THE MALE REPRODUCTIVE SYSTEM

Many of the disorders associated with the female reproductive system are present in the disorders of the male reproductive system. There are at least five postmortem conditions associated with male reproductive system disorders that the embalmer should anticipate:

1. Rapid blood coagulation
2. Ascites
3. Edema
4. Infections
5. Discolorations

As is the case in female reproductive system disorders, infectious reproductive system diseases in males may be associated with rapid blood coagulation that can complicate the embalming processes. The lesions associated with these infectious diseases may cause deformation and discoloration of tissues as well. As indicated in Color Plate 29, pathological disorders like cancer of the scrotum also result in lesions that must be treated during embalming. Topical disinfectants and preservatives may be necessary to treat any lesions on the deceased resulting from reproductive system diseases.

The inflammatory processes associated with reproductive system disorders can result in the accumulation of edematous fluids in the abdomen and pelvis. Although ascites occurs in combination with many disorders, hydrocele is unique to the male reproductive system and presents a particular challenge to the embalmer. Hydrocele, which is the accumulation of fluids in the scrotum, causes gross distention and rapid decomposition. Proper treatment of hydrocele requires thorough aspiration of the scrotum, and the injection of cavity embalming fluids.

Whenever possible, the scrotum itself should not be penetrated to limit potential leakage. Passing the trocar into the scrotum may be possible from within the abdomen and pelvis. To aspirate the scrotum, insert the trocar in the abdomen as usual (i.e., 2 inches superior and 2 inches to the anatomical left of the umbilicus), and then direct the point of the trocar into the scrotum by passing behind the pubic bone. Cavity fluid should be introduced into the scrotum in the same manner.

The scrotum should also be treated with a surface pack to desiccate and firm the tissues, which will help limit the potential leakage of edematous fluids from within the scrotum. Prior to dressing in plastic garments, the anus should be packed, and the male genitals should be treated with embalming powder and covered in an absorbent material such as cotton.

REVIEW QUESTIONS

Matching

1. _____ orchitis
2. _____ cryptorchism
3. _____ hydrocele
4. _____ myalgia
5. _____ prostatitis

a. failure of the testis to descend
b. inflammation of the testicle
c. inflammation of the prostate gland
d. edema in the scrotum
e. pain and tenderness of the muscles

Multiple Choice

1. Which of the following describes the most advanced form of cancer?
   a. stage A
   b. stage B
   c. stage C
   d. stage D
2. Which of the following is not a form of testicular cancer?
   a. cryptorchidism
   b. teratoma
   c. choriocarcinoma
   d. nonseminomas
3. Which of the following disorders only develops in males?
   a. pelvic inflammatory disease
   b. breast cancer
   c. prostate cancer
   d. endometritis

4. When treating hydrocele, which of the following procedures should be followed?

    i. Aspirate the edematous fluid by needle aspiration directly through the scrotum using several points of injection to reach all areas of edematous fluid.

    ii. Hypodermically inject cavity fluid directly into the scrotum using several points of injection to reach all areas of edematous fluid.

    iii. Aspirate the edematous fluid through a trocar inserted in the abdomen and directed toward the affected area.

    iv. Apply topical embalming chemicals directly to the external surface of the affected area.

       a. i and ii

       b. ii and iii

       c. i and iii

       d. iii and iv

5. Which of the following disorders can result from mumps infection in young boys?

    a. prostatitis

    b. orchitis

    c. cryptorchism

    d. hernia

Putting Learning to Work!

The purpose of the following case analysis is to allow you to apply the information you have learned in a real-world situation. Read the case carefully and try to answer the following questions:

    What disorder do you suspect the person had at the time of death?

    What potential embalming complications do you anticipate?

    What precautions should you take as the embalmer to limit the effects of these complications?

Case Analysis

A 67-year-old man died at his home while under home healthcare for his illness. Approximately six months before his death, he found a painless lump in his testicle. He also noticed that his testicle was enlarged, and he experienced a dull ache in his lower abdomen and groin. During your embalming analysis, you notice the presence of severe hydrocele.

Bibliography

Genital herpes. (2001). Retrieved July 26, 2003, from the National Center for HIV, STDs, and TB Prevention, Division of HIV/AIDS Prevention, Centers for Disease Control and Prevention at http://www.cdc.gov/ nchstp/dstd/Fact_Sheets/facts_Genital_Herpes.htm.

Gonorrhea. (2001). Retrieved July 26, 2003, from the National Center for HIV, STD, and TB Prevention, Division of Sexually Transmitted Diseases, Centers for Disease Control and Prevention at http://www.cdc.gov/ nchstp/dstd/Fact_Sheets/FactsGonorrhea.htm.

Human papilloma virus. (1997). Retrieved May 29, 2003, from the Department of Gynecology and Obstetrics, University of Iowa at http://obgyn.uihc.uiowa.edu/Patinfo/Adhealth/hpv.htm.

Inguinal hernia. (2002). Retrieved March 17, 2004, from the National Kidney and Urologic Diseases Information Clearinghouse (NKUDIC), National Institute of Diabetes and Digestive and Kidney Diseases (NIDDK), National Institutes of Health at http://digestive.niddk.nih.gov/ddiseases/pubs/inguinalhernia/.

An introduction to sexually transmitted diseases. (1999). In *Health matters*. Retrieved March 16, 2004, from the National Institute of Allergy and Infectious Diseases, National Institutes of Health at http://www.niaid. nih.gov/factsheets/stdinfo.htm.

Kang, Y. (2002). Orchitis. In *Medical Encyclopedia*. Retrieved July 25, 2003, from the U.S. National Library of Medicine and the National Institutes of Health at http://www.nlm.nih.gov/medlineplus/ency/article/ 001280.htm.

Kazzi, Amin A. (2002). *Hydrocele*. Retrieved March 17, 2004, from eMedicine at http://www.emedicine.com/ emerg/topic256.htm.

Kumar, V., Cotran, R., & Robbins, S. (2003). *Robbins basic pathology* (7th ed.). Philadelphia: Saunders.

Male genital disorders. (2003). Retrieved July 25, 2003, from MedlinePlus, the U.S. National Library of Medicine and the National Institutes of Health at http://www.nlm.nih.gov/medlineplus/malegenitaldisorders.html.

Mayer, R. (2000). *Embalming: History, theory, & practice* (3rd ed.). New York: McGraw-Hill.

Neighbors, M., & Tannehill-Jones, R. (2000). *Human diseases*. Clifton Park, NY: Thomson Delmar Learning.

Pathology for funeral service. (1999). Dallas, TX: Professional Training Schools.

Prostatitis: Disorders of the prostate. (2003). Retrieved March 17, 2004, from the National Kidney and Urologic Diseases Information Clearinghouse (NKUDIC), National Institute of Diabetes and Digestive and Kidney Diseases (NIDDK), National Institutes of Health at http://kidney.niddk.nih.gov/kudiseases/ pubs/prostatitis/.

Shelton, H. (1992). *Boyd's introduction to the study of disease* (11th ed.). Philadelphia: Lea & Febiger.

Testicular cancer. (2003). Retrieved July 25, 2003, from MedlinePlus, the U.S. National Library of Medicine and the National Institutes of Health at http://www.nlm.nih.gov/medlineplus/testicularcancer.html.

Venes, D. (Ed.). (2001). *Taber's cyclopedic medical dictionary* (19th ed.). Philadelphia: F. A. Davis.

CHAPTER 16

Diseases of the Bones and Joints

Learning Objectives

Upon completion of the chapter, review questions, and case analysis, the reader should be able to:

- Compare and contrast osteoporosis, osteomyelitis, osteomalacia, and osteosarcoma.
- Differentiate between osteoarthritis, rheumatoid arthritis, and psoriatic arthritis.
- Discuss restoration options for twisted fingers and swollen knuckles due to diseases of the joints.
- Explain fractures by listing and describing the different types.
- Compare and contrast scoliosis and achondroplasia.
- Describe bursitis as it relates to joint inflammation.
- Explain the impact of diseases of the bones and joints on the condition of the deceased.

Key Terms

bursitis
osteomalacia
osteomyelitis

osteoporosis
rickets
scoliosis

DISORDERS OF THE BONES AND JOINTS

Human remains exhibiting bone disorders are prone to extreme malformation. Traumatic events like automobile accidents can result in fractures of bone that may be restorable through mortuary procedures. Inflammatory diseases of bone may also result in edema and deformation of bones and joints. While reading this chapter, the reader may review the anatomy of the bones and joints by referring to Appendix K.

Osteoporosis

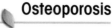

Osteoporosis is loss of bone mass that occurs throughout the skeleton, resulting in a predisposition to bone fracture. Healthy bone constantly remodels itself by taking up structure elements from one area and patching others. In osteoporosis, more bone is resorbed than laid down, and the skeleton loses some of the its strength. Type II osteoporosis, which used to be known as senile osteoporosis, is caused by aging. Aging causes bone loss in both men and women, predisposing them to vertebral and hip fractures.

Type I osteoporosis is a disorder primarily affecting postmenopausal women, but it also affects men. It occurs as a result of the loss of the protective effects of estrogen on bone that takes place after menopause. Although osteoporosis is a condition with variable causes, it may be associated with an increased demand for calcium in women's bodies after menopause. This disorder has a long, slow onset, and it is characterized by loss of bone tissue causing weak, brittle bones.

Fractures of the bones of the hip, spine, and wrist are particularly common among persons with osteoporosis, and the individual's body weight may cause enough force to result in bone fracture. Rather than a fall causing an elderly person to break a hip, it is often likely that a broken hip caused the fall. One characteristic of advanced osteoporosis is severe curvature of the spine. This curvature of the spine, depicted in Figure 16-1, can complicate positioning of the deceased during both embalming and casketing.

Any of the following may increase the risk of developing osteoporosis:

- Having a thin or small frame
- Being Caucasian or Asian
- Having a family history of osteoporosis
- Smoking cigarettes
- Having an eating disorder such as anorexia nervosa or bulimia
- Having a diet low in calcium
- Heavy alcohol consumption
- Having an inactive lifestyle
- Using medications such as corticosteroids and anticonvulsants

The leading cause of osteoporosis is a lack of estrogen, which occurs during menopause, when estrogen levels are lowered. Women over 60 are more prone to osteoporosis because they may have an inadequate intake of calcium and vitamin D in their diets. They are also less likely to participate in weight-bearing exercise such as walking, which strengthens bones. Although swimming is an excellent form of aerobic exercise, it is not a weight-bearing exercise, and bone is strengthened by weight-bearing exercises. In fact, one hazard to astronauts is the immediate loss of bone mass while in space due to weightlessness in the absence of Earth's gravity.

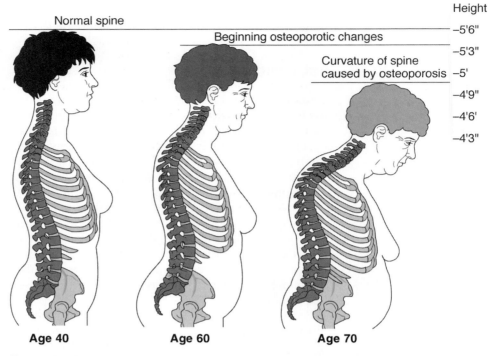

Figure 16-1 Loss of height and curvature of the spine due to osteoporosis.

Osteomyelitis

Osteomyelitis is an inflammatory disorder of bone and bone marrow resulting from pyogenic bacteria, which get their name because they cause pus in the body. The infection associated with osteomyelitis may be localized or it may spread throughout the bone. Two prevalent forms of osteomyelitis are hematogenous osteomyelitis and direct inoculation osteomyelitis.

Hematogenous osteomyelitis is an infection caused by bacteria that migrate from the blood into the bone, which occurs primarily in children. Rapidly growing bones contain many blood vessels. Where the blood vessels make sharp angles at the ends of the bones, the blood flow slows, predisposing these sites to blood clot formation. The slowed blood combined with the clots can result in necrosis of the bone and surrounding tissue as well as the promotion of bacterial growth. Despite its name, acute hematogenous osteomyelitis can have a slow clinical development so gradual as to be well established before becoming apparent.

Direct or contiguous inoculation osteomyelitis is caused by direct contact of the tissue and bacteria during trauma or surgery. Any trauma forcing bacteria into the tissues can result in a focal infection. The focal infection can then spread to the bone causing direct inoculation osteomyelitis. This disorder can result from nosocomial infections after surgical procedures, which implies the potential for funeral service professionals to become infected via needle sticks or other parenteral injury during the embalming process.

In cases of osteomyelitis, the microorganism that causes the infection varies based on the age of the patient and the mechanism of the infection. Osteomyelitis is twice as likely to develop in boys than girls. An abscess typically forms on the shaft side of the epiphyseal plate. In severe cases of osteomyelitis, staphylococci infect the blood clots that form in the bone's blood vessels.

Osteomyelitis is characterized by the following:

- Acute high fever or a slow, unnoticed onset
- Fatigue
- Irritability
- Restriction of movement
- Local edema, redness, and tenderness
- A previously existing acute bacterial infection
- Nonhealing ulcer
- Late-stage sinus drainage due to infection

Osteomalacia and Rickets

Osteomalacia and rickets are both deficiency diseases of the bone. Osteomalacia occurs in adults, and rickets occurs in children. **Osteomalacia** is a disease marked by softening of the bones due to faulty calcification in adulthood, while **rickets** is a disease of infants and young children caused by deficiency of vitamin D and resulting in defective bone growth. Deficiencies in calcium and phosphate in the bone's matrix cause softening of the bone. These deficiencies are typically due to deficiencies in vitamin D in the diet, which is necessary for proper calcification of bone tissue. Other conditions that can cause osteomalacia include hereditary or acquired disorders of vitamin D metabolism, kidney failure, low dietary intake of phosphates, cancer, and medications used to treat seizures. People are at an increased risk for osteomalacia or rickets when they do not get enough sunlight, and when they do not intake enough milk products possibly because of lactose intolerance. Sunlight is necessary for proper utilization of Vitamin D in the body, and lactose intolerance is an inability to digest the milk sugar lactose found in dairy products.

The symptoms of osteomalacia and rickets are as follows:

- Diffuse bone pain, especially in the hips
- Muscle weakness
- Bone fractures with minimal trauma
- Numbness around the mouth
- Numbness of extremities
- Spasms of hands or feet
- Abnormal heartbeat

Arthritis

The most common form of joint disorder is arthritis. Edema associated with arthritis is typically extravascular and is, therefore, not generally removed during the arterial injection of embalming fluids. Surface packs may have little effect on fluid buildup in the joints because the fluid is deep inside the tissues, and surface chemicals are not astringent enough to draw the edema out of the joint. If aggressive surface chemicals were to be utilized, they would not leave aesthetically pleasing results. The major embalming complication associated with arthritis is positioning of the extremities and poor distribution due to deterioration of the joints.

There are numerous forms of arthritis, and all forms of arthritis have the following characteristics in common:

- Redness
- Swelling of the joints
- Lack of flexibility of the joints
- Hardening and stiffening of the joints
- Disfigurement of the joints

Although it is not technically a form of arthritis, embalmers frequently encounter contractures in persons from nursing facilities who have been immobile for long periods. Joints stiffen when they are not moved, and in a short time, the tissues around the joints also stiffen. Joints and tissues surrounding joints that stiffen due to immobility are known as contractures, and contractures as severe as those in Figure 16-2 cannot be removed through normal embalming processes.

Osteoarthritis. Osteoarthritis, or degenerative joint disease, is one of the most common types of arthritis. It is caused by the deterioration of joint cartilage,

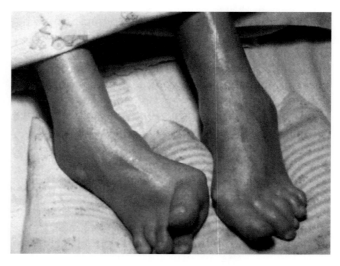

Figure 16-2 Contractures are a complication of immobility.

which causes bones to rub against each other, resulting in pain, inflammation, and loss of movement. Osteoarthritis affects the hands and weight-bearing joints such as the knees, hips, feet, and back. Although age is a risk factor for osteoarthritis, it is not an inevitable part of aging. People with joint injuries due to sports, work-related activity, or accidents may be at increased risk of developing osteoarthritis, and people who are obese may develop osteoarthritis of the knees. Some people may be born with defective cartilage or structure defects in the joints, which can also cause osteoarthritis. It is also believed that osteoarthritis might be genetic—especially when it affects the hands.

Rheumatoid Arthritis. Rheumatoid arthritis is an inflammation of the lining of the joints or internal organs. Rheumatoid arthritis is chronic, affecting many different joints with periodic flare-ups and remissions. This systemic disease affects the entire body and is one of the most common forms of arthritis. It is characterized by the inflammation of the synovial membrane and the cardinal signs of inflammation (i.e., pain, loss of function, heat, redness, and swelling). The inflammatory cells release enzymes that digest bones and cartilage resulting in severe deformities as represented in Figure 16-3. The direct cause of rheumatoid arthritis is unknown, but it is an autoimmune disease. In autoimmune diseases, the body's immune system does not operate as it should and attacks its own otherwise healthy tissues.

Psoriatic Arthritis. A less common form of arthritis is psoriatic arthritis. Psoriatic arthritis is an inflammatory arthritis associated with psoriasis, a chronic skin and nail disease. Psoriatic arthritis may primarily involve the joints of the

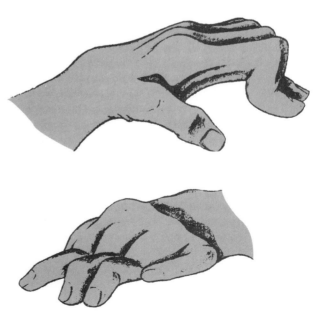

Figure 16-3 Joint changes caused by rheumatoid arthritis.

fingers or toes, joints of the extremities, or the sacroiliac joint and spine. Psoriatic arthritis involving the sacroiliac joint and spine is referred to as psoriatic spondylitis, and it is progressive and severely debilitating. For some people, the joint that is affected changes with successive flare-ups. The exact cause of psoriatic arthritis is unknown, but an interplay of immune system, genetic, and environmental factors are suspected.

Bursitis

Bursitis is inflammation of the bursae in certain joints of the body. There are more than 150 bursae in the body, and their job is to cushion pressure points between the bones and tendons as the muscles move near the joints (Edwards 2003). Bursae are small, fluid-filled sacs, and they become inflamed causing joint pain in cases of bursitis. Commonly affected joints include the shoulders, elbows, and hips. Less common sites of bursitis include the knees, heels, and the base of the big toes. Bursitis pain typically subsides within about a week with treatment, but recurrence is common. Symptoms of bursitis include a dull ache or stiffness in the affected joint, worsening pain on movement of the affected joint, swelling of the affected joint, and heat and redness surrounding the inflamed joint.

Bursitis is typically due to overuse, stress or strain of a joint, or repeated bumping or pressure from kneeling. Less commonly, bursitis may be due to staphylococcal infections, arthritis, or even tuberculosis. Bursitis is a good example of an occupational disorder in many cases. Weaver's bottom is a type of bursitis of the joints in the buttocks, due to prolonged sitting and swaying back and forth on a hard surface, as weavers once did at a weaver's loom. Housemaid's knee is a form of bursitis in which a soft, egg-shaped bump occurs on the front of the knee, resulting from activities like kneeling to install tile or scrub floors, or kneeling in a field or garden. Miner's elbow occurs due to swinging a pick, pushing a vacuum cleaner, throwing a baseball, or other repetitive activities of the elbows. Repeated leaning on the elbows can lead to bursitis as well.

Fractures

There is no difference between a broken bone and a fractured bone. A bone fracture is a break in a bone, and it is accompanied by damage to surrounding tissues. There are two classifications of bone fractures: simple and compound. In a simple fracture the broken bone does not protrude through the skin, but in a compound fracture the bone does protrude through the skin. A compound fracture is also known as an open fracture, which can become infected, causing damage to surrounding tissues as indicated in Color Plate 30. Bone fractures are further classified by the position of the bone fragments. Table 16-1 includes a description of the classification of fractures based on the presentation of bone fragments, while Figure 16-4 offers examples of various fractures.

Besides the obvious trauma-related injuries that can cause bone fractures, there are several causes of bone fracture that can indicate more serious disease conditions. Possible causes of bone fractures include:

- Aging
- Osteoporosis
- Diets deficient in calcium or vitamin D
- Eating disorders such as anorexia and bulimia
- Medications to control seizures or high blood pressure
- Hypogonadism
- Hyperparathyroidism

Bone fractures are often observed in cases of physical abuse including child abuse, elder abuse, and spousal abuse. For example, a common abuse fracture in children is a twisting fracture of the forearm. All bone fractures in children are particularly important to treat because damage to the growth plate may result in permanent deformity.

Bone fractures may also cause any or all of the following:

- Pain
- Swelling
- Bruising
- Limb deformation
- Loss of function in the affected area
- Numbness or tingling
- Paleness of tissues due to blood vessel damage

Table 16–1 Classification of Bone Fractures

Greenstick	The line of fracture does not include the whole bone.
Closed	A fracture without rupture of ligaments or skin.
Compound	An external wound leads down to the site of fracture, or fragments of bone protrude through the skin.
Impacted	One bone fragment is forced into another.
Comminuted	The bone breaks into small pieces.
Spiral	The fracture follows a helical line along and around the course of a long bone. This fracture may indicate child abuse resulting from twisting of the arm.
Depressed	A piece of bone is broken and driven inward.
Colles	A transverse fracture of the distal end of the radius with displacement of the hand backward and outward.
Angulated	Fragments lie at an angle to each other.
Displaced	The fragments separate and are deformed.
Nondisplaced	The two sections of bone keep their normal alignment.
Overriding	Fragments overlap and the total length of the bone is shortened.
Segmental	Fractures occur in two nearby areas with an isolated central segment.
Avulsed	Fragments are pulled from their normal positions by muscles.

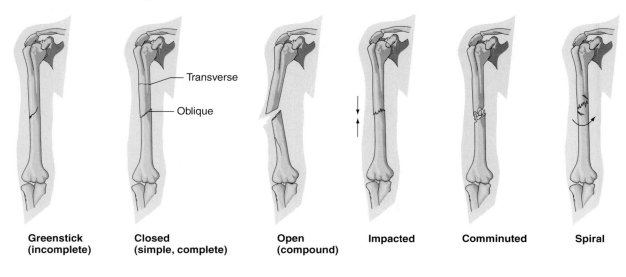

Greenstick (incomplete)   Closed (simple, complete)   Open (compound)   Impacted   Comminuted   Spiral

— Transverse

— Oblique

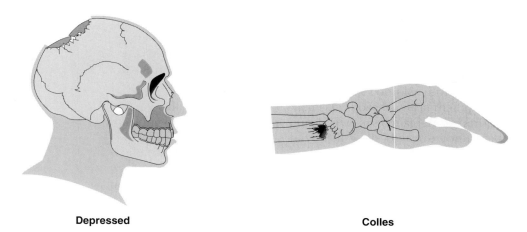

Depressed

Colles

Figure 16-4 Types of fractures.

Scoliosis

Scoliosis is a developmental disorder of the spine in which the spinal column exhibits a lateral curvature. It is often discovered at about the age of eight, when signs become apparent. The cause of scoliosis is unknown, but many theories have been proposed implicating connective tissue disorders, hormone imbalance, and nervous system disorders. Scoliosis runs in families and may be hereditary. Girls are more likely than boys to have scoliosis, and girls with scoliosis grow faster and begin puberty earlier than girls without scoliosis. Treatment consists of casts, braces, traction, or electrical stimulation. Surgery may also be required in severe cases. Figure 16-5 compares scoliosis to two other spinal de-

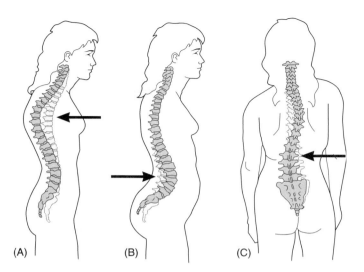

Figure 16-5 Abnormal curvatures of the spine: (A) kyphosis, (B) lordosis, (C) scoliosis.

formities. In cases of kyphosis, the abnormal curvature is in a posterior direction, while in cases of lordosis, the lumbar vertebra curve abnormally toward the anterior of the body.

Scoliosis can cause any or all of the following:

- Uneven shoulders
- Prominent shoulder blade or blades
- Uneven waist
- Elevated hips
- Leaning to one side

Achondroplasia

Achondroplasia is a genetic disorder of bone growth caused either through inheritance or genetic mutation resulting in a condition known as dwarfism. If the pituitary gland secretes excess human growth hormone, it can result in a condition known as gigantism. The word *achondroplasia* is derived from the Greek words meaning "without cartilage formation." It is believed to be one of the oldest birth defects due to its depiction in ancient Egyptian art.

The average overall height of an adult with achondroplasia is about 4 feet tall. Persons with achondroplasia have shortened arms and legs, but their torso is nearly normal size. Their upper arms and thighs are more shortened than their forearms and lower legs. They also may have a large head with a prominent forehead. Their nose usually has a flat bridge. The hands of someone with achondroplasia are short with stubby fingers and a separation between the third and fourth fingers resulting in a trident hand.

Achondroplasia is accompanied by deformed joints and poor muscle tone, which can result in sudden death—often during sleep. These deaths are thought to result from compression of the upper end of the spinal cord that interferes with breathing. The compression is caused by abnormalities in the size and structure of the opening in the base of the skull (foramen magnum) and vertebrae in the neck.

Paget's Disease

Paget's disease is an excessive growth, in the form of hyperplasia, of the bones of the elderly, causing chronic inflammation, thickening, and softening of the bones. Bowing of long bones may also be present. This idiopathic disease is also known as osteitis deformans and is more common in men than women. The progression of Paget's disease includes bone tissue being reabsorbed and synthesis of new bone at abnormally high rates. The new growth of bone tissue can cause compression of the spinal and cranial nerves leading to disability and death. The increased number of blood vessels in the bone leads to increased cardiac output, which may culminate in cardiac failure. The signs of Paget's disease are:

- Pain in the back, hips, and pelvis
- Deafness
- Increased head size
- Headaches
- Heart failure

Osteosarcoma

According to the American Cancer Society, osteosarcoma, which is also known as osteogenic sarcoma, is the most common type of cancer that develops in bone. The cells that cause osteosarcoma produce bone matrix in a similar fashion to healthy osteoblasts, with the exception that the "malignant bone" tissue of an osteosarcoma is not as strong as normal bones. Osteosarcomas can spread to other nearby tissues, and cells from osteosarcoma may fragment from the main tumor and metastasize through the bloodstream to the rest of the body. In 80 percent of osteosarcomas, the tumor is located either at the distal end of the femur or at the proximal end of the tibia where these bones join the knee. The second most common site of osteosarcomas is at the proximal end of the humerus where it joins the shoulder, although osteosarcomas can occur in any bone.

POSTMORTEM CONDITIONS ASSOCIATED WITH DISEASES OF THE BONES AND JOINTS

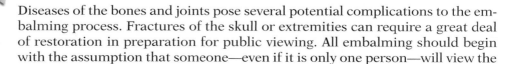

Diseases of the bones and joints pose several potential complications to the embalming process. Fractures of the skull or extremities can require a great deal of restoration in preparation for public viewing. All embalming should begin with the assumption that someone—even if it is only one person—will view the deceased. The seasoned funeral service practitioner realizes, however, that restoration is not always practical or possible. Many crushing injuries to the skull can cause severe distortion of the head. Additionally, even when skull fractures are not apparent on the surface of the head, the embalmer should take extreme caution during the injection of arterial embalming chemicals if skull fracture may have occurred based on the cause and manner of death. Potential skull fractures, even when they are not obvious from the external head, can complicate the arterial injection of embalming chemicals due to the likelihood of facial and cranial swelling during the embalming process. It is advisable to employ an embalming technique known as a "head freeze" in such cases to avoid further distortion of the head when possible.

One of the most common embalming complications related to diseases of the joints is the physical distortion of joints affected by arthritis. Arthritic joints are often swollen and misshapen. The injection of arterial embalming chemicals often does not remove fluids from swollen joints caused by arthritis because the fluids are extravascular. Depending on the situation, it may be advisable to utilize surface embalming techniques as well as the hypodermic treatment of swollen tissues; however, in cases of chronic arthritis, aggressive surface embalming techniques and straightening of deformed joints may not be practical or necessary based on local custom. Certainly any extraordinary methods of embalming and restoration such as incising tendons or dislocation of joints are considered major restorations and require the written permission of the legal next of kin.

The anatomical donation of bones requires a procedure referred to as a bone procurement. During this processes, long incisions are made into the extremities to remove bones in the arms, hips, legs, and feet. The procured bone is used to replace diseased or damaged bone in living recipients. Embalming the remains of bone donors requires specialized embalming procedures and a knowledge of the procurement process. Good relationships between the local procurement team and local funeral service professionals is essential to reduce embalming complications and to foster increased donor participation.

REVIEW QUESTIONS

Matching

1. _____ communicated fracture
2. _____ segmental fracture
3. _____ angulated fracture
4. _____ colles fracture
5. _____ avulsed fracture

a. fragments of bone are pulled from their normal position by muscles

b. a transverse fracture of the distal end of the radius with displacement of the hand backward and outward

c. fractures occur in two nearby areas with an isolated central portion

d. fragments of bone lie at an angle to each other

e. fracture in which the bone breaks into small pieces

Multiple Choice

1. Which of the following is a developmental disorder of the spine in which the spinal column exhibits a lateral curvature?
   a. spina bifida
   b. scoliosis
   c. rickets
   d. cystic fibrosis

2. Which of the following is an inflammatory disorder of the bone marrow resulting from pyogenic bacteria?
   a. osteoporosis
   b. osteomalacia
   c. osteoarthritis
   d. osteomyelitis

3. Which of the following disorders often results in a "humped" back?
   a. osteomyelitis
   b. Down syndrome
   c. osteoporosis
   d. bursitis

4. Which of the following is not a sign of arthritis?
   a. redness
   b. abscess formation in the joints
   c. swelling of the joints
   d. lack of flexibility of the joints

5. Which of the following types of fractures may be indicative of physical abuse?
   a. twisting fracture of the forearm
   b. compound fracture of the finger
   c. impacted fracture of the scapula
   d. depressed fracture of the pelvis

Putting Learning to Work!

The purpose of the following case analysis is to allow you to apply the information you have learned in a real-world situation. Read the case carefully and try to answer the following questions:

What disorder do you suspect the person had at the time of death?

What potential embalming complications do you anticipate?

What precautions should you take as the embalmer to limit the effects of these complications?

Case Analysis

You are embalming the remains of a 16-year-old boy who died suddenly in his sleep. You notice that he is considerably under height for a child his age. You estimate his height to be between 3½ and 4 feet tall. His joints are deformed, and as you check for the presence of rigor mortis, you notice that they are difficult to flex and rotate. The child's torso appears to be of average size for a child his age. There is also a separation between the child's third and fourth fingers.

Bibliography

Achondroplasia. (n.d.). Retrieved May 30, 2003, from the March of Dimes at http://www.marchofdimes.com/professionals/681_1204.asp.

Bassett, G. (1996). The osteochondrodysplasias. In R. Morrissy & S. Weinstein (Eds.), *Lovell and Winter's pediatric orthopaedics* (4th ed., pp. 203–254). Philadelphia: J.B. Lippincott.

Bjerke, H. (2002). *Flail chest*. Retrieved June 9, 2003, from eMedicine at http://www.emedicine.com/med/topic2813.htm.

DeGroot, H. (2003). *Osteoma*. Retrieved May 29, 2003, from http://bonetumor.org/tumors/pages/page12.html.

Edwards, Brooks S. (2003). *Bursitis*. Retrieved March 18, 2004, from the Mayo Clinic at http://www.mayoclinic.com/invoke.cfm?objectid=155B4438-0D8A-42D8-AE93C08753CBE114&dsection=1.

Enneking, W. (1995). Osteosarcoma. In *Musculoskeletal Pathology*. Retrieved May 29, 2003, from http://www.med.ufl.edu/medinfo/ortho/ostsarc.html#A1.

Hendrickson, G. (2001). Bone fracture. In *Injuries Encyclopedia*. Retrieved May 30, 2003, from Discovery-health.com at http://health.discovery.com/diseasesandcond/encyclopedia/3286.html.

King, R. (2002). Osteomyelitis. Retrieved June 1, 2003, from eMedicine at http://www.emedicine.com/emerg/topic349.htm#section~treatment.

Kumar, V., Cotran, R., & Robbins, S. (2003). *Robbins basic pathology* (7th ed.). Philadelphia: Saunders.

Mayer, R. (2000). *Embalming: History, theory, & practice* (3rd ed.). New York: McGraw-Hill.

Neighbors, M., & Tannehill-Jones, R. (2000). *Human diseases*. Clifton Park, NY: Thomson Delmar Learning.

Osteomalacia. (2002). In *Medical Encyclopedia*. Retrieved June 1, 2003, from MedlinePlus, the U.S. National Library of Medicine and the National Institutes of Health at http://www.nlm.nih.gov/medlineplus/ency/article/000376.htm.

Pathology for funeral service. (1999). Dallas, TX: Professional Training Schools.

Scoliosis. (2002). Retrieved June 1, 2003, from the Mayo Clinic at http://www.mayoclinic.com/invoke.cfm?objectid=7DBFF2C2-87DE-43DE-8FB57941FC1AC5F6.

Shelton, H. (1992). *Boyd's introduction to the study of disease* (11th ed.). Philadelphia: Lea & Febiger.

Venes, D. (Ed.). (2001). *Taber's cyclopedic medical dictionary* (19th ed.). Philadelphia: F. A. Davis.

What is osteosarcoma? (2003). Retrieved March 18, 2004, from the American Cancer Society at http://www.cancer.org/docroot/cri/content/cri_2_4_1x_what_is_osteosarcoma_cancer_52.asp?

CHAPTER 17

Diseases of the Endocrine System

Learning Objectives

Upon completion of the chapter, review questions, and case analysis, the reader should be able to:

- Describe the role of the islets of Langerhans in diabetes mellitus.
- Compare and contrast diabetes mellitus and diabetes insipidus.
- Compare and contrast hypothyroidism and hyperthyroidism.
- Compare and contrast hypoparathyroidism and hyperparathyroidism.
- Differentiate between Addison's disease, Cushing's syndrome, and Waterhouse-Friderichsen syndrome.
- Compare and contrast acromegaly, giantism, dwarfism, and cretinism/myxdema.
- Differentiate between Graves' disease and goiters.
- Explain the impact of diseases of the endocrine system on the condition of the deceased.

Key Terms

acromegaly
Addison's disease
cretinism
Cushing's syndrome
goiter

Graves' disease
hyperthyroidism
myxedema
polyuria

A number of processes may disturb the functions of the endocrine system. Some of the malfunctions may result from failure to properly secrete or synthesize hormones, failures in the appropriate interactions between hormones and their target organs, and the failure of target organs to respond to hormonal stimuli. In general, endocrine disorders can be classified as diseases in which hormones are either underproduced or overproduced, or as diseases associated the development of lesions within the endocrine system. While reading this chapter, the reader may review the anatomy of the endocrine system by referring to Appendix L.

DISEASES OF THE PANCREAS

Diabetes Mellitus

Diabetes mellitus is categorized as either Type I (insulin-dependent diabetes) or Type II (non-insulin-dependent diabetes). Diabetics may have a sweet smell to their breath due to the presence of acetone in the body. It is a metabolic disorder in which the carbohydrates that break down into sugars in the digestive system are not digested effectively because of a lack of appropriate insulin production in the pancreatic islets (the islets of Langerhans). When left untreated, diabetes mellitus can lead to coma and death. Diabetes can cause blindness, carbuncles of the legs and feet, and ulcers of the feet (Figure 17-1). Amputation of parts of

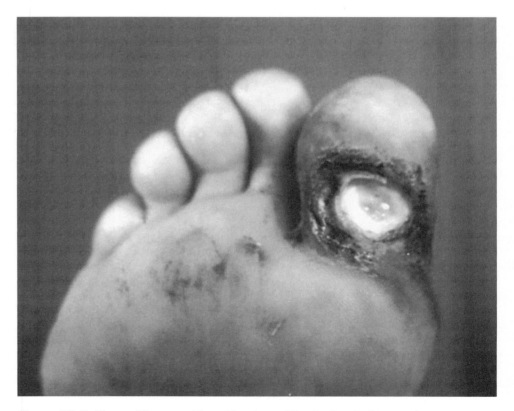

Figure 17-1 Ulcer of the great toe. (Courtesy of the Centers for Disease Control and Prevention, Atlanta, GA.)

the lower extremities is not uncommon, and diabetes mellitus can also cause renal failure and cardiac disorders. Diet, exercise, and proper medication are essential aspects of the treatment of diabetes. Diabetes mellitus can cause a variety of complications, including the following:

- Elevated blood sugar levels
- Excessive urination (**polyuria**)
- Excessive thirst
- Increased appetite

Cancer of the Pancreas

Most pancreatic cancers begin in the ducts that carry pancreatic juices. When cancer of the pancreas metastasizes outside the pancreas, cancer cells are often found in nearby lymph nodes, the peritoneum, the liver, and the lungs. Pancreatic cancer is sometimes called a silent disease because early pancreatic cancer often does not cause symptoms. Later in its progress, pancreatic cancer is characterized by:

- Pain in the upper abdomen or upper back
- Jaundice
- Dark urine
- Weakness
- Loss of appetite
- Nausea
- Vomiting
- Weight loss

Cancer of the pancreas is extremely difficult to control with current treatments, and many patients' only option is medication that is still in the clinical trial stage. The mortality rate for pancreatic cancer is high.

DISEASES OF THE PITUITARY GLAND

Acromegaly

Acromegaly is hyperfunction of the anterior lobe of the pituitary gland after ossification has been completed. The name *acromegaly* comes from the Greek words for "extremities" and "enlargement." It is a chronic disease characterized by elongation and enlargement of bones of the extremities and certain head bones, especially the frontal bone and the jaws (see Color Plate 31). Acromegaly appears slowly over time and is caused by overproduction of human growth hormone within the anterior portion of the pituitary gland. In most cases of acromegaly in adults, the overproduction of growth hormone is caused by a benign tumor of the pituitary gland known as an adenoma. The characteristics of acromegaly are:

- Abnormal growth of the hands and feet
- Enlargement of the nose and lips

- Thickening of the soft tissues of the face
- Protrusion of the brow and lower jaw
- Increased space between the teeth
- Sleepiness
- Moodiness
- Thick, coarse, oily skin
- Deepening of the voice due to enlarged sinuses and vocal cords
- Snoring due to upper airway obstruction
- Excessive sweating and skin odor
- Impaired vision
- Abnormalities of the menstrual cycle in women
- Breast discharge in women
- Impotence in men.
- Diabetes mellitus
- High blood pressure
- Polyps of the colon that can develop into cancer

Giantism and Dwarfism

The pituitary gland is responsible for secreting several hormones, one of which is somatotropin, which is also known as human growth hormone. Overstimulation of the pituitary produces an excess amount of growth hormone and can result in abnormal growth of the body, a condition known as giantism, or gigantism. This form of giantism must begin in childhood, otherwise, the bones have already ossified and will no longer grow to excessive lengths. If the hypersecretion of growth hormone from the pituitary gland occurs in adulthood, the condition is known as acromegaly, as previously described.

If the pituitary fails to secrete sufficient amounts of growth hormone during the growth years, growth may be stunted resulting in a condition referred to as dwarfism. Although dwarfism may be caused by hyposecretion of human growth hormone, a variety of other causes may also be at fault, for example, heredity, nutritional deficiencies, renal insufficiency, or diseases of the skeleton.

Diabetes Insipidus

Diabetes insipidus and diabetes mellitus are different diseases. Diabetes mellitus is caused by a disorder of the pancreas, while diabetes insipidus is caused by a disorder between the pituitary gland and the kidneys. Diabetes insipidus is an uncommon condition resulting from the inability of the kidneys to conserve water. This function of the kidney is controlled by the release of antidiuretic hormone from the pituitary gland. Antidiuretic hormone is actually produced by the hypothalamus and is then stored and released by the pituitary gland.

The most pronounced symptoms of diabetes insipidus are extreme thirst and excessive urination. The sensation of thirst causes people with diabetes insipidus to drink large amounts of fluids to compensate for water lost in the urine.

Diabetes insipidus is caused by damage to the hypothalamus or pituitary gland as a result of surgery, infection, tumors, or head injury. It may also be caused by defects in the kidney that can be inherited in male children from their mothers (Brown 2003). Other diseases like polycystic kidney and the effects of drugs like lithium and amphotericin B may cause diabetes insipidus as well.

DISEASES OF THE THYROID GLAND

Cretinism/Myxedema and Hypothyroidism

Cretinism is a hypothyroid condition of infants and children in which the thyroid gland does not secrete sufficient quantities of thyroid hormones. It is characterized by arrested physical and mental development, dystrophy of the bones, and lowered basal metabolism. Among children who were not born with the disorder, it is largely the result of an iodine deficiency in the diet

Myxedema is the clinical manifestations of hypothyroidism that includes an infiltration of the skin by a thick, gelatinous substance formed from the bonding of water and mucopolysaccharides, which gives the skin a waxy or coarsened appearance. Myxedema can refer to hypothyroidism in children, but it is more prevalently used to refer to conditions of hypothyroidism in adults. Like cretinism, myxedema usually results from an iodine deficiency in the diet, although it may result from surgical removal of the thyroid gland or excessive use of thyroid drugs. The symptoms of myxedema are enlargement of the tongue, coarse and thickened edematous skin, slow speech, puffiness of hands and feet, dryness of the hair, mental apathy, drowsiness, and sensitivity to cold. Both cretinism and myxedema are treated with thyroid hormone replacement therapy.

Graves' Disease and Hyperthyroidism

Graves' disease is a distinct type of hyperthyroidism caused by an autoimmune attack on the thyroid gland. It is the leading cause of an overactive thyroid gland, which is a disorder referred to as **hyperthyroidism**. The disorder affects women seven times more often than men, and the peak age for developing Graves' disease is between 25 and 40.

Graves' disease is an autoimmune disorder in which antibodies are produced that stimulate growth of the thyroid gland. The excessive growth results in the excess secretion of thyroid hormone. Similar antibodies may cause excessive growth of the tissues in the eye and the skin on the front of the lower leg. The following are commonly associated with Grave's disease:

- Fatigue
- Weight loss
- Restlessness
- Tachycardia (rapid heart beat)
- Changes in libido (sex drive)
- Muscle weakness
- Heat intolerance

- Tremors
- Enlarged thyroid gland
- Increased sweating
- Blurred or double vision
- Nervousness and irritability
- Swelling, redness, and discomfort of the eyes
- Hair changes
- Erratic behavior
- Increased appetite
- Decrease in menstrual cycle
- Increased frequency of stools

One of the most common signs of Graves' disease is hyperplasia of the eyeballs, which is known as exophthalmia, as shown in Figure 17-2. Grave's diseases is sometimes referred to as exophthalmic goiter due to the presence of both protrusion of the eyes and the presence of a goiter.

 ## Goiter

Hyperthyroidism may result in the formation of a **goiter**, which is the excessive growth of the thyroid gland due to a lack of iodine in the diet. Graves' disease and goiters are more prevalent in developing countries that do not add iodine to

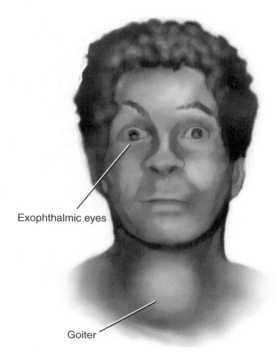

Exophthalmic eyes

Goiter

Figure 17-2 Hyperthyroidism.

their salt, as is done in the United States. Goiters are most likely to occur in geographic areas where the soil, water, and food supply lack sufficient iodine. Such conditions are common in mountainous regions of the world like the Himalayas and the Andes.

A goiter is an enlargement of the thyroid gland that is not associated with inflammation or cancer (Jain 2003). A simple goiter occurs when the thyroid gland enlarges to overcome deficiencies in the production of thyroid hormone. The two forms of simple goiters are endemic goiters and sporadic goiters.

Endemic goiters are also known as colloid goiters, and they are generally the result of a lack of iodine in the diet. Iodine is essential in the production of thyroid hormone, and people residing in geographic areas away from the sea coast are unable to ingest sufficient quantities of iodine in their diets because the soil in these regions of the world is deficient in iodine. Endemic goiters are more common in central Asia and central Africa; they are rare in the United States due to the use of iodized table salt. In contrast to endemic goiters, sporadic goiters, which are also known as nontoxic goiters, have an unknown cause, but they may result from the use of certain medications like lithium and aminoglutethimide.

DISEASES OF THE PARATHYROID

Hyperparathyroidism and Hypoparathyroidism

Hyperparathyroidism and hypoparathyroidism are two conditions in which the parathyroid glands overproduce and underproduce hormones, respectively. The parathyroid glands regulate the level of calcium in the body's tissues. The overproduction of hormones from the parathyroid gland, which is referred to as hyperparathyroidism, is characterized by weakness, weight loss, fatigue, muscle atrophy, bone pain, gastrointestinal distress, pancreatitis, kidney stones, and the presence of adenomas.

The underproduction of parathyroid hormone, or hypoparathyroidism, causes numbness of the extremities and the mouth. It also causes muscle cramps of the hands and feet, irritability, and depression. Chvostek's sign and Trousseau's sign are tests used in the diagnosis of parathyroid disorders. Chvostek's sign is a twitching of the muscles of the mouth, nose, or eyelids that is evoked by tapping the facial nerve. Trousseau's sign occurs when a blood pressure cuff is inflated above the individual's systolic pressure for over two minutes causing spasms of the wrist. These nervous reactions are known as tetany and are indicative of decreased levels of calcium in the tissues.

DISEASES OF THE ADRENAL GLANDS

Addison's Disease

Addison's disease is a rare endocrine disorder, occurring when the adrenal glands fail to produce enough of the hormones cortisol or aldosterone. Addison's disease is also known as chronic adrenal insufficiency or hypocortisolism and was first identified in 1849 by Dr. Thomas Addison. The characteristics of Addison's disease are:

- Weight loss
- Muscle weakness
- Dizziness and fainting due to low blood pressure
- A bronze darkening of the skin of persons with light complexions
- Milky-white patches on the skin of persons with dark complexions
- Nausea
- Vomiting
- Diarrhea
- Sudden, penetrating pain in the back, abdomen, or legs

The bronze discoloration associated with Addison's disease is most visible on scars, skin folds, lips, mucous membranes, and pressure points such as the elbows, knees, knuckles, and toes. In cases of Addison's disease, the use of highly concentrated formaldehyde embalming fluids is contraindicated because it may result in severely darkened discolorations of the tissues.

About 70 percent of reported cases of Addison's disease are autoimmune disorders, in which the adrenal cortex is gradually destroyed by the body's own immune system. Tuberculosis accounts for about 20 percent of cases of primary adrenal insufficiency in developed countries. Other less common causes of adrenal insufficiency include chronic fungal infections, metastasis of cancer cells to the adrenal glands, and amyloidosis.

A condition similar to Addison's disease may also occur if individuals who have taken a glucocorticoid hormone, such as prednisone, for a long time suddenly stop taking the medication. Glucocorticoid hormones are used to treat inflammatory illnesses like rheumatoid arthritis, asthma, and ulcerative colitis. Prednisone blocks the release of hormones that stimulate the pituitary gland to secrete other hormones that result in the production of cortisol in the adrenal cortex. Without the continued use of prednisone, the body cannot produce sufficient quantities of cortisol.

Cushing's Syndrome

Cushing's syndrome is an iatrogenic disorder of the adrenal glands due to chronic glucocorticoid hormone therapy. Prednisone is a commonly prescribed steroid for the management of chronic diseases, and its long term use can cause Cushing's syndrome. Unlike Addison's disease, which results from a deficiency in cortisol from the adrenal cortex, Cushing's syndrome results from excesses of the hormone cortisol. Cushing's may also result from tumors of the adrenal glands or the pituitary gland. Color Plate 32 pictures a woman with a characteristic "moon face" resulting from steroid therapy. Cushing's syndrome is characterized by the following:

- A rounded face due to excess fat deposits (moon face)
- Obesity in the upper body
- Mental retardation and obesity in children

- Purple stretch marks on the skin
- Translucent, thin skin
- Muscle weakness
- Easy bruising
- High blood pressure
- Destruction of bone tissue
- Diabetes mellitus
- Impaired immune function
- Excessive facial hair in men and women
- Balding in women
- Kidney stones
- Perforations of the viscera
- Fungal infections

Waterhouse-Friderichsen Syndrome

Waterhouse-Friderichsen syndrome is a failure of the adrenal glands to secrete appropriate levels of corticosteroids due to bleeding within the adrenal cortex. The disease usually affects children, and it is characterized by a septic bacterial infection with a rapidly deteriorating progression leading to cardiovascular collapse and death. The disorder typically manifests with congestion of the blood vessels and insufficient levels of platelets disrupting proper blood clotting. Massive hemorrhaging ensues, which results in a pinpoint red rash of the skin along with bruising over the body. Because the adrenal gland is highly vascular, it may be the site of massive hemorrhaging and necrosis. If a bacterial infection known as meningococcemia occurs during anticoagulant therapy, after surgery, or during pregnancy, it may lead to an acute adrenal crisis resulting in sudden death.

POSTMORTEM CONDITIONS ASSOCIATED WITH ENDOCRINE GLAND DISORDERS

Several of the disorders associated with the endocrine system can complicate the embalming processes. There are four postmortem conditions associated with endocrine gland disorders with which the embalmer should be familiar:

1. Edema
2. Discoloration
3. Deformities
4. Circulatory disturbances

The presence of edema is always of great concern to the embalmer for several reasons. First, excess fluids in the tissues of the deceased will dilute the arterial embalming fluid being injected. The primary dilution of arterial embalming fluid occurs when the concentrated arterial fluid is mixed with water in the tank of the embalming machine. Secondary dilution occurs when the injected arterial fluid mixes with the fluids (i.e., blood, lymph, edematous fluids) in the deceased's remains. The primary dilution is controlled by the embalmer, but the degree of secondary dilution is not under the embalmer's direct control. It may be necessary, therefore, to utilize several injection points with different strengths and quantities of embalming solution.

Disorders like Waterhouse-Friderichsen may result in severe hemorrhaging that culminates in a rashlike stain or bruising of the skin. Other disorders such as Addison's disease may result in both areas of excess pigmentation and areas of depigmentation. The use of astringent embalming fluids containing a high concentration of formaldehyde, or the use of astringent surface embalming chemicals, may further discolor the tissues. Not only may the discolorations be extravascular, disturbances in circulation may further complicate the embalming process.

Deformities related to endocrine disorders such as acromegaly, which result in excess thickening of facial tissues, may be permanent, especially given their slow, insidious onset. The physical changes associated with the long-term use of steroids may also cause permanent changes. The characteristic moon face and upper body corpulence cannot be removed through embalming procedures. The proper positioning, of the deceased is probably of greater importance in cases of deformity than are attempts at restoration. Remember, any major restoration requires written permission from the legal next of kin.

REVIEW QUESTIONS

Matching

1. _____ acromegaly
2. _____ diabetes insipidus
3. _____ Cushing's syndrome
4. _____ cretinism
5. _____ Addison's disease

a. results from the kidneys' inability to conserve water
b. characterized by a bronze discoloration of the body
c. hypothyroidism in children
d. caused by an overproduction of human growth hormone in adults
e. due to chronic glucocorticoid hormone therapy

Multiple Choice

1. Which of the following is a disorder occurring when the adrenal glands fail to produce enough of the hormones cortisol or aldosterone?
   a. Cushing's syndrome
   b. Graves' disease
   c. hypoparathyroidism
   d. Addison's disease
2. Which of the following results from an excess of the hormone cortisol?
   a. Cushing's syndrome
   b. Addison's disease
   c. Graves' disease
   d. Down syndrome

3. A goiter is an excessive growth of which of the following glands?
   a. pineal
   b. parathyroid
   c. thyroid
   d. adrenal

4. Which of the following is characterized by arrested physical and mental development, dystrophy of the bones, and lowered basal metabolism?
   a. hyperparathyroidism
   b. Waterhouse-Friderichsen syndrome
   c. hyperthyroidism
   d. cretinism

5. Which of the following is not associated with hypoparathyroidism?
   a. Chvostek's sign
   b. aldosterone
   c. Trousseau's sign
   d. tetany

Putting Learning to Work!

The purpose of the following case analysis is to allow you to apply the information you have learned in a real-world situation. Read the case carefully and try to answer the following questions:

What disorder do you suspect the person had at the time of death?

What potential embalming complications do you anticipate?

What precautions should you take as the embalmer to limit the effects of these complications?

Case Analysis

A 59-year-old man died in the critical care unit of a local hospital. He is approximately 40 pounds overweight, and he has lost his vision in his left eye. He took dialysis due to chronic renal failure, and his right foot is amputated just below the ankle. His lower legs and left foot are wrapped in bandages. After removing the bandages, you notice that his legs are a blackish-purple color and covered with pustules, which appear to extend deep into the tissues.

Bibliography

Adler, G. (2001). *Cushing's syndrome*. Retrieved June 1, 2003, from eMedicine at http://www.emedicine.com/emerg/topic117.htm.

Brown, Todd T. (2003). Diabetes insipidus. In *Medical Encyclopedia*. Retrieved March 18, 2004, from MedlinePlus, the U.S. National Library of Medicine and the National Institutes of Health at http://www.nlm.nih.gov/medlineplus/ency/article/000377.htm.

Corrigan, E. (1989). *Addison's disease*. Retrieved June 1, 2003, from the National Institutes of Health, National Institute of Diabetes and Digestive and Kidney Diseases at http://www.niddk.nih.gov/index.htm.

Corrigan, E. K. (1997). *Cushing's fact sheet*. Retrieved May 29, 2003, from the Cushing's Support and Research Foundation at http://world.std.com/~csrf/factsheet.html#cushing.

Ezzat, S., Forster, M., Berchtold, P., Redelmeier, D., Boerlin, V., & Harris, A. (1994). Acromegaly: Clinical and biochemical features in 500 patients. *Medicine, 73*(5), 233–240.

Jain, Tarun. (2003). Goiter. In *Medical Encyclopedia*. Retrieved March 18, 2004, from MedlinePlus, the U.S. National Library of Medicine and the National Institutes of Health at http://www.nlm.nih.gov/medlineplus/ency/article/001178.htm.

Karakousis, P., Page, K., Varello, M., Howlett, P., & Stieritz, D. (2001). Case report: Waterhouse-Friderichsen syndrome after infection with group A Streptococcus. *Mayo Clinic Procedures 76*, 1167–1170.

Khoury, G., & Deeba, S. (2001). *Pancreatitis*. Retrieved June 7, 2003, from eMedicine at http://www.emedicine.com/EMERG/topic354.htm.

Kumar, V., Cotran, R., & Robbins, S. (2003). *Robbins basic pathology* (7th ed.). Philadelphia: Saunders.

Mayer, R. (2000). *Embalming: History, theory, & practice* (3rd ed.). New York: McGraw-Hill.

Melmed, S. (1990). Acromegaly. *New England Journal of Medicine, 322*, 966–977.

Neighbors, M., & Tannehill-Jones, R. (2000). *Human diseases*. Clifton Park, NY: Thomson Delmar Learning.

Pathology for funeral service. (1999). Dallas, TX: Professional Training Schools.

Shelton, H. (1992). *Boyd's introduction to the study of disease* (11th ed.). Philadelphia: Lea & Febiger.

Sowaka, J., Gurwood, A., & Kabat, K. (2001). Pituitary adenoma. In *Handbook of Ocular Disease Management*, Jobson Publishing. Retrieved May 29, 2003, from http://www.revoptom.com/handbook/SECT54a.HTM.

Tonsillitis/tonsillectomy. (2003). Retrieved July 24, 2003, from MedlinePlus, the U.S. National Library of Medicine and the National Institutes of Health at http://www.nlm.nih.gov/medlineplus/tonsilstonsillectomy.html.

Venes, D. (Ed.). (2001). *Taber's cyclopedic medical dictionary* (19th ed.). Philadelphia: F. A. Davis.

CHAPTER 18

Diseases of the Integument

Learning Objectives

Upon completion of the chapter, review questions, and case analysis, the reader should be able to:

- Describe the pathogenesis of abscesses.
- Differentiate between a chancre and a gumma in cases of syphilis.
- Compare and contrast psoriasis and eczema.
- Describe the warning signs of skin cancer.
- Discuss the progression of bedsores.
- Differentiate between acne, seborrhoreic dermatitis, and vitiligo.
- Explain the impact of diseases of the integument on the condition of the deceased.

Key Terms

chancre
decubitus ulcers
eczema

gumma
psoriasis
vitiligo

 ## DISORDERS OF THE INTEGUMENT

Disorders of the integument are common and range from discolorations that are primarily of cosmetic concern to life threatening malignant melanomas. Although many integumentary disorders affect the skin, others are characteristic of more serious systemic disorders. Lesions of the integument are extremely important for the funeral service professionals to recognize, as they can indicate the existence of infectious diseases. Color Plate 33 is a photograph of an infected fingernail. Such infectious lesions are covered in Part Two of this text, but this chapter discusses noninfectious pathologies of the integument and the lesions they cause. While reading this chapter, the reader may review the anatomy of the integumentary system by referring to Appendix M.

 ## Acne

Acne is the term for blackheads, whiteheads, and pimples on the skin. It affects humans throughout their lifetime, and, although it is not a life threatening condition, it can cause serious and permanent scarring. A lesion is a physical change in body tissues caused by disease or injury, and Table 18-1 lists and describes some of the lesions associated with sebaceous glands involved in acne.

Acne starts between the ages of 10 and 13 and usually lasts for 5 to 10 years. Men are more likely than women to have severe, longer-lasting forms of acne. Women are more likely to have acne caused by cosmetics and intermittent acne due to hormonal changes associated with their menstrual cycle. Acne lesions are most common on the face, but they can also occur on the neck, chest, back, shoulders, scalp, and extremities.

 ## Abscess

An abscess is a localized collection of pus that is walled off by a membrane formed by the body's immune system cells—specifically, by macrophages—in any body part. It results from invasion of a pyogenic bacterium or other pathogen. A pyogenic bacterium is one that causes pus to form. *Staphylococcus aureus* is a common cause of skin abscesses, which themselves are fairly common. Skin abscesses are often the result of wounds that tear the skin, and they are more common in impaling or penetrating injuries that drive infectious microorganisms into deeper tissues.

Abscesses can disrupt surrounding tissues' ability to function due to the resulting inflammation, which includes swelling and inflammatory exudates. If the infectious microorganisms in the abscess spread through the surrounding

Table 18-1 Lesions Associated with Acne

Comedo	A sebaceous follicle plugged with sebum, dead cells, hairs, and bacteria. A comedo in an open pore is called a blackhead, and a comedo under the skin is a whitehead.
Papule	A small solid lesion slightly elevated above the surface of the skin.
Pustule	A dome-shaped lesion containing pus consisting of white blood cells, dead skin cells, and bacteria.
Macule	A temporary red spot left by a healed acne lesion.
Nodule	A solid, dome-shaped inflammatory lesion that extends deep into the skin and causes scarring.
Cyst	A saclike lesion containing semiliquid material consisting of white blood cells, dead cells, and bacteria. Cysts are larger than pustules and extend deep into the skin. They are painful and result in scarring.

tissue and bloodstream to the remainder of the body, a fatal infection can develop.

Syphilis

Syphilis is described in greater detail in Part Two of this book, but it is important to mention in this chapter due to the skin lesions that signal the presence of this sexually transmitted disease. In the primary stage of syphilis, a lesion known as a chancre is commonly present at the site of the bacterial infection. A **chancre** is a hard, primary ulcer due to syphilis infection appearing approximately two to three weeks after infection. Chancres are common on the external genitalia, on the mouth, and on the anus. During the secondary stage of syphilis, ulcerations of the mucous membranes, particularly the mouth, are present in addition to a reddish or copper-colored skin rash. In the tertiary stage of syphilis, a rubberlike skin lesion known as a gumma may be present. A **gumma** is an infectious lesion due to tertiary syphilis consisting of a central necrotic mass surrounded by an inflammatory zone and fibrous deterioration of the tissues. During embalming, each of these lesions requires topical disinfectants preservatives.

Seborrheic Dermatitis

Seborrheic dermatitis, which is also known as seborrhea, is a disorder of the sebaceous glands of the scalp, face, and trunk. In addition to sebum, this skin disorder has been linked to a fungus (*Pityrosporum ovale*) and immune system abnormalities. The symptoms of seborrhea are aggravated by humidity, scratching, change in seasons, and emotional stress. Seborrhea may be as mild as dandruff or as severe as thick crust formation over the scalp, which is known as cradle cap.

Seborrheic dermatitis may appear in combination with systemic disorders like Parkinson's disease or AIDS. Seborrhea is common on the scalp of infants, which is believed to be the result of hormones in the uterus. Among the elderly, cradle cap is due to a fungal infection. The embalmer must be extremely cautious when washing, drying, brushing, or combing the hair because the scalp and hair are quite fragile in cases of seborrhea, which is pictured in Color Plate 34.

Psoriasis

Psoriasis is a chronic, inflammatory skin disease, characterized by red, thickened areas with silvery scales, most often on the scalp, elbows, knees, and lower back (see color Plate 35). Although the cause of psoriasis is unknown, it is believed that an abnormality in the functioning of white blood cells triggers an immune system response that causes the skin cells to shed prematurely. This shedding is accompanied by excessive growth of the skin, which causes the psoriatic plaques to form.

There are many types of psoriasis, but most may be exacerbated by trauma to the skin such as cuts or sunburns. Psoriasis can also be activated by infections such as strep throat or by certain medications. Flare-ups are also common during dry winter months, when the skin is exposed to less sunlight. Psoriasis of the nails may cause the nail to fall from the nail bed.

Treatments depend on the severity of psoriasis, but may include steroids, scalp treatments with coal tar or cortisone, application of a synthetic form of vitamin D (calcipotriene), topical retinoid creams, ultraviolet light therapy, an anticancer drug (methotrexate), and a drug that inhibits rejection after organ transplant (cyclosporine).

Eczema

Eczema is a general term for a variety of inflammatory skin conditions. It is characterized by dry, red, extremely itchy patches on the skin that may ooze an inflammatory exudate (see Color Plate 36). Among infants, eczema occurs on the forehead, cheeks, forearms, legs, scalp, and neck. In children and adults, eczema occurs on the face, neck, and the insides of the elbows, knees, and ankles. Skin affected by eczema may become easily infected.

Vitiligo

Vitiligo is an idiopathic disorder in which the melanocytes stop producing pigment and are destroyed. The loss of pigment results in white, patchy spots on the affected part, which can occur anywhere on the body. The patches are more common on areas of the skin exposed to greater sunlight such as the hands, feet, arms, face, and lips. Other common areas include the mouth, eyes, nostrils, navel, and genitalia. People with certain autoimmune diseases such as hyperthyroidism or pernicious anemia appear to develop vitiligo.

Skin Cancer

There are many types of skin cancers (see Chapter 7). Many of them begin with a change in the appearance of a skin mole, which is also known as a melanocytic nevus. Moles are pigmented epithelial tumors on the skin, and changes in them may be precancerous. The appearance of new moles, changes in the color of moles, lumpy or painful moles, moles that are crusty, moles that bleed, or moles that ooze fluids can all signal the presence of skin cancers. Additionally, the appearance of a red "halo" around a mole may indicate a precancerous lesion. Both squamous cell carcinoma and basal cell carcinoma are examples of skin cancer described in Chapter 7. Skin cancers are often attributable to long-term exposure to the sun's ultraviolet rays.

Bedsores

Bedsores are preventable pressure sores that are technically known as **decubitus ulcers**. With proper care, bedsores should not occur. They occur when a person's weight compresses tissue between the bed or wheelchair and a superficial bone. The compressed tissue receives inadequate blood flow, and it becomes necrotic and infected. Bedsores begin as a mild pink discoloration at the site of pressure, which resolves with no aftereffect when the pressure is removed. However, they can progress into a deep wound extending to a bone or internal organ.

Bedsores form from pressure due to immobility. Persons who are paralyzed or suffer from muscular or neural disorders that prevent them from moving must be repositioned approximately every two hours to prevent bedsores from forming. Bedsores may also occur from friction by rubbing against bed sheets, casts, or braces. Areas of the body in which bones are superficial and covered with little tissue are more likely to develop decubitus ulcers.

Like most wounds, bedsores are classified by stage of development, as described in Table 18-2. It is important to note that bedsores do not skip stages. A stage three or four bedsore began as a stage one wound, but was not diagnosed or treated due to inadequate professional care. Funeral service professionals may find bedsores on the deceased when untrained family members, rather than professional healthcare providers, care for individuals who are immobile. Stage three and four bedsores will require surface embalming chemicals, aspiration of pus, and treatment to reduce odor. The bedsores pictured in Figure 18-1 are stage four.

Table 18-2 Stages and Treatment of Bedsores

Stage	Description	Treatment
Stage 1	Initial stage in which the skin is unbroken, red, and superficial.	Improved nutrition including the prevention of dehydration is the first step toward prevention of bedsores. The cause of the pressure should also be removed. Padding is available to help cushion the area and reduce pressure.
Stage 2	A partial layer of the skin is injured and a blister is probably present.	The wound is cleaned and covered to prevent infection.
Stage 3	The bedsore extends through all layers of the skin and is at a high risk of infection.	A bedsore at this stage requires medical treatment that includes antibiotics and pharmaceuticals to aid in the healing process.
Stage 4	The bedsore has reached the underlying muscle and bone. It is necrotic and infected.	The surgical removal of the necrotic tissue is likely, and aggressive treatment of the infection is required to keep it from becoming a fatal blood poisoning. Amputation of the affected area may be necessary.
Stage 5	Older classification in which the wound is extremely deep, possibly involving organs.	The treatment is the same as stage 4 bedsores.

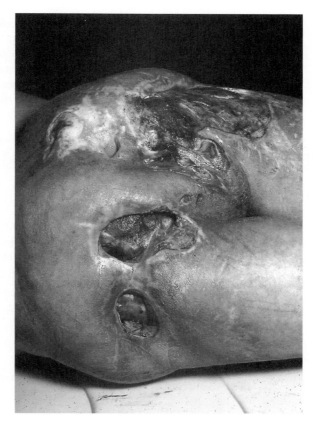

Figure 18-1 Stage 4 decubitus ulcers. (Reprinted with permission from Vincent J. DiMaio and Dominick DiMaio, 2001, *Forensic pathology*, 2nd ed. Copyright CRC Press, Boca Raton, FL.)

POSTMORTEM CONDITIONS ASSOCIATED WITH DISORDERS OF THE INTEGUMENT

Disorders of the integument are likely to complicate the embalming process because they are visible during the visitation and funeral. There are five post-mortem conditions associated with disorders of the integument:

1. Discolorations
2. Dehydration (dryness/scales)
3. Lesions
4. Pigmentation or depigmentation
5. Swelling due to inflammation

Proper treatment of the deceased will require the removal of lesions, the reduction of discolorations, the treatment of inflamed areas, and the application of cosmetics to mask the visible signs of the disorder. Depending on the severity and extent of the lesions, the embalmer may need to employ restorative art techniques that qualify as major restorations. Remember that major restorations always require permission from the legal next of kin. Proper topical disinfection and the plasticization of nonintact lesions is integral to the inhibition of the spread of microbial agents and possible leakage.

REVIEW QUESTIONS

Matching

1. _____ seborrhea
2. _____ macule
3. _____ psoriasis
4. _____ bedsore
5. _____ chancre

a. disorder in which plaques form on the skin
b. a hard, primary ulcer due to syphilis infection appearing approximately two to three weeks after infection
c. a lesion associated with acne
d. also known as cradle cap
e. also known as a decubitus ulcer

Multiple Choice

1. Which of the following disorders of the integument is characterized by depigmentation of the skin?
   a. psoriasis
   b. vitiligo
   c. eczema
   d. acne
2. Which of the following is a localized collection of pus that results from invasion of a pyogenic bacterium or other pathogen?
   a. abscess
   b. chancre
   c. gumma
   d. papule
3. Which of the following is related to the application of cosmetics or hormonal changes?
   a. syphilis
   b. seborrhea
   c. acne
   d. eczema
4. Which of the following is noted by the presence of silvery scales on the skin?
   a. eczema
   b. vitiligo
   c. seborrhea
   d. psoriasis

5. Which of the following lesions is indicative of the tertiary stage of syphilis?

    a. a chancre

    b. a red rash on the soles of the feet

    c. a gumma

    d. a cold sore

Putting Learning to Work!

The purpose of the following case analysis is to allow you to apply the information you have learned in a real-world situation. Read the case carefully and try to answer the following questions:

    What disorder do you suspect the person had at the time of death?

    What potential embalming complications do you anticipate?

    What precautions should you take as the embalmer to limit the effects of these complications?

A 28-year-old woman died suddenly while playing golf. She received CPR from a friend on the golf course, and she was treated in the ambulance and in the emergency room for heart failure. While conducting the case analysis, you notice red splotches on her face. She also has thick scales on the knuckles of her right hand. In addition, she has silvery, dry patches on her elbows and behind her ears on her scalp. Her forehead appears to have dry scales near the hairline. She also is missing two toenails from digits four and five on her left foot.

Bibliography

Kumar, V., Cotran, R., & Robbins, S. (2003). *Robbins basic pathology* (7th ed.). Philadelphia: Saunders.

Mayer, R. (2000). *Embalming: History, theory, & practice* (3rd ed.). New York: McGraw-Hill.

Neighbors, M., & Tannehill-Jones, R. (2000). *Human diseases*. Clifton Park, NY: Thomson Delmar Learning.

Pathology for funeral service. (1999). Dallas, TX: Professional Training Schools.

Seldon, S. (2001). Seborrheic dermatitis. Retrieved May 29, 2003, from eMedicine at http://www.emedicine. com/derm/topic396.htm.

Shelton, H. (1992). *Boyd's introduction to the study of disease* (11th ed.). Philadelphia: Lea & Febiger.

Venes, D. (Ed.). (2001). *Taber's cyclopedic medical dictionary* (19th ed.). Philadelphia: F. A. Davis.

CHAPTER 19

Diseases of the Lymphatic System

Learning Objectives

Upon completion of the chapter, review questions, and case analysis, the reader should be able to:

- Describe the pathogenesis of tonsillitis.
- Describe the pathogenesis of lymphangitis.
- Describe the pathogenesis of splenomegaly.
- Describe the pathogenesis of lymphadenopathy.
- Describe the pathogenesis of lymphoma.
- Explain the impact of diseases of the lymphatic system on the condition of the deceased.

Key Terms

lymphadenopathy
lymphangitis
lymphoma

splenomegaly
tonsillitis

DISORDERS OF THE LYMPHATIC SYSTEM

This chapter describes some of the most significant pathological disorders of the lymphatic system. It also includes some important infectious diseases, each of which is described in greater detail in Part Two. While reading this chapter, the reader may review the anatomy of the lymphatic system by referring to Appendix N.

Tonsillitis

Tonsillitis is an inflammation of the tonsils caused by an infection. The tonsils become enlarged, red, and often spotted or coated by microorganisms, which appear yellow, gray, or white. Tonsillitis can begin as sudden sore throat and painful swallowing; it can progress into severe respiratory difficulties. Tonsillitis is contagious and can spread through contact with the throat or nasal fluids of infected persons. At one time, removing tonsils from the throat, called a tonsillectomy, was a common practice. Healthcare professionals have since discovered the importance of the tonsils in the immune system, and tonsillitis is now treated with antibiotics.

Lymphangitis

Lymphangitis is an inflammatory disorder of the lymph vessels, characterized by local and systemic pain. It commonly results from a bacterial infection of the skin known as cellulitis, or from a skin abscess. The presence of lymphangitis suggests that an infection is progressing, and that bacteria may have migrated to the bloodstream. This fatal condition may be confused with blood clots in the veins of the legs, which is a disorder known as *thrombophlebitis*. Lymphangitis may spread within hours, and antibiotic treatment should begin immediately if it is to be controlled. The characteristics of lymphangitis are:

- Red streaks extending from the infected area to the axillary space or groin
- Throbbing pain along the affected area
- Fever and chills
- Anorexia
- Headache
- Muscle aches

Splenomegaly

Splenomegaly is an enlargement of the spleen beyond its normal size. The spleen is involved in the production of red blood cells, white blood cells, and functions in the lymphatic and immune systems. Common causes of splenomegaly include viral, parasitic, and bacterial infections, cirrhosis of the liver, inflammation of the gall bladder, cystic fibrosis, anemia, leukemia, lymphomas, and sickle cell anemia. Rupture of the enlarged spleen is possible in cases of infectious mononucleosis, and appropriate limitations on activity may help prevent trauma that might cause the spleen to rupture. If the spleen is surgically removed, the procedure is known as a splenectomy.

Lymphadenopathy

The enlargement of lymph nodes is known as **lymphadenopathy**. The increased size is caused by proliferation of lymphocytes and leukocytes within the node or by the presence of a tumor in the node. Most frequently, lymphadenopathy occurs as a result of local, regional, or systemic infections. It can also be due to cancer, inflammation of the thyroid, autoimmune diseases like rheumatoid arthritis, or drug reactions. Lymphadenopathy is more common in young children because their immune systems are responding more frequently to newly encountered infections. In the United States, some possible causes of lymphadenopathy include infectious mononucleosis, cytomegalovirus infections, upper respiratory infections, and HIV infection. Internationally, however, lymphadenopathy is more commonly due to tuberculosis, typhoid fever, trypanosomiasis, schistosomiasis, and various fungal infections.

Lymphoma

Lymphoma is a cancer of the lymphatic system, causing some of the cells in the lymphatic system to grow abnormally and out of control. Because there is lymph tissue throughout the body, the cancer cells may spread to other organs, or even into the bone marrow. There are two broad categories of lymphoma known as Hodgkin's lymphoma and non-Hodgkin's lymphoma. All lymphomas that are not Hodgkin's lymphomas are grouped together and referred to as non-Hodgkin's lymphoma.

Hodgkin's lymphoma, which is also known as Hodgkin's disease, was first described in 1666 by Marcelle Malpighi, an Italian professor of medicine. In 1832, an English physician named Thomas Hodgkin provided the first documentation of actual cases of this idiopathic lymphatic cancer. The primary difference between Hodgkin's disease and non-Hodgkin's lymphoma is the presence of a specific abnormal cell: Reed-Sternberg cells. B-cells should produce antibodies that guide the immune system in defense of invading bacteria, but Reed-Sternberg cells are a malignant, nonfunctional form of B lymphocyte. Like most cancers, chemotherapy and radiation therapy are the two main methods of treating Hodgkin's disease. Complications due to Hodgkin's lymphoma include pain after drinking alcohol, night sweats, loss of appetite, weight loss, fever, and general itching over the entire body.

Non-Hodgkin's lymphoma is actually a collection of many varied lymphomas. Most arise within a lymph node, but some arise in areas other than nodes, such as the jaw or brain. Until recently, science was not able to make fine distinctions among the subtypes of non-Hodgkin's lymphoma. However, advances in molecular genetics have shown that non-Hodgkin's lymphoma is actually many diseases. Some of the non-Hodgkin's lymphomas more closely resemble leukemia than they do the Hodgkin's lymphomas. As more becomes known, some lymphomas that were categorized as non-Hodgkin's lymphomas may be reclassified with other cancers.

POSTMORTEM CONDITIONS ASSOCIATED WITH DISEASES OF THE LYMPHATIC SYSTEM

There are four postmortem conditions associated with diseases of the lymphatic system that can potentially complicate the embalming process:

1. Edema
2. Emaciation

3. Dehydration

4. Metastasis

Since one of the crucial functions of the lymphatic system is to filter the lymph and return it to the bloodstream, any disorder of the lymphatic system is prone to cause fluid disruptions such as edema and dehydration. Both the disruption of the circulation of lymph and the debilitating effects of lymphatic diseases can prevent nutrients from reaching the tissues leading to emaciation. In cases of lymphatic cancers, metastasis of tumor cells can cause systemic tissue damage and impede the thorough embalming of the deceased.

REVIEW QUESTIONS

Matching

1. _____ tonsillitis
2. _____ lymphangitis
3. _____ splenomegaly
4. _____ lymphadenopathy
5. _____ lymphoma

a. can occur due to a bacterial infection known as cellulitis
b. enlargement of the spleen
c. inflammation of the tonsils
d. cancer of the lymphatic system
e. enlargement of the lymph nodes

Multiple Choice

1. Which of the following disorders is characterized by red streaks extending from the infected area to the axillary space or groin?

a. leukemia
b. lymphadenopathy
c. lymphoma
d. lymphangitis

2. Which of the following refers to a collection of many varied lymphomas?

a. non-Hodgkin's
b. Hodgkin's
c. lymphadenopathy
d. leukemia

3. Which of the following diseases is the result of a proliferation of lymphocytes and leukocytes within a lymph node or by the presence of a tumor in a lymph node?

a. lymphoma
b. splenomegaly
c. lymphangitis
d. lymphadenopathy

4. An infection of the tonsils in which the tonsils become inflamed is known as which of the following?
   a. lymphoma
   b. tonsillitis
   c. lymphangitis
   d. Hodgkin's lymphoma
5. Which of the following may occur in cases of sickle cell anemia?
   a. lymphangitis
   b. lymphoma
   c. splenomegaly
   d. lymphadenopathy

Putting Learning to Work!

The purpose of the following case analysis is to allow you to apply the information you have learned in a real-world situation. Read the case carefully and try to answer the following questions:

　　　What disorder do you suspect the person had at the time of death?

　　　What potential embalming complications do you anticipate?

　　　What precautions should you take as the embalmer to limit the effects of these complications?

Case Analysis

A middle-aged woman died from an undiagnosed disease. She refused medical treatment for her illness due to religious reasons. Members of her religion came to her home to pray for her and to meet the needs of her husband and five children. They describe her illness as being characterized by fever, night sweats, chills, and a total lack of energy. They thought it was especially strange that she complained of itching.

　　During your case analysis, you notice that the woman has a large swollen neck. She also has swelling in her axillary spaces. As you remove her clothing, it is obvious that the woman has lost a great deal of weight because she is emaciated, and her clothes are far too large for her. She also has a large swollen area on the left side of her groin. Her legs are swollen, and when you remove her socks, you notice they have left indentations in her swollen ankles.

Bibliography

Fisman, D. H. (2001). Lymphadenitis and lymphangitis. In *Medical Encyclopedia*. Retrieved June 5, 2003, from MedlinePlus, the U.S. National Library of Medicine and the National Institutes of Health at http://www.nlm.nih.gov/medlineplus/ency/article/001301.htm.

Johnsonton, L. (1999). *Non-Hodgkin's lymphomas: Making sense of diagnosis, treatment, and options.* Sebastopol, CA: O'Reilly & Associates.

Kumar, V., Cotran, R., & Robbins, S. (2003). *Robbins basic pathology* (7th ed.). Philadelphia: Saunders.

Learning about lymphoma. (2002). Retrieved May 29, 2003, from the Lymphoma Research Foundation at http://www.lymphoma.org/site/PageServer?pagename=lymphoma.

Lymphatic diseases. (2003). Retrieved July 24, 2003, from MedlinePlus, the U.S. National Library of Medicine and the National Institutes of Health at http://www.nlm.nih.gov/medlineplus/lymphaticdiseases.html.

Lymphoma.com. (n/d). Retrieved June 5, 2003, from http://www.lymphoma.com.

Mayer, R. (2000). *Embalming: History, theory, & practice* (3rd ed.). New York: McGraw-Hill.

Neighbors, M., & Tannehill-Jones, R. (2000). *Human diseases*. Clifton Park, NY: Thomson Delmar Learning.

Pathology for funeral service. (1999). Dallas, TX: Professional Training Schools.

Shelton, H. (1992). *Boyd's introduction to the study of disease* (11th ed.). Philadelphia: Lea & Febiger.

Sills, R., & Jorgenson, S. (2002). *Lymphadenopathy*. Retrieved June 5, 2003, from eMedicine at http://www.emedicine.com/PED/topic1333.htm.

Venes, D. (Ed.). (2001). *Taber's cyclopedic medical dictionary* (19th ed.). Philadelphia: F. A. Davis.

PART TWO

MICROBIOLOGY

ABFSE Subject Description

This section encourages a survey of the basic principles of microbiology. It relates these principles to funeral service education especially as they pertain to sanitation, disinfection, public health, and embalming practice. The development and use of personal, professional, and community hygiene and sanitation is discussed.

ABFSE Objectives:

Upon satisfactory completion of this course in microbiology, the learner should be able to:

- Explain basic microbial morphology and physiology.
- Demonstrate an understanding of host–parasite relationships and interactions, and the requirements of successful parasitism.
- Describe and demonstrate knowledge of personal and environmental disinfection and decontamination procedures by proper use of chemical disinfection and sterilization techniques.
- Describe the fundamentals of the infectious processes and specific and nonspecific defense mechanisms against disease.
- Explain the methods of transmission of infectious diseases and describe the control procedure of these diseases with special emphasis on protection to the embalmer, the funeral director, and the public.
- Differentiate between the indigenous microorganisms and pathogens or opportunists causing disease commonly associated with the human host and dead human remains.

CHAPTER 20

Introduction to Microbiology

Learning Objectives

Upon completion of the chapter and review questions, the reader should be able to:

- Describe the theory of spontaneous generation.
- Explain the germ theory of disease.
- Discuss how microorganisms are named.
- List the divisions of microbiology.
- Compare and contrast the pathogenic microorganisms described in this chapter.
- Compare and contrast enkaryotic and prokaryotic cells.
- Discuss Edward Jenner's role in the history of vaccination.
- Describe the magic bullet.
- Discuss how kingdoms are related to naming microorganisms.

Key Terms

bacteria
bacteriology
chlamydia
fungi
mycology
mycoplasma
prions

protozoa
protozoology
rickettsia
rickettsiology
virology
virus

SPONTANEOUS GENERATION

Before the 19th century, it was commonly believed that life forms could spontaneously appear from nonliving matter. This spontaneous generation was believed to occur most frequently from dead and decaying matter. A 17th-century plan for spontaneously generating mice called for sweaty underwear and husks of wheat to be placed in an open-mouthed jar. After about 21 days, it was believed that the sweat from the underwear would penetrate the wheat husks, changing them into mice. Although such antiquated beliefs may seem ridiculous by modern standards, they were in line with the religious and cultural beliefs of the time.

In 1668, Francesco Redi challenged the theory of spontaneous generation. The common belief that decaying meat gave rise to maggots was rejected by Redi's experiment. Redi believed that maggots arose from the eggs left on meat by flies. To test his hypothesis, Redi left meat in a variety of places including sealed flasks. As predicted, maggots only developed on meat on which flies could lay eggs. The sealed flasks of meat contained no maggots.

This experiment did not change peoples' beliefs in spontaneous generation completely, and even Redi continued to believe that spontaneous generation occurred under certain circumstances. Surprisingly, the development of the microscope initially strengthened the theory of spontaneous generation. Scientists of the period argued that to see spontaneous generation in action, one needed only to place hay in water and observe it under the microscope to see the new creations, which they called "animalcules."

In 1745, John Needham, an English clergyperson, tested the theory of spontaneous generation. After boiling chicken broth, he poured it into flasks and sealed the flasks. Soon, the broth became clouded with microorganisms. Later, Lazzaro Spallanzani argued that spontaneous generation had only occurred in Needham's experiment because microorganisms had been introduced from the air, when the chicken broth was poured into the flasks. Spallanzani duplicated Needham's experiment but altered it slightly. He placed the broth in flasks, sealed the flasks, removed the air from the flasks creating a vacuum, and then boiled the broth. Although the experiment did not result in the growth of microorganisms, scientists simply assumed that air was required for spontaneous generation to occur.

It was not until 1859 that the theory of spontaneous generation was dispelled, and scientists began to recognize that life forms could not simply appear from nowhere. Louis Pasteur entered a contest, sponsored by The French Academy of Sciences, with an alteration of both Needham's and Spallanzani's experiments (see Figure 20-1).

Pasteur boiled broth in a flask and then heated the glass neck of the flask until he could bend it into an S-shape. This shape allowed air to reach the broth, but the airborne microorganisms settled into the curved neck of the flask due to gravity. After no microorganisms grew in the broth, Pasteur tipped the flasks, allowing the broth to reach the curved neck of the flask. Soon, the broth was full of microorganisms, which finally proved that the theory of spontaneous generation was incorrect, and that microorganisms were everywhere—even in the air.

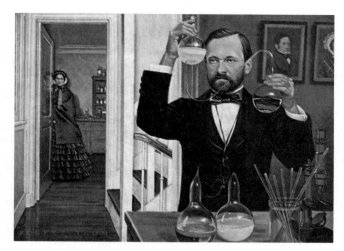

Figure 20-1 Louis Pasteur. (Courtesy of Park-Davis and Company, copyright 1957.)

The implications of the inadequacy of the theory of spontaneous generation are critical to modern beliefs about the origin, transmission, and control of
disease. The modern medical community accepts Rudolph Virchow's 1858 theory of biogenesis, which is based on the principle that no life-form can spontaneously appear. Living cells can only arise from preexisting living cells. It is,
therefore, possible to control the spread of microorganisms and impact conditions of disease. Modern aseptic techniques—the techniques used to prevent
contamination by unwanted microorganisms—are the standard practice in
laboratories and medical procedures, including embalming.

VACCINATION

It has only been since the early 1900s that medical science has recognized that
microorganisms cause disease. Before then, germ theory was not accepted by
the scientific community, and most effective treatments for disease were simply a matter of trial and error, with little or no understanding that microorganisms caused disease.

Edward Jenner trained in London as an army surgeon before returning to
his native Gloucestershire in the West of England, where he spent his entire career as a country doctor. In 1798, Jenner tried to find a way to protect people
from smallpox. The smallpox epidemic spread throughout Europe and devas-
tated the American colonies, killing about 90 percent of the Native American
population, when the colonists brought the virus from Europe.

Building on a previously developed method of vaccination against smallpox
used in Turkey, and his own observation that milkmaids who had developed
cowpox were immune to smallpox, Jenner inoculated healthy volunteers with
material scraped from cowpox blisters. After a mild illness due to the inoculation, the volunteers did not develop cowpox again, and they did not contract
smallpox. The process became known as vaccination from the word *vacca* for
"cow."

GERM THEORY OF DISEASE

At one time, it was a common religious belief that disease was a punishment for crimes and sin. In those days, people believed that disease came from foul odors from sewage, the wrath of a deity, or poisonous vapors from swamps. In contrast, the theory that microorganisms cause disease is known as the germ theory of disease.

In 1665, Robert Hooke reported that the smallest structural forms of life were "little boxes," or "cells," as he called them. Hooke observed these small structures through a compound microscope, which used two sets of lenses. His observations formed the basis of cell theory, which contends that all living beings are composed of individual cells. Between 1674 and 1683, Anton van Leeuwenhoek reported the observation of microorganisms—or "animalcules" as they were known at the time—in rainwater, lake water, on the surface of human teeth, in the gut of horseflies, and in human diarrhea (see Figure 20-2).

The theory of spontaneous generation was not dismissed overnight by the theory of biogenesis, and the gradual acceptance of germ theory was not generally established until about 1900. In 1835, Agostino Bassi proved that a particular type of silkworm disease was caused by a fungus. In the 1840s, Ignaz Semmelweis demonstrated that childbirth fever—which was known as childbed fever at the time—could be spread among patients by physicians who did not disinfect their hands. Later, in 1865, Louis Pasteur found that a protozoan caused a silkworm disease that threatened the silk industry throughout Europe.

In the 1860s, Joseph Lister applied the germ theory of disease to the treatment of his patients during medical procedures (see Figure 20-3). Although disinfectants were unknown at the time, Lister recognized that carbolic acid, or phenol, killed microorganisms, so he began treating surgical wounds with a solution of it. Many people died from surgical wound infections prior to Lister's

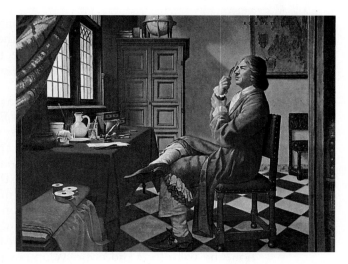

Figure 20-2 Anton van Leeuwenhoek. (Courtesy of Parke-Davis and Company, copyright 1957.)

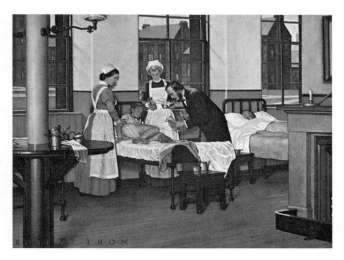

Figure 20-3 Joseph Lister. (Courtesy of Parke-Davis and Company, copyright 1957.)

discovery, and phenol is still a common component of many chemicals used in the modern embalming facility.

In 1876, Robert Koch established the causation of disease by microorganisms. As anthrax killed numerous cattle and sheep throughout Europe, Koch and other scientists were attempting to discover a method of containing the spread of the disease. Koch discovered the existence of rod-shaped bacteria (*Bacillus anthracis*) in the blood of cattle that had died of the disease. After culturing the bacteria on nutrients, Koch injected samples of the culture into healthy animals, which then developed the disease. After comparing the bacteria found in the healthy animals with the bacteria from the animals that had originally died of the disease, Koch observed that the bacteria were the same within the two sets of blood cultures. For the past century, scientists have used a sequence of steps to determine the specific microorganisms that cause a specific disease based on Koch's original steps. These steps are now known as Koch's postulates:

1. The microorganism must be present in every case of the disease.
2. The microorganism must be isolated from the host with the disease and grown in pure culture.
3. The specific disease must be reproduced when a pure culture of the microorganism is inoculated into a healthy susceptible host.
4. The microorganism must be recoverable from the experimentally infected host.

THE MAGIC BULLET

Once the germ theory of disease gained acceptance, and scientists agreed that disinfectants could control microorganisms outside the body, it was logical to hypothesize that microorganisms should be able to be controlled within the diseased body as well. The idea that a chemical, which was a "magic bullet," could be used to destroy a disease-causing microorganism in the body, without harming the infected person, was the foundation of modern pharmaceutical treatments.

Paul Ehrlich was a German physician who studied the staining of animal tissues as a medical student. The theories and methods Ehrlich described in his dissertation are the basis of many of the staining techniques in use today in microbiology labs around the world. In 1899, Ehrlich was appointed as the director of the Institute of Experimental Therapy in Frankfurt-am-Main, Germany. In this position, he began searching for a "magic bullet" that would treat syphilis.

Drawing on the work in his dissertation, Ehrlich established the principles of modern chemotherapy by studying the chemical constitution of drugs, their chemical action, and their action on the cells of the disease-causing microorganism for which they were developed. These pharmaceutical agents were designed to go straight to the microorganism and destroy it without harming the cells of the infected host. Table 20-1 lists several common microorganisms, their related pharmaceutical treatments, and their modes of action.

Table 20-1 Some Disease-Causing Microorganisms, Their Related Drug or Antibiotic Treatments, and Their Modes of Action

Disease	Bacteria	Drug or Antibiotic Treatment	Mode of Action
Anthrax	*Bacillus anthracis*	Erythromycin	Interferes with protein synthesis
		Penicillin	Inhibits cell-wall synthesis
		Tetracycline	Interferes with protein synthesis
Boils, carbuncles, pneumonia, septicemia	*Staphylococcus aureus*	*Lincomycin*	*Inhibits protein synthesis*
		Penicillin	*Inhibits cell-wall synthesis*
		Vancomycin	*Inhibits cell-wall synthesis*
Botulism	*Clostridium botulinum*	Kanamycin	Induces abnormal protein synthesis
		Penicillin	Inhibits cell-wall synthesis
Cholera	*Vibrio cholerae*	Chloramphenicol	Interferes with protein synthesis
		Streptomycin	Produces abnormal protein synthesis
Diphtheria	*Corynebacterium diphtheriae*	Lincomycin	Inhibits protein synthesis
		Penicillin	Inhibits cell-wall synthesis
Gangrene, wound infections, gastroenteritis	*Clostridium perfringens* and any *Salmonella* species	Kanamycin	Induces abnormal protein synthesis
		Penicillin	Inhibits cell-wall synthesis
		Ampicillin	Inhibits cell-wall synthesis
		Chloramphenicol	Interferes with protein synthesis
		Tetracycline	Interferes with protein synthesis
		Clindamycin	Interferes with protein synthesis
Gonorrhea	*Neisseria gonorrhoeae*	Penicillin	Inhibits cell-wall synthesis
		Tetracycline	Interferes with protein synthesis
		Sulfisoxazole	
Leprosy	*Mycobacterium leprae*	Kanamycin	Induces abnormal protein synthesis
		Novobiocin	Affects DNA formation

Table 20-1 Continued

Meningitis	Neisseria meningitidis Haemophilis influenzae	Penicillin	Inhibits cell-wall synthesis
	Cryptococcus neoformans	Amphotericin B	Damages cell wall
Pertussis (whopping cough)	Bordetella pertussis	Ampicillin	Inhibits cell-wall synthesis
		Penicillin	Inhibits cell-wall synthesis
		Tetracycline	Interferes with protein synthesis
Plague	Yersinia pestis	Streptomycin	Produces abnormal protein synthesis
		Tetracycline	Interferes with protein synthesis
Pneumonia	Klebsiella pneumoniae	Colistin	Causes cell membrane deterioration
	Streptococcus pneumoniae	Kanamycin	Induces abnormal protein synthesis
		Neomycin	Induces abnormal protein synthesis
		Penicillin	Inhibits cell-wall synthesis
Rocky Mountain spotted fever	Rickettsia rickettsii	Chloramphenicol	Interferes with protein synthesis
		Tetracycline	Interferes with protein synthesis
Strep throat, scarlet fever, rheumatic fever	Streptococcus pyogenes	Erythromycin	Interferes with protein synthesis
		Lincomycin	Inhibits protein synthesis
		Penicillin	Inhibits cell-wall synthesis
Syphilis	Treponema pallidum	Erythromycin	Interferes with protein synthesis
		Penicillin	Inhibits cell-wall synthesis
		Tetracycline	Interferes with protein synthesis
Tetanus (lockjaw)	Clostridium tetani	Kanamycin	Induces abnormal protein synthesis
		Penicillin	Inhibits cell-wall synthesis
Thrush	Candida albicans	Amphotericin B	Damages cell wall
Tuberculosis	Mycobacterium tuberculosis	Isoniazid	Competitive inhibition
		Streptomycin	Produces abnormal protein synthesis
Typhoid fever	Salmonella typhi	Ampicillin	Inhibits cell-wall synthesis
		Chloramphenicol	Interferes with protein synthesis
		Tetracycline	Interferes with protein synthesis
Urinary infections	Escherichia coli	Ampicillin	Inhibits cell-wall synthesis
		Kanamycin	Induces abnormal protein synthesis
		Sulfonamides	Competitive inhibition

By 1907, Ehrlich and his assistants had tried hundreds of chemicals in the treatment of syphilis with limited success. During this period, however, they discovered the usefulness of arsenic-based drugs against protozoan infections that caused trypanosomiasis (African sleeping diseases). Although the 606th drug in a series had already been rejected as a treatment for syphilis, Ehrlich had an assistant test this arsenic-based drug again on rabbits that had been infected with the spirochete that causes syphilis (*Treponema pallidum*). Ehrlich also found that the 914th drug tested also effectively treated syphilis. After testing both drugs hundreds of times, Ehrlich reported that salvarsan and neosalvarsan were effective treatments for syphilis.

By the late 1930s, researchers had determined that many synthetic drugs were effective agents in the treatment of infectious diseases. Many of the most significant drugs were derivatives of dyes, based on Ehrlich's early studies as a medical student. At about the same time, sulfa drugs were also determined to be capable of destroying disease-causing microorganisms.

It should be noted, however, that no drug is a "magic bullet" in the treatment of disease. All medications have side effects on the body, and the mixing of medications with other prescription medications, with illicit drugs (e.g., marijuana, cocaine, heroin), or with alcohol produces an interaction effect that can prove to be deadly. Even nonprescription drugs, herbal remedies, and vitamin and mineral supplements can interact with prescription medications.

For the embalmer, it is of particular importance to recognize the effect of prescription medications on the condition of the human remains and the interaction effect pharmaceutical agents may have on the embalming process in the presence of embalming chemicals. In the modern age of nuclear medicine, it is important for the embalmer to be familiar with the hazards inherent in the preparation of human remains related to radioactive chemicals, which are primarily used in the diagnosis and treatment of cancer.

Not all medications are synthetic. The first antibiotic was discovered by accident in 1928, by Alexander Fleming, when his culture plates were contaminated by mold. Unlike the sulfa drugs and arsenic-based drugs that had specifically been studied for their effects against microorganisms, the natural ability of this fungus to inhibit the growth of bacterial cells was unexpected. The specific mold was later named penicillin, and it was originally produced on corn and decomposing cantaloupe in Illinois. Before World War II, approximately 400 million units of penicillin had been produced. By the end of the war, U.S. companies were producing 650 billion units each month.

NAMING MICROORGANISMS

Microbiology is defined as the study of microorganisms and their effect on other living organisms, but the word can be broken down even further. *Micro-* is a prefix that means "extremely small," while the root word *bio* means "life." So combining the prefix *micro-* with the root word *bio* literally means "extremely small life."

To study extremely small life-forms and the way they influence others, scientists use some rather large words. For example, everyone has had a pimple. They are caused by the presence of tiny life-forms within the skin. The body reacts to the presence of these life-forms, and pus is produced, causing the area to become inflamed, resulting in pain, swelling, and redness. The name of one of the tiny life-forms found on the skin that contributes to pimple formation is *Staphylococcus aureus*. This Latin name looks quite intimidating at first, but it becomes much easier to understand after learning its prefixes, root words, and suffixes.

The word *coccus* means "shaped like a sphere or ball." The word *staphyl* means "clustered together" similar to grapes, and the word *aureus* means "a golden-yellow color." The combination of these terms results in the words

Staphylococcus aureus, which is something that looks similar to a bunch of gold-colored grapes. Knowing what the words mean is the biggest part of understanding microorganisms.

Assume for a minute that aliens have just arrived on Earth. It is their job to describe all of the life-forms that they observe. They would notice immediately that trees do not look like humans and that flowers do not look like horses. Perhaps they would decide to make some broad categories called plants and animals. They might then decide to start categorizing the animals. Some of the animals have fur and others do not. Some of the animals stand on two legs and others walk on all four. Some animals are brown and some are black. Some animals are tall and others are short. Animals may be large, or they may be small. All of these characteristics and many more would likely be included in the aliens' descriptions of animals on Earth.

In 1673, Anton van Leeuwenhoek saw red blood cells for the first time through a microscope, and he was in the same position as the fictitious aliens on Earth. Early scientists wanted to differentiate one microorganism from another, so they began to describe them in ever-smaller groups by their characteristics. Those same basic groups are still in use today, and they form the backbone of an understanding of all life forms.

EUKARYOTIC CELLS VERSUS PROKARYOTIC CELLS

Since every living organism has cellular properties, there are two broad categories of cells, eukaryotic cells and prokaryotic cells. Eukaryotes are usually distinguished from other forms of life by the presence of nuclei and a cytoskeleton. Most human cells are eukaryotic. Their cytoskeleton comprises a variety of proteins. The cytoskeleton provides shape for the cell and support for membrane-bound organelles. The nuclei contain genetic information organized into discrete chromosomes and contained within a membrane-bounded compartment.

The most evident organelle in most cells is the nucleus, and it is from the presence of this organelle that the eukaryotes get their name. Most cells have a single nucleus, some have thousands, while still others, like mature red blood cells have none—but they can all be shown to derive from cells with nuclei. The nucleus is bounded by a membranous envelope called a nuclear envelope. The envelope is perforated by nuclear pores that allow compounds to pass between the nucleus and the surrounding cytoplasm. Some eukaryotes, called protists, have more than one kind of nucleus—using one to retain a copy of the genetic material for purposes of reproduction and another to regulate activities. Within the nucleus, the genes are located on a number of chromosomes. The total amount of DNA in a nucleus measuring less than one hundredth of a millimeter across may stretch to over a meter.

The major, and extremely significant, difference between prokaryotes and eukaryotes, is that eukaryotes have a nucleus and membrane-bound organelles, while prokaryotes do not. The word *eukaryote* means "true nucleus," while the word *prokaryote* means "before nucleus." The DNA of prokaryotes floats freely around the cell, while the DNA of eukaryotes is held within the nucleus. The organelles of eukaryotes allow them to exhibit much higher levels of intracellular division of labor than is possible in prokaryotic cells. Eukaryotic cells are, on average, ten times the size of prokaryotic cells. The DNA of eukaryotes is much more complex and, therefore, much more extensive than the DNA of prokaryotes. Prokaryotes have a cell wall composed of peptidoglycan, which is a single large polymer of amino acids and sugar. Many types of eukaryotic cells also have cell walls, but none are made of peptidoglycan. The cells of animals, plants, protozoa and most algae are typically eukaryotic, while the cells of bacteria and cyanobacteria (blue-green algae) are prokaryotic.

KINGDOMS

There are five kingdoms used to classify all biological forms, which include all of the eukaryotes and the prokaryotes. The five kingdoms are Monera (or Prokaryotae), Protista, Fungi, Plantae, and Animalia. These five kingdoms classify all forms of life by their shared characteristics and are divided into successively smaller groups. Each group classifies the particular life-form from the larger group. The order of classification is kingdom, division or phylum, class, order, family, genus, and species. The genus and species are the most important for the naming of microorganisms.

Monera is the only kingdom composed of prokaryotic organisms, which have a cell wall and lack both membrane-bound organelles and multicellular forms. The most ancient eukaryotic kingdom, protists, includes a variety of eukaryotic forms. Protists are best defined as eukaryotes that are not fungi, animals, or plants. Fungi are a eukaryotic, multicellular group of cells with multiple nuclei enclosed within cell walls. Plants are immobile, multicellular eukaryotes that produce their food by photosynthesis and have cells encased in cellulose cell walls. Animals are multicellular eukaryotes capable of mobility at some stage during their lives, and their cells lack cell walls.

Microorganisms have a first and a last name just like people. It is customary in Western cultures to write the given name first and the surname last, with each being capitalized, while in some Eastern cultures a person's last name is written first and the first name is written last. Microorganisms are named by two names as well.

Each microbe has both a first name, referring to its genus, and a second name, referring to its species. The genus is always capitalized and the species is lowercase. So, the microorganism that causes blood poisoning is named *Staphylococcus aureus*. Its genus is *Staphylococcus,* and its species is *aureus*. (Technically, the species is binomial requiring both names [Upton 2004], but that rule will not be followed in this explanation.) The name is written in italics out of custom because it is not English. Since the names are so long, it is also customary that they be abbreviated after they are written once. It would be appropriate after writing the full name once to refer to the *Staphylococcus aureus* microorganism as *S. aureus,* and readers would all know that the *S.* stands for *Staphylococcus.* The species name is not abbreviated, however.

Just as the name Henrietta Wilcox describes a person by a given name and a family name, the bacterium that causes blood poisoning is named *Staphylococcus aureus,* reflecting its genus and species. Just as Henrietta Wilcox's family name associates her with a group of ancestors with shared biological character-istics, microorganisms of the same genus have certain characteristics that they share in common. For example, dogs all belong to the genus *Canis*. All dogs have certain similarities, and those similarities are inferred in the term *Canis*.

Staphylococci all share their shape and arrangement in common. Regard-less of the specific species, microorganisms of the genus *Staphylococcus* are spheres, clustered together like grapes. The species name then adds a specific characteristic to the genus. In the example of *Staphylococcus aureus*, the species *aureus* suggests that the arrangement of spheres in a grape cluster are gold col-ored. This naming system of genus and species allows scientists to differentiate one microorganism from another.

DIVISIONS OF MICROBIOLOGY

Five important divisions of microbiology are:

1. Bacteriology
2. Rickettsiology
3. Virology
4. Protozoology
5. Mycology

Bacteriology is the study of bacteria. **Rickettsiology** is the study of rickettsia. **Virology** is the study of viruses. **Protozoology** is the study of protozoa, and **mycology** is the study of fungi. The remainder of this chapter describes each of these microorganisms as they relate to human diseases.

PATHOGENIC MICROORGANISMS

Not all microorganisms cause disease. There are many microorganisms ben-eficial to both humans and the environment. Beneficial microorganisms are used to make food, in treating infections, in water treatment facilities, and in the human digestive tract. However, there are also many microorganisms that cause disease in both human and in nonhuman animals. Microorgan-isms that cause disease in humans are known as pathogenic microorganisms, or pathogens. The microorganisms discussed in this text that are of major health importance to humans include bacteria, mycoplasmas, rickettsia, chlamydia, viruses, protozoa, fungi, and prions.

Bacteria

Bacteria are defined as prokaryotic, one-celled microorganisms of the king-dom Monera, existing as free-living organisms or as parasites, multiplying by binary fission, and having a large range of biochemical properties. Pathogenic bacteria are living, disease-causing microorganisms. The majority of infectious diseases described in this book are caused by bacteria. Bacteria are relatively small and must be viewed individually with a microscope, but they are about

10 times as large as a virus. When they are grown in a proper nutrient source, they form colonies containing billions of bacterial cells that can be seen without a microscope.

Mycoplasmas

The **mycoplasma** is the smallest and simplest self-replicating bacterium, being intermediate in size between viruses and bacteria. Mycoplasmas have no cell wall, unlike other prokaryotes, and they are the smallest free-living organism presently known. Colonies of mycoplasma may grow in a characteristic fried-egg shape. Mycoplasma contain double-stranded DNA, with a total of between 500 and 1,000 genes. The nutritional requirements of mycoplasmas are also quite exacting, with some feeding on urea and others thriving only in the presence of certain cholesterols. Mycoplasmas cause a variety of urogenital tract infections as well as respiratory diseases such as AIDS-related infection, primary atypical pneumonia, stillbirths, infertility, spontaneous abortion, and urinary tract infections. Mycoplasmas produce hydrogen peroxide, which has been shown to damage the cell membranes of human cells. Repeated infection of mycoplasmas are usually required before the symptoms of disease appear in the host.

Rickettsias

Another type of bacteria that can cause disease is the rickettsias. **Rickettsia** is a genus of rod-shaped, gram-negative, intracellular parasitic bacteria. Rickettsia, however, may be rod-shaped, sphere-shaped, or may change shapes. Rickettsia can only reproduce within a host cell, which makes them similar to viruses. In morphological and in limited biochemical aspects, however, they resemble bacteria and are, therefore, classified as such. They are extremely small and usually spread by arthropod vectors, such as lice, fleas, ticks, or mites. Except for *Rickettsia prowazekii*, which causes epidemic typhus, rickettsias do not contain flagella. Rickettsia must have living cells to replicate, and are obligate parasites, meaning they cannot survive outside of the host cell. Rickettsias are dependent on the rich cytoplasm of host cells due to the bacteria's uniquely permeable and unstable cell membrane.

Rickettsias typically infect the epithelial lining of the intestinal tract of the arthropod vector and are excreted through the vector's feces. These bacteria are commonly transmitted from the arthropod vector to humans through bites. In infected humans, rickettsia are commonly found in the small blood vessels of the brain, heart, and skin. Localized blood clot formation leads to the loss of plasma, decreased blood volume, and fatal shock. It is also speculated that rickettsia produce a toxin. Although rickettsial infections are commonly treated with drugs like tetracycline, their growth is actually increased in the presence of other drugs such as sulfonamides.

Chlamydia

Chlamydia are a group of nonmotile, gram-negative, intracellular parasites that can cause disease in humans. Although chlamydial diseases manifest in a similar manner to viral diseases, chlamydia are not viruses, they are bacteria that replicate in the cytoplasm of host cells. The spherically shaped chlamydial cell contains no flagella or capsule; however, it does contain a rigid cell wall and often a cell membrane consisting of a large quantity of lipids. Chlamydia are believed to be dependent on host cells because the bacteria lack a source of energy production, and, therefore, require the ATP found in the cytoplasm of the host cell.

In humans, chlamydia can cause infections of the eye and genitourinary infections by infecting the mucous membranes in those areas. There are also over 100 species of birds that naturally carry chlamydia including pigeons, ducks, chickens, turkeys, finch, and seabirds. If the chlamydia from these birds are passed to humans, they can infect the mucous lining of the respiratory tract. In addition, chlamydia can cause infections of the liver, kidney, and heart of humans, as well as spontaneous abortion in pregnant women.

Protozoa

Protozoa are of the kingdom Protista and are one-celled eukaryotes, although some may be colonial with various mechanisms of motility. Even though protozoa lack a cell wall, they may have rigid forms that change based on their development through their life course. Although the majority of protozoa are free-living organisms with no disease-causing potential in humans, certain protozoa do cause serious diseases. There are more protozoa in the world than any other microorganism, and they play an important role in consuming both bacteria and multicellular organisms. There are four classifications of protozoa, which includes the flagellates, amoebae, sporozoans, and the ciliates. Protozoa are responsible for such diseases as amebic dysentery, malaria, toxoplasmosis, African sleeping disease, giardiasis, trichomoniasis, brain infections, and infections of the skin and lungs.

Fungi

The study of fungi is referred to as mycology. **Fungi** are a group of often filamentous unicellular and multicellular organisms lacking chlorophyll and usually bearing spores. Yeasts, molds, and dimorphic fungi are the three fundamental categories of fungi. A fungus that typically has a capsule and is unicellular is known as a yeast, while molds are fungi that are filamentous and multicellular. Dimorphic fungi alternate between unicellular and multicellular forms.

Since fungi lack chlorophyll, they often grow on decomposing matter and are called saprophytes. Depending on the variety, fungi may produce either sexually or asexually through budding or reproductive spore formation. Some fungi produce toxins that are harmful to humans. Although yeast is an ingredient of both beer and bread, some yeasts cause disease. Molds are essential in the production of life-saving drugs like penicillin, and they flavor cheese, but the variety that grows on peanuts (*Aspergillus*) can be toxic to humans. Almost all the world's commercial penicillin is produced from the fungus *Penicillium chrysogenum* pictured in Figure 20-4. Note the consistently round patterns of the cultures, which is indicative of fungus. Other types of microorganisms grow in other patterns.

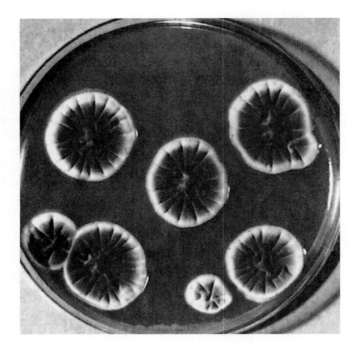

Figure 20-4 Almost all of the world's penicillin is produced from a form of *Penicillium chrysogenum*. (Courtesy of Pfizer, Inc.)

Human fungal diseases are categorized by the level of tissue penetration. Superficial mycoses penetrate the least and are found only in the outermost layers of the skin and hair. Cutaneous mycoses are fungal infections of the skin, hair, and fingernails such as ringworm, jock itch, and athlete's foot. The cutaneous mycoses are caused by dermatophytes, and they occur deeper in the integument than the superficial mycoses. Subcutaneous mycoses occur deep in the integument and may include the deeper-lying structures such as the fascia, muscle tissue, and bone. Subcutaneous mycoses are often the result of trauma to the integument, and they frequently require surgical removal. Systemic mycoses, which include histoplasmosis, blastoplasmosis, coccidioidomycoses, and fungal meningitis, spread throughout the body and generally originate in the tissues of the lungs.

Persons with suppressed immune systems are more susceptible to opportunistic fungal diseases, which can result as a secondary infection due to treatment for their original disorder. The elderly, children, persons with AIDS, persons with diabetes, and persons receiving chemotherapy for cancer could all be described as having suppressed immune systems. Fungal infections can be fatal and are often extremely difficult to manage. They can also be passed from the deceased to the living through a variety of means.

Viruses, Viroids, and Prions

The smallest category of disease-causing microorganism is the virus. A **virus** is an intracellular, infectious parasite, capable of living and replicating only in living cells. Viruses range between 20 and 300 nanometers in size. A nanometer is one billionth of a meter, which is approximately the length of a yardstick. Since there are about 25 million nanometers in an inch, approximately 84,000 of the largest viruses could be lined up side-by-side in an inch. Viruses come in a variety of shapes and sizes, with some resembling two parallel lines and others resembling two conjoined balls. Figure 20-5 depicts a more complexly shaped virus called a *bacteriaphage,* which looks like an alien spaceship's landing craft, with its six legs, head, and tail.

Viruses can infect almost any living cell, including bacteria, fungi, parasites, plants, animals, and, of course, human cells. They are basically a piece of genetic material wrapped in protein, and they contain only one type of nucleic acid, either DNA or RNA. They multiply inside living cells by using the cell's own structures to produce more infected cells. There are many ways to classify viruses, and no single way has proven satisfactory. Table 20-2 lists some of the families of viruses that contain human pathogens. They are classified by nucleic acid, size, shape, and substructure of the virus, as illustrated in Figure 20-6.

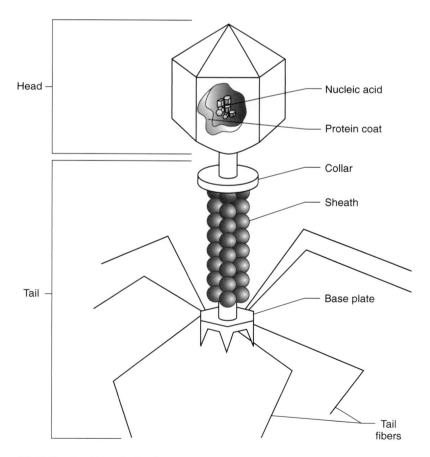

Figure 20–5 Typical bacteriophage.

Table 20-2 Virus Groups That Cause Disease in Humans

Virus Group	Examples of Diseases	Description
Poxvirus	Smallpox	Large, brick-shaped virus containing DNA
Herpesvirus	Cold sores, shingles, chickenpox	Medium-size, 20-sided virus containing DNA
Adenovirus	Conjunctivitis	Medium-size, cube-shaped virus containing DNA
Rhabdovirus	Rabies	Bullet-shaped virus containing RNA
Arbovirus	Equine encephalitis	Carried by arthropods (e.g., ticks, mites, fleas)

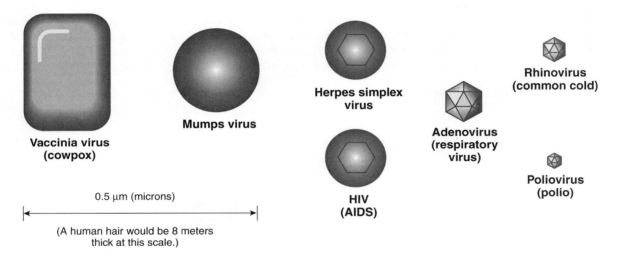

Vaccinia virus
(cowpox)

Mumps virus

Herpes simplex
virus

HIV
(AIDS)

Adenovirus
(respiratory
virus)

Rhinovirus
(common cold)

Poliovirus
(polio)

0.5 μm (microns)

(A human hair would be 8 meters
thick at this scale.)

Figure 20-6 Virus morphology.

Viruses lack enzymes like ATP for producing energy, so they are dependent on their host cells. Some viruses are sensitive to disinfectants due to the presence of lipids in their coverings. For example, HIV, the virus that causes AIDS, can be inactivated by a solution of 10 percent household bleach in water. Both detergents and ether are capable of inactivating many viruses by simply dissolving their lipid coverings. This effect is not unlike the ability of dish soap to dissolve fat from a dirty skillet.

A viroid is similar to a virus, except viroids contain only RNA, and they do not have a protein coat. Just like viruses, viroids are intracellular parasites that cannot survive outside the host cell. Both viruses and viroids create an immune reaction response in humans. And, even though the majority of diseases caused by viroids occur in plants, hepatitis D is a disease of the human liver caused by a viroid. The viroid that causes hepatitis D is actually enclosed in the capsule of the hepatitis B virus, which embalmers can contract through blood-to-blood exposure with the deceased. One case of hepatitis B was reportedly contracted by a forensic pathologist whose knuckles scraped against the deceased's exposed rib cage during an autopsy.

Prions are small proteinaceous, infectious particles that are resistant to most procedures that modify nucleic acids. Unlike viruses and viroids, prions do not contain either DNA or RNA, and they do not cause an immune system response in humans. Prions consist entirely of proteins that are produced by human genes and are, therefore, obligate intracellular parasites, just like viruses and viroids. Viruses, viroids, and prions are all nonliving agents, hence they can only multiply inside living cells.

Diseases caused by prions are collectively known as spongiform encephalopathies because they leave holes in the brain tissue that resemble a sponge. Prion-related diseases may be either inherited or develop sporadically and be transmitted through blood-to-blood contact. The common denominator among all prion disorders is the presence of amyloid deposits in the tissues. Amyloid is a general term for any intracellular or intercellular starchlike protein deposit. These deposits stain easily with Congo red dye and appear homogenous, waxy, and translucent.

Amyloid degeneration also occurs in non-prion-related pathological disorders like tuberculosis, osteomyelitis, leprosy, Hodgkin's disease, and various cancers. Prion diseases such as scrapie and mad cow disease (bovine spongiform encephalopathy) are found in sheep and cows, respectively. Prions are suspected causes of human disease such as Creutzfeldt-Jakob disease, variant Creutzfeldt-Jakob disease, kuru, Gerstmann-Straussler syndrome, Alzheimer's disease, fatal familial insomnia, and Down syndrome (Del Bo et al. 2003).

REVIEW QUESTIONS

Matching

1. _____ Anton van Leeuwenhoek
2. _____ Joseph Lister
3. _____ Robert Koch
4. _____ Louis Pasteur
5. _____ Edward Jenner

a. recognized that phenol killed microorganisms
b. used cowpox as a vaccine for smallpox
c. helped save the European silk industry by identifying the protozoan that cased a silkworm disease
d. reported microorganisms in rainwater, lake water, on the surface of human teeth, in the gut of horseflies, and in the feces of human diarrhea
e. established the causation of disease by microorganisms

Multiple Choice

1. The belief that life-forms can spontaneously appear from nonliving matter is known as which of the following?
   a. germ theory
   b. spontaneous generation
   c. cell theory
   d. magic bullet theory

2. When first seen by scientists through a microscope, microorganisms and cells were referred to as which of the following?

a. cells

b. little boxes

c. vacca

d. animalcules

3. Which of the following refers to the theory that the growth of microorganisms can be controlled because living cells can only arise from preexisting living cells?

a. theory of biogenesis

b. spontaneous generation

c. cell theory

d. germ theory

4. Which of the following refers to the theory that microorganisms cause disease?

a. theory of biogenesis

b. spontaneous generation

c. cell theory

d. germ theory

5. Which of the following refers to the theory that all living beings are composed of individual cells?

a. theory of biogenesis

b. spontaneous generation

c. cell theory

d. germ theory

Bibliography

Abedon, S. (2003). *Eukaryotic microorganisms and parasites*. Retrieved July 26, 2003, from lecture notes for Micro 509 at the Ohio State University at http://www.mansfield.ohio-state.edu/~sabedon/black11.htm.

Campbell, W. (2002). *The germ theory calendar*. Retrieved June 26, 2003, from http://germtheorycalendar.com/.

Chamberlain, N. (2000a). *Introduction to microbiology*. Retrieved July 25, 2003, from the Kirksville College of Osteopathic Medicine at http://www.kcom.edu/faculty/chamberlain/Website/intmic.htm.

Chamberlain, N. (2000b). *Rickettsia, chlamydia, mycoplasma*. Retrieved July 15, 2003, from Kirksville College of Osteopathic Medicine at http://www.kcom.edu/faculty/chamberlain/Website/Lects/RICKETT.HTM#ri.

Del Bo, R., Comi, G. P., Giorda, R., Crimi, M., Locatelli, F., Martinelli-Boneschi, F., Pozzoli, U., Castelli, E., Bresolin, N., & Scarlato, G. (2003). The 129 codon polymorphism of the prion protein gene influences earlier cognitive performance in Down syndrome subjects. *Journal of Neurology, 250*(6), 688–692.

Dobell, C. (Ed.). (1960). *Antony van Leeuwenhoek and his "little animals."* New York: Dover Publications.

Edmonds, P. (1978). *Microbiology: An environmental perspective*. Basingstoke Hampshire, England: Macmillan Publishing.

Ehrlich, Paul biography. (n.d.). Retrieved June 26, 2003, form the Nobel e-Museum: http://www.nobel.se/medicine/laureates/1908/ehrlich-bio.html.

Fleming discovers penicillin. (1998). In *People and Discoveries, A Science Odyssey*. Retrieved June 26, 2003, from WGBH, PBS Online at http://www.pbs.org/wgbh/aso/databank/entries/dm28pe.html.

Fogel, R., & Rogers, P. (2000). *Penicillin: The first miracle drug*. Retrieved July 25, 2003, from the University of Michigan at http://www.herb.lsa.umich.edu/kidpage/penicillin.htm.

Ford, B. (1991). *The Leeuwenhoek legacy*. London: Biopress, Bristol, and Farrand Press.

Frobisher, M., Hinsdill, R., Crabtree, K., & Goodheart, C. (1974). *Fundamentals of microbiology*. Philadelphia: Saunders.

Gale, J. (2003). Bacteria. In *Watersheds*. Retrieved June 30, 2003, from the North Carolina State University Water Quality Group at http://h2osparc.wq.ncsu.edu/info/bacteria.html.

Gaudy, A., & Gaudy, E. (1980). *Microbiology for environmental scientists and engineers*. New York: McGraw-Hill.

Grover-Lakomia, L., & Fong, E. (1999). *Microbiology for Health Careers* (6th ed.). Clifton Park, NY: Thomson Delmar Learning.

Jacobs, F. (1985). *Breakthrough: The true story of penicillin*. New York: Dodd, Mead & Company.

Levine, R., & Evers, C. (1998). *The slow death of spontaneous generation (1668–1859)*. Retrieved June 26, 2003, from Access Excellence, The National Health Museum at http://www.accessexcellence.org/AB/BC/Spontaneous_Generation.html.

Lienhard, J. (1997). *Ignaz Philipp Semmelweis*. Retrieved July 25, 2003, from the University of Houston at http://www.uh.edu/engines/epi622.htm.

Lister, Joseph (1827–1912). (n/d). Retrieved July 25, 2003, from the BBC at http://www.bbc.co.uk/education/medicine/nonint/indust/dt/indtbi5.shtml.

Mahon, C., & Manuselis, G. (2000). *Textbook of Diagnostic Microbiology* (2nd ed.). Philadelphia: Saunders.

Mayer, R. (2000). *Embalming: History, theory, & practice* (3rd ed.). New York: McGraw-Hill.

Neighbors, M., & Tannehill-Jones, R. (2000). *Human diseases*. Clifton Park, NY: Thomson Delmar Learning.

Nester, E., Anderson, D., Roberts, C., Pearsall, N., & Nester, M. (2001). *Microbiology: A human perspective* (3rd ed.). Boston: McGraw Hill.

Pathology for funeral service. (1999). Dallas, TX: Professional Training Schools.

Razin, S. (n.d.). Mycoplasmas. In *Medical Microbiology*, 4th ed. Retrieved July 15, 2003, from the University of Texas Medical Branch. At Galveston, TX at http://gsbs.utmb.edu/microbook/ch037.htm.

Razin, S., & Barile, M. (Eds.). (1985). *The mycoplasmas*, volume 4. Orlando, FL: Academic Press.

Rhee, S. (1998). *Louis Pasteur (1822–1895)*. Retrieved July 25, 2003, from Access Excellence, The National Health Museum at http://www.accessexcellence.org/AB/BC/Louis_Pasteur.html.

Rottem, S., & Kahane, I. (Eds.). (1993). *Mycoplasma cell membranes*. New York: Plenum Press.

Scott, P., & Pierce, J. (1996). *Edward Jenner and the discovery of vaccination*. Retrieved June 26, 2003, from the Thomas Cooper Library, University of South Carolina at http://www.sc.edu/library/spcoll/nathist/jenner.html.

Shelton, H. (1992). *Boyd's introduction to the study of disease* (11th ed.). Philadelphia: Lea & Febiger.

Stewart, K., & Stewart, D. (1998). *Bacteria and their characteristics*. Retrieved June 30, 2003, from the Food Safety Management Course, Stewart Enterprises at http://www.saturnnet.com/stewartent/webdoc201.htm.

Tortora, G., Funke, B., & Case, C. (1998). *Microbiology: An introduction* (6th ed.). Menlo Park, CA: Benjamin/Cummings Publishing.

Upton, Steve J. (2004). Biology 625 Animal Parasitology lecture notes. Retrieved March 14, 2004, from the Department of Biology at Kansas State University at http://www.ksu.edu/parasitology/classes/625intro.html.

Venes, D. (Ed.). (2001). *Taber's cyclopedic medical dictionary* (19th ed.). Philadelphia: F. A. Davis.

Virchow, Rudolph (1821–1902). (2003). Retrieved July 25, 2003, from the Department of Diagnostic Medicine/Pathobiology at Kansas State University at http://www.vet.ksu.edu/depts/dmp/personnel/faculty/virchowbioe.htm.

CHAPTER 21

Anatomy of Bacteria

Learning Objectives

Upon completion of the chapter and review questions, the reader should be able to:

- Explain how bacteria multiply.
- Compare and contrast the cell wall and the cell membrane.
- Describe the significance of both the capsule and the ability to form endospores in relationship to some bacteria's ability to withstand environmental changes.
- Compare and contrast flagella, pili, and fimbriae as means of motility.
- Explain gram staining and the significance it has on the characteristics of bacteria.
- Discuss the purpose of fluid suspensions and smearing as related to microscopy.
- Explain how morphology is used in the study of microorganisms.
- Compare and contrast the cytoplasm of eukaryotes and prokaryotes.

Key Terms

bacillus	flagella
coccus	morphology
diplobacilli	staphylococci
diplococci	streptobacilli
endospore	streptococci

BACTERIA

Bacteria and other microorganisms differ substantially in their anatomical and physiological attributes from human cells. This chapter describes the anatomy of bacteria and other microorganisms in such a way as to emphasize the role different structures play in the microorganism's function. The chapter concludes with a brief description of how microscopes and stainings are used to see these microscopic structures.

Binary Fission

Binary fission, which is also known as simple transverse fission, is a method of asexual reproduction in bacteria, in which the cell splits into two parts, each of which develops into a complete individual. The process of binary fission can occur relatively quickly, producing multiple generations of a single bacterial cell within a brief period of time resulting in a mass of bacteria. A bacterial colony is a visible group of bacteria growing on a solid medium, presumably arising from a single microorganism. It requires approximately 1 million bacteria before a colony is visible without a microscope, and some bacteria are capable of reproducing once every 20 minutes under perfect conditions, although perfect conditions are almost never met.

Morphology

Bacteria come in all shapes and sizes, and studying those differences is called morphology. The **morphology** of bacteria refers to their size, shape, and arrangements. The three basic shapes of the bacteria discussed in this book are (1) those shaped like a sphere, (2) those shaped like a rod, (3) and those with a spiral shape. Bacteria have three basic arrangements. They may be connected in (1) pairs, they can be formed in a (2) chain, or they can be arranged together forming a pattern similar to a (3) cluster of grapes.

There are other arrangements and shapes of bacteria that are not discussed because they are beyond the scope of this text, but the embalmer should be aware that many shapes exist. For example, bacteria may be shaped like either stars or squares known as *Stella* and *Haloarcula*, respectively. Although most bacteria are monomorphic, meaning they have only one shape, some important disease-causing bacteria like *Cornybacterium* are pleomorphic, meaning they can have many shapes.

As mentioned, the bacteria described in this text are typically shaped as spheres, rods, or spirals. Bacteria with a spherical shape include the word **coccus** in their names. The plural of coccus is cocci. The spheres can be arranged in pairs called **diplococci**. The spheres may also be arranged in a chain referred to as **streptococci**, or the spheres may be shaped like a cluster of grapes called **staphylococci**. Cocci are illustrated in Figure 21-1. Cocci cause diseases like strep throat, food poisoning, scarlet fever, wound infection, and toxic shock syndrome.

Some bacteria are shaped like a rod, and they include the word **bacillus** in their names (Figure 21-2). The plural of bacillus is bacilli. If the rods are paired together they are called **diplobacilli**, and if the rods take the shape of a chain they are called **streptobacilli**. Bacilli cause diseases like typhoid, diphtheria, and lockjaw.

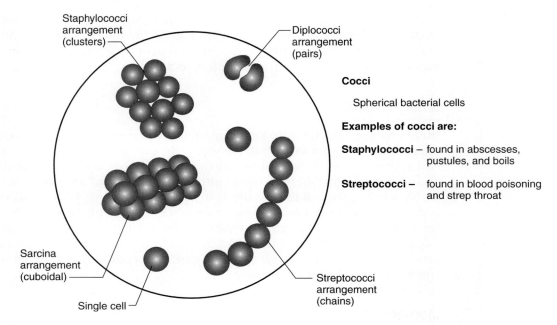

Figure 21-1 Cocci.

Labels in figure:
- Staphylococci arrangement (clusters)
- Diplococci arrangement (pairs)
- Sarcina arrangement (cuboidal)
- Single cell
- Streptococci arrangement (chains)

Cocci

Spherical bacterial cells

Examples of cocci are:

Staphylococci – found in abscesses, pustules, and boils

Streptococci – found in blood poisoning and strep throat

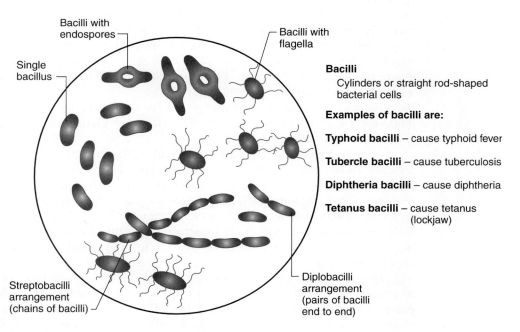

Figure 21-2 Bacilli.

Labels in figure:
- Bacilli with endospores
- Bacilli with flagella
- Single bacillus
- Streptobacilli arrangement (chains of bacilli)
- Diplobacilli arrangement (pairs of bacilli end to end)

Bacilli

Cylinders or straight rod-shaped bacterial cells

Examples of bacilli are:

Typhoid bacilli – cause typhoid fever

Tubercle bacilli – cause tuberculosis

Diphtheria bacilli – cause diphtheria

Tetanus bacilli – cause tetanus (lockjaw)

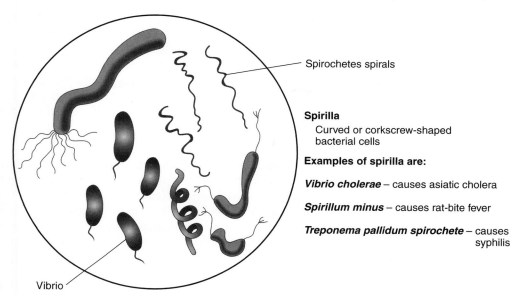

Figure 21-3 Spirilla.

Spiral or helical-shaped bacteria are named spirilla and resemble corkscrews (Figure 21-3). Bacteria that look like curved rods are called *vibrios*. Spirochetes are surrounded by an axial filament that allows them to control their movements by turning like corkscrews. Two important spirochetes are *Treponema pallidum* and *Borrelia burgdorferi,* which cause syphilis and Lyme disease, respectively.

Cell Wall Versus Cell Membrane. Almost all prokaryotic cells have cell walls. The cell wall of bacteria is a semirigid structure that provides the cell with its shape. The cell wall's primary purpose is to prevent bacteria from rupturing when the osmotic pressure inside the cell differs greatly from the osmotic pressure outside the cell. The body defends itself from certain bacteria by forming antibiotics that attack the cell wall. Some eukaryotic cells in plants, algae, and fungi have cell walls that are less complex and less rigid than those of prokaryotes, but most eukaryotic cells do not contain a cell wall.

Not all bacteria have cell walls. The smallest known bacteria that can grow and reproduce outside the living host cell are mycoplasmas. The most common type of lung infection of individuals between the ages of 5 and 35 is a disease known as primary atypical pneumonia, caused by a bacterium known as *Mycoplasma pneumoniae,* which does not have a cell wall. Certain pharmaceutical agents are not effective in the treatment of primary atypical pneumonia because they attack the cell wall of bacteria.

The cell membrane, which is also known as a plasma membrane or a cytoplasmic membrane, lines the inside of the cell wall of many bacteria. It is composed of some proteins, but mostly of phospholipids, which are repeating units of fats and clusters of phosphorus. The cell membrane is selectively semi-permeable, which means that certain molecules and ions may pass through the membrane while others are restricted. A variety of antimicrobial agents, including soaps, alcohols, and quaternary ammonium compounds, are capable of killing bacterial cells by targeting the phospholipids in the cell membrane. Once the cell membrane is damaged, the contents of the bacterial cell are exposed and the cell dies.

Cytoplasm.   In eukaryotic cells, the term *cytoplasm* generally refers to the many functional organelles inside the cell. In contrast, the cytoplasm of prokaryotic cells does not contain functional organelles; instead, it refers to the internal matrix of the material inside the cell membrane. Cytoplasm is about 80 percent water that is rich in enzymes, carbohydrates, and lipids, and it resembles a thick, cloudy, elastic fluid. In addition, the cytoplasm of prokaryotic cells contains a much higher concentration of inorganic ions than the cytoplasm of eukaryotic cells.

Within the cytoplasm's nuclear area are both the bacterial chromosome and the plasmids. The nuclear area is not bound by a nuclear envelope, but contains the bacterial chromosome, which is a single, long, circular molecule of double-stranded DNA. The plasmids are small, circular, double-stranded DNA molecules that the bacterial cell can actually pass along to other bacterial cells. Plasmids are independent of the bacterial chromosome and can carry a variety of genetic materials that could produce toxins or increase resistance to certain antibiotics. Plasmid DNA is used for genetic engineering and cloning.

Glycocalyx and Capsules.   Bacteria are single-celled, prokaryotic microorganisms that contain specialized structures with specific functions, as illustrated in Figure 21-4. Prokaryotic cells secrete a sticky, gelatinous coating, called a *glycocalyx*, that surrounds the cell wall. This outer coating on prokaryotic cells differs greatly between different species, and is known as a *capsule* only when it is organized and firmly attached externally to the cell wall. If the glycocalyx is unorganized and only loosely attached to the cell wall, it is known as a *slime layer*.

The capsule on some species of bacteria allows the cell to survive through adverse circumstances. For example, encapsulated *Streptococcus pneumoniae* is able to produce pneumonia in humans, while unencapsulated *S. pneumoniae* is typically destroyed by the body's immune system and, therefore, does not cause pneumonia in most cases. Another group of bacteria known as *Klebsiella pneumoniae* also is protected from the body's immune system by its capsule, but the capsule on *K. pneumoniae* also allows it to adhere to the surfaces in the mucus membranes of the respiratory tract. In extreme circumstances, some bacteria like *Streptococcus mutans* is capable of digesting the sugars in its own capsule as a source of nutrients.

Motility.   Many bacterial cells also contain structures that allow them to move about, which is known as motility. Some bacterial cells are flagellated, mean-

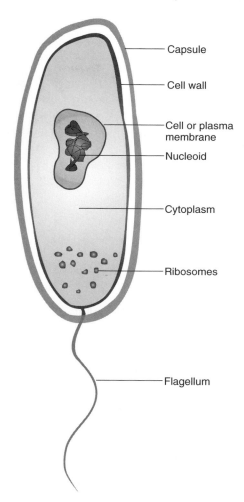

Capsule

Cell wall

Cell or plasma membrane

Nucleoid

Cytoplasm

Ribosomes

Flagellum

Figure 21–4 Basic prokaryotic bacterial cell with a flagellum.

ing that they have **flagella**, which are long, whiplike, filament-containing appendages that propel the bacteria. A monotrichous bacterium has one flagellum; an amphitrichous bacterium has one flagellum at either end of its cell; a lophotrichous bacterium has two or more flagella on either end of its cell; and, a peritrichous bacterium has flagella distributed over its entire cell. Figure 21-5 illustrates these four groups of flagellated bacteria.

The flagella of prokaryotic bacterial cells function differently from the flagella of eukaryotic cells. For example, human sperm propel themselves through fluids with a wavelike motion of their attached flagella. In contrast, prokaryotic

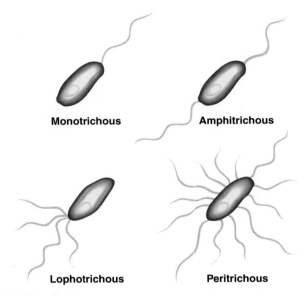

Figure 21-5 Flagellated bacteria.

cells spin the flagellum at its point of attachment in either a clockwise or counterclockwise direction. By changing the direction of spin of their flagella, bacterial cells are capable of controlling their direction of movement (Figure 21-6). Motility is a great advantage to certain bacteria because it allows them to move away from unfavorable environments toward more favorable environments.

Some bacterial cells are covered with structures known as fimbriae and pili, which are shorter, thinner, and straighter than flagella. Unlike flagella, which provide cells with motility, fimbriae and pili allow bacteria to attach to surfaces. A few fimbriae can occur at the ends of the cells, or hundreds may be distributed over the entire cell. Pili, which are longer than fimbriae, differ from fimbriae in that there are usually only one or two pili on a bacterial cell, and they allow bacterial cells to join together to transfer DNA from one cell to another.

A sexually transmitted disease known as gonorrhea is caused by the bacteria, *Neisseria gonorrhoeae*. The bacteria must form colonies on the body's mucus membranes before the disease gonorrhea occurs. *N. gonorrhoeae* are covered with fimbriae, and when they are genetically mutated so that they are not covered with fimbriae, they do not colonize on the mucous membranes and, therefore, do not cause gonorrhea.

Endospores

When the survival of bacteria is threatened, the bacterial cell may form an endospore, which is also known as a spore. An **endospore** is a thick-walled cell produced by a bacterium to enable it to survive unfavorable environmental

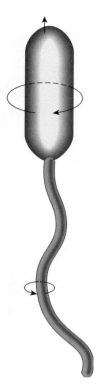

Figure 21-6 Movement of a flagellum as it propels a bacterium through a liquid.

conditions. Basically, the cell forms a highly resistant form of itself that can survive for thousands of years. Figure 21-7 pictures the tough outer wall of spores, which explains their resistance. An endospore is not part of the reproductive process because the number of bacteria is not increased by the presence of spores.

When the endospore germinates, changing back into the fully developed bacterium from which it came, it is known as a vegetative bacterium. The vegetative bacterium may then form a new endospore within its cell membrane if triggered to do so, and the cycle repeats itself, allowing bacteria to be extremely resistant under different environmental conditions.

Under conditions of starvation, especially the lack of carbon and nitrogen sources, an endospore may form within the bacterium. The process of forming an endospore is called sporulation, and this ability to package only its most essential components into a spore form allows bacteria to be extremely resistant. Endospores are resistant to antibiotics, most disinfectants, and physical agents such as radiation, boiling, and drying.

Although the endospores themselves are generally harmless until they germinate into a vegetative state, endospores are involved in the transmission of

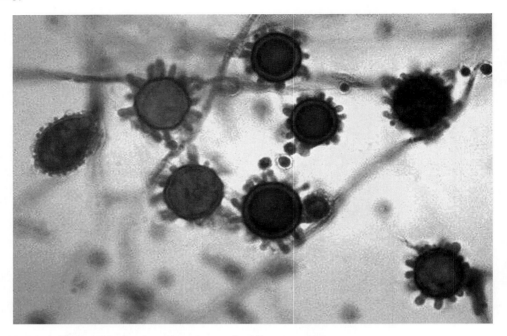

Figure 21-7 Note the tough outer wall of these spores. (Courtesy of the Centers for Disease Control and Prevention, Atlanta, GA.)

some diseases to humans. Infections transmitted to humans by endospores include anthrax, caused by *Bacillus anthracis*; tetanus, caused by *Clostridium tetani*; botulism, caused by *C. botulinum*; and gas gangrene, caused by *C. perfringens*.

Endospores are extremely important to embalmers because they are resistant to disinfectants. Embalming is fundamentally the disinfection, preservation, and restoration of human remains. The primary difference between disinfection and sterilization is that endospores are destroyed during sterilization, and endospores are not destroyed during disinfection. Since human remains are not sterilized, only disinfected, the presence of endospores is probable. This means that it is possible for disease to be spread from the deceased to the living by transmission of endospores.

Endospores also remain on countertops, embalming tables, embalming instruments, and other inanimate objects after terminal disinfection, unless these accessory instruments and equipment are sterilized or treated with sporicides. This is why it is so important for embalmers to always wear personal protective equipment in the embalming facility, where access must be restricted and limited only to essential personnel. The embalming room is never a place to socialize with other embalmers, and equipment that has entered the embalming room should not be utilized in other areas without first being sterilized.

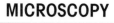

MICROSCOPY

Because microorganisms can have a variety of different structures, microbiologists use a number of methods to see them through a microscope. Since bacteria have unique characteristics such as different forms of motility and different structures, the scientist must first determine which structures should be observed and then utilize the appropriate technique to see them with the microscope. If the appropriate technique is not chosen, the bacterial structures appear transparent and motile bacteria would have to be motionless. There are two basic techniques used to observe the morphology of microorganisms through light microscopy. The living specimen may be observed by suspending it in some fluid such as water, or smears of the specimen may be dried, fixed, and stained on a piece of glass called a slide.

Fluid Suspensions

If the scientist wants to observe the structures of microorganisms while they are alive to see them move, the specimen is suspended in a fluid. One way to suspend microorganisms in a fluid is to use a hanging-drop technique, and the other method is to use a wet-mount technique. The hanging-drop and wet-mount techniques are used to observe the morphology of spiral bacteria, to observe the movement of bacteria, to observe cell inclusion bodies like fatty materials, or to observe cellular reproduction.

The wet-mount technique begins with a ring of petroleum jelly on the coverslip and then a drop of the specimen is added to the center of the coverslip. Then the glass slide is placed on the coverslip and the two are gently pressed together so they are sealed. When the slide is turned over, it can be placed on the microscope and the specimen can be observed through the coverslip. The petroleum jelly prevents airflow from disturbing the microorganisms. The wet-mount technique is best suited to the observation of large microbes such as fungi, protozoans, and yeasts. When suspended in fluid, both motile and non-motile bacteria exhibit Brownian movement, which is a rapid motion due to the movement of the liquid's molecules against the bacteria. Motile bacteria may dash about, spin, or move in a wavelike fashion.

Smearing

To observe the morphology of microorganisms, a thin layer of bacteria called a smear is typically prepared on a glass slide. A smear is prepared by using a special technique to place bacteria from a bacterial colony culture onto the slide with an inoculating loop, which is a loop of wire affixed to a handle. The specimen is allowed to dry on the slide. The bacteria is fixed to the slide by heating it so that the proteins in the bacteria coagulate and stick to the slide. The bacteria that have been fixed to the slide are not dead; the fixing simply prevents them from falling off the slide as it is handled. After drying and fixing the smear, it is typically stained so that the desired structures may be visualized with the microscope.

Staining

A common dye used to observe DNA or RNA in a cell is methylene blue. Both methylene blue and crystal violet are classified as basic dyes because the dye's ions have a positive charge and stain alkaline structures in cells. Acidic dyes such as acid fuchsin, Congo red, and eosin have a negative charge on the dye ion and are used to stain positively charged cellular proteins. Fats in cells are observable with a stain called Sudan black. All of these simple stains are designed to stain the entire cell so that its structure can be seen more clearly, while differential staining is far more complex because multiple stains are employed to stain certain parts of the cell.

Dr. Hans Christian Gram, a Danish physician working in a morgue in Berlin, developed Gram staining in 1884. Gram staining is one of the most important and widely used methods of classifying bacteria into two groups: gram-positive or gram-negative.

Gram staining occurs through a four-part process:

1. A purple dye is added to the bacteria fixed on a slide and all bacteria that are able to absorb this dye are stained purple.
2. A dilute solution of iodine is added, creating a less soluble dye-iodine complex.
3. An organic solvent such as ethanol is added to remove the purple dye-iodine complex from some but not all of the bacteria depending on the genus of the bacteria.
4. A red dye such as safranin is then applied, staining all the bacteria.

Bacteria that appear red had the dye-iodine complex removed during the process and are called gram-negative bacteria. Those bacteria that appear purple, due to masking of the red dye by the purple dye, are considered gram-positive bacteria.

Gram-positive bacteria have cell walls that are composed of few lipids, while gram-negative bacteria contain a high concentration of lipids in their cell walls. Gram-positive bacteria are more permeable to basic dyes, while gram-negative bacteria are less permeable to basic dyes. Gram-positive bacteria tend to have more complex nutritional requirements than gram-negative bacteria. Gram-positive bacteria are generally more resistant to physical treatment and exposure to some enzymes than gram-negative bacteria. Gram-positive bacteria are killed easily by penicillin and sulfonamide drugs, while gram-negative bacteria are more susceptible to streptomycin and tetracycline.

The proper staining method must be chosen to observe the desired structures on cells. Both the bacteria that cause tuberculosis, *Mycobacterium tuberculosis,* and the bacteria that cause leprosy, *M. leprae* are difficult to stain. The genus *Mycobacterium* is effectively stained with a solution to which 3 percent concentrated acid has been added, and it is, therefore, known as an acid-fast stain. Rickettsias cause such diseases as epidemic typhus, endemic typhus, Rocky Mountain spotted fever, and Q fever. Rickettsias are best observed after staining them in the cytoplasm of the host cell through a technique known as Giemsa staining. This method is also valuable in the examination of the Protozoan parasite that causes malaria, *Plasmodium malariae.* Capsule staining is useful in the examination of one cause of pneumonia known as *Streptococcus pneumoniae,* and bacterial endospores may be observed only with specialized spore stains. Flagella on bacteria are extremely fine, and deposits of tannic acid salts are applied prior to staining them to increase their diameter, so they can be observed under a light microscope. The correct choice of stain is an important part of the examination of any specimen.

REVIEW QUESTIONS

Matching

1. _____ bacillus
2. _____ flagella
3. _____ spirochete
4. _____ capsule
5. _____ morphology

a. bacteria that are surrounded by an axial filament and have a shape similar to a flexible corkscrew
b. an organized and firmly attached outer coating on some prokaryotic cells
c. bacteria shaped like a rod
d. the study of the size, shape, and arrangement of microorganisms
e. long, whiplike, filament-containing appendages that propel bacteria

Multiple Choice

1. Which of the following is a method of asexual reproduction in bacteria in which the cell splits into two parts, each of which develops into a complete individual?
   a. sporulation
   b. binary fission
   c. endospore formation
   d. vegetation
2. Bacteria shaped like a sphere are known as which of the following?
   a. coccus
   b. bacillus
   c. spirilla
   d. spirochete
3. Which of the following refers to bacteria with a spiral or helical shape?
   a. spirochete
   b. vibrio
   c. spirillum
   d. streptobacilli

4. Which of the following is a sticky, gelatinous coating that surrounds the cell wall of prokaryotic cells?

   a. flagella

   b. fimbriae

   c. pili

   d. glycocalyx

5. Which of the following is not a characteristic of gram-positive bacteria?

   a. They have a cell wall composed of few lipids.

   b. They are more permeable to basic dyes.

   c. They have less complex nutritional requirements.

   d. They are killed easily by penicillin and sulfonamide drugs.

Bibliography

Chamberlain, N. (2000a). *Introduction to microbiology*. Retrieved July 25, 2003, from the Kirksville College of Osteopathic Medicine at http://www.kcom.edu/faculty/chamberlain/Website/intmic.htm.

Chamberlain, N. (2000b). *Rickettsia, chlamydia, mycoplasma*. Retrieved July 15, 2003, from Kirksville College of Osteopathic Medicine at http://www.kcom.edu/faculty/chamberlain/Website/Lects/RICKETT.HTM#ri.

Edmonds, P. (1978). *Microbiology: An environmental perspective*. Basingstoke Hampshire, England: Macmillan Publishing.

Frobisher, M., Hinsdill, R., Crabtree, K., & Goodheart, C. (1974). *Fundamentals of microbiology*. Philadelphia: Saunders.

Gale, J. (2003). Bacteria. In *Watersheds*. Retrieved June 30, 2003, from the North Carolina State University Water Quality Group at http://h2osparc.wq.ncsu.edu/info/bacteria.html.

Gaudy, A., & Gaudy, E. (1980). *Microbiology for environmental scientists and engineers*. New York: McGraw-Hill.

Grover-Lakomia, L., & Fong, E. (1999). *Microbiology for health careers* (6th ed.). Clifton Park, NY: Thomson Delmar Learning.

Mahon, C., & Manuselis, G. (2000). *Textbook of diagnostic microbiology* (2nd ed.). Philadelphia: Saunders.

Maniloff, J., McElhaney, R., Finch, L., & Baseman, J. (Eds.). (1992). *Mycoplasmas: Molecular biology and pathogenesis*. Washington, D.C.: American Society for Microbiology.

Mayer, R. (2000). *Embalming: History, theory, & practice* (3rd ed.). New York: McGraw-Hill.

Neighbors, M., & Tannehill-Jones, R. (2000). *Human diseases*. Clifton Park, NY: Thomson Delmar Learning.

Nester, E., Anderson, D., Roberts, C., Pearsall, N., & Nester, M. (2001). *Microbiology: A human perspective* (3rd ed.). Boston: McGraw-Hill.

Pathology for funeral service. (1999). Dallas, TX: Professional Training Schools.

Rottem, S., & Kahane, I. (Eds.). (1993). *Mycoplasma cell membranes*. New York: Plenum Press.

Shelton, H. (1992). *Boyd's introduction to the study of disease* (11th ed.). Philadelphia: Lea & Febiger.

Stewart, K., & Stewart, D. (1998). *Bacteria and their characteristics*. Retrieved June 30, 2003, from the Food Safety Management Course, Stewart Enterprises at http://www.saturnnet.com/stewartent/webdoc201.htm.

Todar, K. (2002). Bacteria of medical importance. In *Todar's online textbook of bacteriology*. Retrieved July 18, 2003, from the Department of Bacteriology, University of Wisconsin-Madison at http://www.bact.wisc.edu/microtextbook/disease/overview.html.

Tortora, G., Funke, B., & Case, C. (1998). *Microbiology: An introduction* (6th ed.). Menlo Park, CA: Benjamin/Cummings Publishing.

Venes, D. (Ed.). (2001). *Taber's cyclopedic medical dictionary* (19th ed.). Philadelphia: F. A. Davis.

Wassenarr, T. (n/d). *Images of bacteria*. Retrieved July 25, 2003, from the Virtual Museum of Bacteria at http://www.bacteriamuseum.org/niches/features/morphology.shtml.

CHAPTER 22

Physiology of Bacteria

Learning Objectives

Upon completion of the chapter and review questions, the reader should be able to:

- Explain the nutrient requirements for the survival of microorganisms.
- Explain the oxygen requirements for the survival of microorganisms.
- Differentiate between optimal temperature, minimum temperature, and maximum temperature as related to microbial growth.
- Describe the role of osmotic pressure in microbial control.
- Compare and contrast between microbial associations.
- Explain the moisture requirements for the survival of microorganisms.
- Describe the role of pH in microbial control.

Key Terms

antagonism	mutualism
autotrophic	parasitism
commensalism	psychrophiles
facultative	saprophytes
heterotrophic	symbiosis
mesophiles	synergism
microaerophilic	thermophiles

REQUIREMENTS FOR THE SURVIVAL OF MICROORGANISMS

Regardless of size, every life-form has certain requirements that must be met to maintain life. From the smallest single-celled amoeba, to the largest multicellular whale, all life-forms have some essential similarities when it comes to maintaining life. They all have food, oxygen, moisture, temperature, pH, light, and osmotic pressure requirements. A large part of controlling the spread of disease is understanding the survival requirements of different microorganisms and then changing the microorganism's environment so that those requirements are not met; thus, the microorganism dies, and it can no longer cause disease (although the death and destruction of certain microbes by the body allows them to release injurious poisons).

Nutrients

Although all microorganisms must have some source of nutrients to survive, different microorganisms have different food requirements. Some microorganisms are capable of meeting their nutrient requirements without an external nutrient source, while others require specific nutrients from specific types of food sources. Still others are capable of adjusting to changes in the availability of external nutrient sources in their environment. They can support their growth by feeding on alternate internal nutrient resources when an external nutrient source is unavailable.

Autotrophic bacteria are self-nourishing bacteria capable of growing in the absence of organic compounds. Autotrophic organisms are capable of obtaining nutritional value from the carbon in carbon dioxide. One of the largest groups of autotrophic bacteria are the cyanobacteria. They receive their name from their appearance as blue-green algae; however, they are not algae, and they may be red or pink as well as blue-green. The red color of the Red Sea is due to cyanobacteria. The scum that exists near the edges of ponds is the result of autotrophic bacteria, and it can cause disease in humans if ingested.

Autotrophic bacteria produce about 20 percent of the Earth's oxygen and are capable of converting inorganic carbon dioxide into the nutrients they need through photosynthesis. Just like plants, autotrophic bacteria use light and carbon dioxide to produce their own food. Cyanobacteria are responsible for the continuation of the nitrogen cycle because they can convert atmospheric nitrogen into its organic form, which most life-forms in the world require for survival. By and large, autotrophic bacteria do not cause disease in humans, but they do cause some human diseases like swimmer's itch. They also participate in the decomposition of human remains.

Heterotrophic bacteria require complex organic food from a carbon source to grow and develop. Heterotrophic bacteria are the cause of numerous diseases in humans. Some heterotrophs are able to survive on a wide variety of organic compounds. For example, *Pseudomonas* is a genus of bacteria that is commonly associated with secondary infections in burn patients. These heterotrophic bacteria can survive on over 90 different organic compounds, including naphthalene, which is the active ingredient in moth balls and is also a solvent used in refinishing furniture to remove paint, stain, varnish, lacquer, and other finishing compounds. Not all heterotrophic bacteria cause disease, however. Some beneficial heterotrophs are integral to the process of fermentation, producing wine, bread, cheese, beer, and sauerkraut. There are three categories of heterotrophic bacteria: strict (obligate) saprophytes, strict (obligate) parasites, and facultative bacteria.

Strict **saprophytes** are organisms that only survive on dead or decaying organic matter. Strict parasites are completely dependent on their living host for the nutrients they need to survive. All viruses, viroids, and prions are obligate parasites because they lack the internal structures to produce energy or utilize food sources. **Facultative** bacteria can adapt to differing sources of nutrition. As food sources in the environment change, facultative bacteria simply feed on the new food sources or produce their own nutritional sources.

Oxygen

Just as all organisms have food requirements, all organisms have oxygen requirements. The oxygen requirements for microorganisms range from those that absolutely cannot survive if any oxygen is present, to those that must have an oxygen-rich environment. There are five classification of bacteria based on their oxygen requirements: obligate (strict) aerobes, obligate (strict) anaerobes, microaerophilic organisms, facultative organisms, and aerotolerant organisms.

Obligate aerobes are microorganisms that can only live in the presence of oxygen, because they need oxygen to metabolize sugars. If oxygen is not present, they are unable to produce energy. Certain intestinal diseases are caused by obligate aerobes like *Escherichia coli* and *Campylobacter jejuni*. Two genera of bacteria that are typically strict aerobes are *Bacillus* and *Pseudomonas*.

Obligate anaerobes are microbes that can only survive in an environment devoid of oxygen. In fact, some forms of oxygen, such as hydrogen peroxide, can be toxic to these bacteria, and some forms of oxygen can denature their enzymes. The anaerobic bacteria *Listeria* and *Clostridium botulinum* are common culprits in cases of food poisoning, and *C. perfringens* is an anaerobic bacterium directly involved in the decomposition of human remains.

Oxygen requirements are not always an either–or proposition, some bacteria survive in varying amounts of free oxygen. **Microaerophilic** microorganisms require little free oxygen (about 2 percent to 10 percent), and facultative bacteria are capable of adjusting to changes in oxygen levels in their environment. Diseases such as meningococcal meningitis, gonorrhea, and stomach ulcers are caused by the microaerophilic bacteria *Neisseria meningitidis, N. gonorrhoea,* and *Helicobacter pylori,* respectively. Aerotolerant organisms can grow in the presence or absence of oxygen. They differ from facultative bacteria in that they are indifferent to oxygen, and they do not gain any benefit from its presence. The diseases strep throat, rheumatic fever, scarlet fever, and puerperal sepsis are all caused by the same aerotolerant bacteria, *Streptococcus pyogenes.*

Moisture Requirements

All microorganisms require moisture, but the amount necessary for growth varies between species. Each microorganism has a maximum, optimum, and minimum amount of water necessary to sustain life. Generally, bacteria that can cause disease in humans require fairly high levels of moisture to grow, while molds and yeasts that can cause human diseases can grow in lower moisture levels. That is why most bacterial diseases occur in the body's tissues, while fungal diseases occur with greater frequency on the surface of the body.

Temperature

Temperature is a factor in the growth of microorganisms. There are three broad categories of bacteria based on their temperature requirements for growth: psychrophiles, mesophiles, and thermophiles. Organisms do not necessarily fit perfectly into each of these three categories, as some bacteria may grow at the extreme ends of each range. The organisms may also grow a little faster or a little slower based on the temperature. Each organism has its own minimum, maximum, and optimum temperature for growth. The minimum temperature is the temperature below which bacterial growth will not take place, while the maximum temperature is the temperature above which bacterial growth will not take place. The optimum temperature is the temperature at which the bacteria grow best.

Psychrophiles are bacteria that prefer cold, thriving at temperatures between 0°C and 25°C (32°–77°F). **Mesophiles** are bacteria that prefer moderate temperatures and grow best between 25°C and 40°C (77°–104°F). **Thermophiles** are bacteria that grow best at high temperatures, between 40°C and 70°C (104°–158°F). Some bacteria grow in the extremely high temperatures found inside of volcanoes at 105°C and 110°C (212°–230°F).

These variations in temperature preferences explain why some bacteria only grow in certain parts of the body. For example, the bacteria that cause leprosy and syphilis both prefer slightly cooler temperatures than that of the body's core, so they grow on the fingertips, toes, lips, and other cooler places on the body and not on the body's internal organs. A treatment for syphilis used to be giving the patient malaria so that the fevers associated with malaria would kill the bacteria that caused the syphilis.

Variations in temperature preferences of different bacteria are important to the embalmer because changes in body temperature occur before and after death influencing the rate of decomposition of the human remains. The deceased may have had a fever before death, resulting in what is known as agonal fever, or the deceased's body temperature may have cooled before death, which is known as agonal algor.

The natural cooling of the human remains occurs at the average rate of four degrees Fahrenheit the first hour after death and one degree Fahrenheit each hour thereafter, until room temperature is met. Placing the deceased in a refrigeration unit reduces bacterial decomposition by retarding the growth of mesophilic bacteria. Although some embalmers refer to these refrigeration units as freezers, that terminology is technically incorrect because their temperature is just above freezing. If the deceased's body were frozen, cellular damage would occur, and the arterial embalming would be inhibited.

pH

One important measure in the ability of organisms to survive in different environments is the pH of those environments. The pH scale is used to indicate pH, which refers to the concentration of hydrogen ions present. The pH scale ranges from 0 to 14, with 0 being extremely acidic and 14 being extremely alkaline (basic). A substance is neutral if its pH level is 7. The human body is slightly alkaline with a pH of 7.4. Bacteria that cause disease in humans thrive at this neutral pH, although many can survive as long as the pH level of their cytoplasm does not change.

Bacteria like *Helicobacter pylori*, which cause stomach ulcers, are able to survive the acids produced by the stomach because they contain an enzyme that allows them to split the urea found in the stomach into ammonia and carbon dioxide. The stomach acids are neutralized by the presence of the ammonia in the area of the bacteria, allowing the bacteria to survive. Yeasts and molds also grow well in an acidic environment, such as that found in the vagina.

Light

Light also affects microbial growth, depending on the type of microbe. For example, yeasts and molds do not contain chlorophyll, so they cannot utilize light to produce energy; therefore, they tend to prefer dark areas for maximum growth. The cyanobacteria are capable of converting light into a food source and thrive in its presence. Still other bacteria are destroyed by ultraviolet light.

Osmotic Pressure

Osmotic pressure can be defined as the pressure required to prevent the net flow of water across a semipermeable membrane, such as the cell membrane found in bacteria. When the fluids outside of the bacterial cell contain high concentrations of salt, the water inside the bacterium is drawn into the external fluid. This condition results in the cell membrane being drawn away from the rigid cell wall, and the cell membrane then collapses upon itself, effectively killing the bacterium. As the salt concentration outside the bacterial cell increases, the bacterium attempts to compensate by producing certain amino acids that help maintain the necessary water levels inside the bacterial cell. So, small changes in osmotic pressure may be compensated for by the bacterium, but larger changes result in its death. As a general rule, molds and yeasts are capable of withstanding greater changes in osmotic pressure than other microorganisms. Figure 22-1 illustrates the effects of osmotic pressure on a red blood cell.

The use of salts as a method of preserving meats, such as pork and fish, has occurred throughout humankind's history because high concentrations of salt retards microbial growth and inhibits decomposition of proteins. Sugar may also be used with a similar preservative effect in products like honey, which are naturally resistant to the decomposition effects of many bacteria. Osmotic pressure

Hypertonic Solution

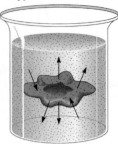

Hypotonic Solution

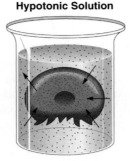

⁑ Water molecules

Isotonic Solution

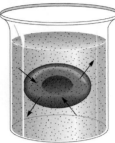

Hypertonic solution (seawater)
A red blood cell will shrink and
wrinkle up because water molecules
are moving out of the cell.

Hypotonic solution (freshwater)
A red blood cell will swell and burst
because water molecules are moving
into the cell.

Isotonic solution (human blood serum)
A red blood cell remains unchanged
because the movement of water molecules
into and out of the cell are the same.

Figure 22–1 The effects of osmotic pressure on a cell.

is high in many embalming fluids, which is one of the reasons that it retards microbial decomposition and decreases the spread of infectious disease from the deceased to the public.

MICROBIAL ASSOCIATIONS

Most microorganisms do not grow in isolation. Consider the nonliving viruses, viroids, and prions as examples. These intracellular parasites depend on a living host cell to provide the structures they lack to gain nourishment from their environment and to reproduce. In contrast to the nonliving microorganisms, multicellular molds contain the necessary structures for reproduction, but many are saprophytes that must have dead organic material as a carbon source because they lack the chlorophyll to produce energy themselves. The different types of associations microorganisms form with other organisms are related to both the formation of disease in humans and the decomposition of human remains. Although the following types of associations are important, it is equally important to recognize that in the real world it is not always possible to distinguish the level of benefit or harm any organisms receives from its associations.

When two or more different species of organisms live together in close association, the arrangement is known as **symbiosis**. Symbiotic relationships are distinguished by the degree to which the host organism is harmed. In a symbiotic relationship known as **mutualism**, two different species live in close association to the mutual benefit of each other. For example, E. coli exist in the human digestive tract, where they synthesize vitamin K and certain B vitamins. There they are also capable of breaking down cellulose found in foods like the outer covering of beans and kernels of corn, which would otherwise be indigestible for humans. Both the human being and the E. coli benefit from the symbiotic relationship, and neither is harmed, although the potential for harm exists because E. coli can cause disease if given the right circumstances.

Another symbiotic relationship, known as **commensalism**, exists when one organism gains some benefit, such as protection or nourishment, and the host is not harmed. Commensalism differs from mutualism in that both organisms gain a benefit in mutualistic relationships, but only one organism gains a benefit during commensalism. There are numerous bacteria that live on the surface of the skin, which neither benefit nor harm the human host. Additionally, the normal microorganisms within the digestive tract in the human body are benefited without harming the human host. An example of commensalism between larger organisms is the symbiotic relationship between remoras and sharks. Remoras have small sucking devices on their dorsal fin that allow them to attach to sharks. The sharks are not harmed, and the remoras save energy by not having to swim, and they get to eat the scraps when the sharks feed. This is an example of commensalism because the host shark gains no benefit and the remoras do gain benefits from the relationship.

Another type of symbiotic relationship is that of **parasitism**. In parasitic relationships, the host is harmed, while the parasite receives some benefit. All living organisms, including humans, can act as hosts for parasites. Typically, the host is a macroscopic organism, while the parasites are microscopic organisms such as bacteria, fungi, viruses, and protozoan. Occasionally, parasites are much larger multicellular organisms, like roundworms and flatworms.

When a symbiotic relationship produces a unique effect, it is referred to as a synergistic effect. A **synergism** occurs when the harmonious action of two microorganisms produces an effect that neither could produce alone. Synergistic infections due to animal bites, especially human bites, can be some of the most destructive to human tissues. Although the bacteria present normally in the mouth are not individually harmful, when they are forced into the tissues by the crushing powers of the jaws, they can develop into a serious infection. Certain enzymes are released from some bacteria that increase the rate of growth of other bacteria. At the same time, aerobic bacteria are utilizing available oxygen, so that anaerobic bacteria can grow where they normally could not. The combined effects of synergistic infections can result in irreversible tissue damage, which any one of the involved bacterial species could not have caused alone.

If all microorganisms were able to replicate without restraint, the world would quickly become oversaturated with microorganisms. One way that the growth of microorganisms is controlled is through the presence of antagonistic microorganisms. **Antagonism** is a mutual opposition or contrary action, and in the case of microbial relationships, the term refers to the inhibition of one microorganism's growth by the presence of another.

Normal flora, which are also known as normal microbiota, are the microorganisms present in the body that do not cause disease. They are on the skin and in the ears, eyes, mouth, nose, throat, urethra, intestines, and anus. Antagonism occurs when the normal flora inhibit the growth of other microorganisms by competing for nutrients or space, or by producing toxins that kill the microorganisms. The *lactobacilli* in the human vagina reduce the pH level to such an acid environment that other microorganisms are frequently incapable of growth, thus, reducing the risk of vaginal infections.

REVIEW QUESTIONS

Matching

1. _____ autotrophic bacteria
2. _____ heterotrophic bacteria
3. _____ obligate aerobes
4. _____ mutualism
5. _____ antagonism
4. _____ mutualism

a. microorganisms that can only live in the presence of oxygen
b. the inhibition of one microorganism's growth by the presence of another
c. self-nourishing bacteria capable of growing in the absence of organic compounds
d. two different species live in close association to the mutual benefit of each other
e. bacteria that require complex organic nutrients from a carbon source to grow and develop

Multiple Choice

1. Which of the following refers to organisms that only survive on dead or decaying organic matter?
   a. obligate anaerobes
   b. strict parasites
   c. obligate saprophytes
   d. autotrophic microbes

2. Which of the following terms describes the need for viruses, viroids, and prions to live only in a host cell due to their lack of internal structures that produce energy or utilize nutrients?
   a. heterotrophs
   b. microaerophilic
   c. saprophytes
   d. obligate parasites

3. Which of the following are bacteria that prefer moderate temperatures and grow best between 25°C and 40°C (77°–104°F)?
   a. psychrophiles
   b. mesophiles
   c. thermophiles
   d. facultative

4. Which of the following types of microorganisms would be most likely to survive in the dry air of the American Southwest?
   a. bacteria
   b. viruses
   c. prions
   d. fungi

5. Why do yeast infections occur more frequently in the vagina than other areas of the body?
   a. The vagina is more acidic and supports the growth of the fungi that cause yeast infections.
   b. The fungi causing yeast infections require more moist areas of the body to grow.

c. The fungi that cause yeast infections only grow on the penis and are spread sexually.

d. The fungi that cause yeast infections are indigenous to the vagina and cannot survive anywhere else.

Bibliography

Chamberlain, N. (2000a). *Introduction to microbiology*. Retrieved July 25, 2003, from the Kirksville College of Osteopathic Medicine at http://www.kcom.edu/faculty/chamberlain/Website/intmic.htm.

Chamberlain, N. (2000b). *Rickettsia, chlamydia, mycoplasma*. Retrieved July 15, 2003, from Kirksville College of Osteopathic Medicine at http://www.kcom.edu/faculty/chamberlain/Website/Lects/RICKETT.HTM#ri.

Edmonds, P. (1978). *Microbiology: An environmental perspective*. Basingstoke Hampshire, England: Macmillan Publishing.

Frobisher, M., Hinsdill, R., Crabtree, K., & Goodheart, C. (1974). *Fundamentals of microbiology*. Philadelphia: Saunders.

Gaudy, A., & Gaudy, E. (1980). *Microbiology for environmental scientists and engineers*. New York: McGraw-Hill.

Grover-Lakomia, L., & Fong, E. (1999). *Microbiology for health careers* (6th ed.). Clifton Park, NY: Thomson Delmar Learning.

Mahon, C., & Manuselis, G. (2000). *Textbook of diagnostic microbiology* (2nd ed.). Philadelphia: Saunders.

Mayer, R. (2000). *Embalming: History, theory, & practice* (3rd ed.). New York: McGraw-Hill.

Neighbors, M., & Tannehill-Jones, R. (2000). *Human diseases*. Clifton Park, NY: Thomson Delmar Learning.

Nester, E., Anderson, D., Roberts, C., Pearsall, N., & Nester, M. (2001). *Microbiology: A human perspective* (3rd ed.). Boston: McGraw-Hill.

Pathology for funeral service. (1999). Dallas, TX: Professional Training Schools.

Shelton, H. (1992). *Boyd's introduction to the study of disease* (11th ed.). Philadelphia: Lea & Febiger.

Stewart, K., & Stewart, D. (1998). *Bacteria and their characteristics*. Retrieved June 30, 2003, from the Food Safety Management Course, Stewart Enterprises at http://www.saturnnet.com/stewartent/webdoc201.htm.

Todar, K. (2002). Bacteria of medical importance. In *Todar's online textbook of bacteriology*. Retrieved July 18, 2003, from the Department of Bacteriology, University of Wisconsin-Madison at http://www.bact.wisc.edu/microtextbook/disease/overview.html.

Tortora, G., Funke, B., & Case, C. (1998). *Microbiology: An introduction* (6th ed.). Menlo Park, CA: Benjamin/Cummings Publishing.

Venes, D. (Ed.). (2001). *Taber's cyclopedic medical dictionary* (19th ed.). Philadelphia: F. A. Davis.

CHAPTER 23

Control of Microorganisms

Learning Objectives

Upon completion of the chapter and review questions, the reader should be able to:

- Differentiate between disinfection, sterilization, and antisepsis.
- List and describe the physical methods of controlling microorganisms presented in this chapter.
- Describe the factors influencing the effectiveness of chemical agents used to control microbial growth.
- List and describe the chemical methods of controlling microorganisms covered in this chapter.
- Compare and contrast carbolic acid, cresols, and hexachlorophene.

Key Terms

antisepsis
bactericides
disinfection
fungicides
germicides

insecticides
larvicides
sporicides
sterilization
viricides

 ## LEVELS OF CONTROL

Controlling the growth of microorganisms is one of the most important aspects of the embalming process, which has been defined as the temporary disinfection, preservation, and restoration of human remains. Controlling the growth of microorganisms is reflected in the first two aspects of the embalming process: disinfection and preservation. To protect the embalmer and the public from the possible transmission of disease-causing microorganisms from the human remains, embalmers must be knowledgeable of both the physical and chemical methods of controlling the growth of infectious organisms. In addition, if the deceased is to be successfully preserved, embalmers must retard the growth of microorganisms that contribute to the decomposition of the human remains.

There are three levels in controlling the growth of microorganisms: sterilization, disinfection, and antisepsis. **Sterilization** offers the highest level of microbial growth control. It is the process of completely removing or destroying all life-forms, endospores, or their products on or in a substance.

Disinfection is the destruction of pathogenic agents by chemical or physical means by applying the disinfectant to an inanimate object. Disinfection offers less control of the growth of microorganisms. The process of disinfection does not inactivate microbial endospores; however, it does kill most vegetative microorganisms. During disinfection, the number of microorganisms is reduced to the point that they no longer present a serious health hazard.

Antisepsis is the process by which microbial growth is inhibited on living tissue to prevent infection. Disinfectants are applied to inanimate objects, while antiseptics are applied to living tissue. Sanitization is the reduction of the microbial population to a safe level as determined by public health standards. There are both physical and chemical methods of controlling microbial growth.

PHYSICAL METHODS OF CONTROLLING MICROORGANISMS

The physical methods of controlling the growth of microorganisms include scrubbing, heat, cold, and ultraviolet light. In the embalming room, embalmers attempt to control the growth of microorganisms contaminating equipment, instruments, and the deceased.

Scrubbing

Whether trying to disinfect work surfaces and instruments, or whether trying to reduce the number of disease-causing microorganisms on the deceased, visible materials must first be removed to control the growth of microorganisms. Scrubbing is a manual process by which microorganisms are removed from a surface. Even the best sterilizers, disinfectants, and antiseptics will not effectively control the growth of microorganisms if the equipment, instruments, and deceased are covered in visible contaminants.

It should be noted that scrubbing should be vigorous and forceful on inanimate objects, but human remains should never be treated with great force due to the possible damage that can occur to the tissues of the body. The skin, hair, nails, and other body parts of the deceased can be damaged during aggressive scrubbing, which may lead to disruptions in the integument. If the skin is not intact, microorganisms can spread from the tissues of the deceased to the public, and microorganisms in the environment could invade the deceased's tissues, promoting accelerated decomposition. Embalming the deceased results in changes in the tissue that render the embalmed body an unsuitable food source for pathogenic microorganisms. Eruptions in the skin may also lead to leakage of body fluids, which can damage the deceased's clothing and the interior of the casket.

Temperature

Temperature is another physical method by which the growth of microorganisms can be controlled. Heat can be used to control the growth of microorganisms by incineration, dry heat, and moist heat, which are forms of boiling, free-flowing steam, and steam under pressure, respectively. Heat kills microorganisms by denaturing the proteins they contain, and proteins are denatured more easily when they are wet. The opposite extreme to heat, which is cold, can also be an effective means of controlling microbial growth.

The *thermal death point* is the lowest temperature at which all microorganisms are killed in 10 minutes. The *thermal death time* is the minimum time it takes to kill all microorganisms present. And the *decimal reduction time* is the time in minutes it takes to kill 90 percent of the present microorganisms.

Incineration. Incineration is used most frequently in funeral homes to treat hazardous waste. The biohazardous waste generated by a funeral home is typically removed by a hazardous waste handler, who gathers waste from several producers and transports it to a hazardous waste treatment facility. A common method of treating these large quantities of hazardous waste is incineration because it reduces the amount of waste to a more manageable quantity and form, ashes.

If incineration is to be an effective means of controlling microbial growth, all of the waste matter must be incinerated. To achieve this end, the waste matter must remain in the combustion chamber a sufficient time and at a high enough temperature for it to mix with the available oxygen to combust completely. If the waste matter does not burn completely, or if portions of the waste matter do not get enough oxygen to support combustion, it is possible that microorganisms will survive in those undercombusted materials. Incineration is a form of sterilization because both the vegetative bacteria and the bacterial endospore are inactivated during incineration.

Cremation. Cremation is a form of incineration. Human remains are placed inside the combustion chamber, which is also known as a retort, and a temperature of approximately 1600°F (871°C) is maintained until the remains have undergone complete combustion. The cremated remains are devoid of soft tissues and are completely sterilized. After cremation, they can no longer harbor infectious disease-causing microorganisms that could spread to the public or the crematory operator.

Dry Heat. There are several reasons why different forms of heat are good methods of controlling the growth of microorganisms. Heat kills microorganisms by coagulating the proteins they contain and breaking hydrogen bonds within the microorganisms. Fried eggs are an example of the coagulation of proteins by heat. The liquid egg white first becomes thick and gelatinous, and then it becomes firm and dry as the heat causes the proteins in the egg white to coagulate.

Although heat cannot be used to sterilize or even disinfect every surface because the object may not be able to withstand the heat, it is generally preferred to chemical methods of decontamination, which may leave behind a toxic residue. Dry heat requires much more exposure time than moist heat methods of decontamination. Dry heat is less effective than moist heat because proteins do not denature as easily when they are dry. As a comparison, 200°C (392°F) for 1.5 hours of dry heat is equivalent to 121°C (250°F) for 15 minutes of moist heat for killing the same amount of microorganisms.

Moist Heat. The three methods of moist heat decontamination are boiling, free-flowing steam, and steam under pressure. Boiling has been used since ancient times as a means of controlling microbial growth. At sea level, water boils at 100°C (212°F), and it takes approximately 10 minutes to sterilize water that does not contain endospores. Boiling kills vegetative bacteria, most viruses, and fungi. Boiling does not guarantee that endospores are killed, especially considering that water boils at less than 100°C above sea level. The endospores of the bacteria *Clostridium botulinum* and *C. perfringens* can survive many hours of boiling.

Another method of decontaminating objects such as instruments and equipment is through free-flowing steam. In a process known as fractional sterilization, items are placed in free-flowing steam for 30 minutes on successive days. On the first day, the items are introduced to the steam, which kills the vegetative bacteria but not the endospores. The materials are incubated overnight to allow the endospores to germinate into vegetative cells. On the second day, the objects are introduced to the free-flowing steam again, which kills the new vegetative cells. The objects are allowed to incubate overnight again, allowing any remaining endospores to germinate. On the third day, the objects are introduced to the free flowing steam again, and the new vegetative cells are destroyed.

Steam under pressure is the most effective form of controlling microbial growth because pressure, temperature, and length of exposure can be controlled. Figure 23-1 shows an autoclave, which is a piece of equipment that works like a pressure cooker. Water, or a liquid chemical, is placed into the autoclave. The items that need to be decontaminated are placed onto a tray inserted into the autoclave. The autoclave door is then closed and sealed, and the autoclave is set on a timer for a certain temperature and pressure.

Because the steam in an autoclave is under pressure, higher temperatures can be reached in a shorter time than can be achieved by simple boiling. The pressure also allows the steam to penetrate the objects to achieve greater decontamination. Steam produced by boiling water at sea level is 100°C (212°F), while steam produced at a higher pressure of 15 pounds per square inch is 121°C (250°F). Bacterial endospores are killed at the latter temperature but not the former. The requirement to kill bacterial endospores is 15 psi (pounds per square inch), at 121°C, for 15 minutes.

Cold. At the opposite temperature extreme, cold can be an effective means of controlling microbial growth. Both refrigeration and freezing are commonly

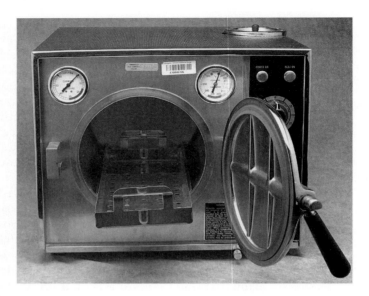

Figure 23-1 An autoclave.

used to preserve food by reducing microbial growth in cold environments. Refrigeration units in morgues are also used to cool human remains to a temperature that retards microbial growth. It is important to note, however, that cold temperatures do not destroy all vegetative cells or endospores. Cold temperatures inhibit the growth of microorganisms, which can begin multiplying again when they are introduced to warm temperatures. For example, in homicide cases in which the victim's body is discarded in a body of water, the decomposition of the remains is retarded during cold months but begins once the water warms. In warm weather, the microorganisms are not destroyed by the cold water, and they begin to digest the body's tissues, producing gases that cause the body to float to the surface.

Light

Ultraviolet (UV) light is a form of nonionizing radiation that can effectively control the growth of microorganisms placed directly in its path. It inhibits microbial growth by damaging the cell's genetic material. When exposed directly to UV light, some microorganisms develop bonds between adjacent thymines in their DNA. Thymines are aromatic bases, known as pyrimidines, produced by the body to form nucleic acids, which contain genetic material. The sun contains UV light; however, much of it is filtered by the Earth's ozone and never reaches the surface in a form that kills microorganisms. For UV light to be effective, the microorganism must be exposed to it directly. Even paper prevents UV light from penetrating enough to kill microorganisms, and many microorganisms contain pigments resistant to the detrimental effects of UV light.

CHEMICAL METHODS OF CONTROLLING MICROORGANISMS

Chemical antimicrobial agents fall into one of two broad categories based on their suffix. Those antimicrobial agents that end in the suffix *–cide* are agents that will kill a particular type of microorganism, while those that end in the suffix *–static* will prevent the growth of a particular type of microorganism. **Germicides** kill a variety of different types of microorganisms, but not necessarily their spores. **Bactericides** kill bacteria but not necessarily their spores. **Fungicides** kill both fungi and their spores. **Viricides** kill viruses. **Insecticides** kill insects, and **larvicides** kill larvae, which are the wormlike forms of newly hatched insects. Figure 23-2 pictures a technician applying a chemical antimicrobial agent to instruments as a method of terminal disinfection. **Sporicides**, agents that kill bacterial and mold spores, can also be used during the process of terminal disinfection of embalming instruments and equipment.

Factors Influencing Chemical Agents

Several factors influence the effectiveness of antimicrobial agents used to control microbial growth. Some of the most significant of those factors are:

- Nature of the disinfectant
- Concentration of the disinfectant
- Nature of the material to be disinfected
- Number of microorganisms present

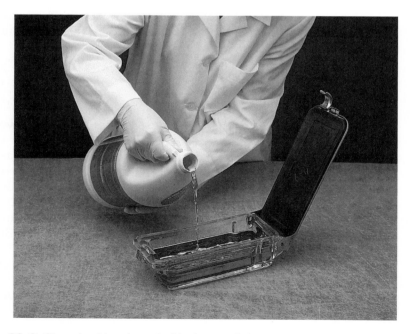

Figure 23–2 Chemical treatment of instruments to control microbial growth.

- Type of microorganism present
- Length of exposure to disinfectant
- Temperature of the disinfectant during exposure
- Disinfectant's pH during exposure

Larger populations of microorganisms take longer to kill than smaller populations. It is more difficult to control microbial growth when different species of microorganism are present on the object being decontaminated. Another factor influencing microbial growth is the state of development of the cells. Vegetative bacterial cells are easier to destroy than bacterial endospores. Higher concentrations of the antimicrobial agent are also generally more efficient, but the relationship is not linear. So, more antimicrobial agent does not necessarily mean that more microbes will be killed. In fact, sometimes adding more of a particular antimicrobial agent will induce growth in other types of microbes.

The longer the length of exposure of the microbe to the antimicrobial agent, the greater the number of microorganisms that will be killed. Higher temperatures will usually increase the effectiveness of the microbial agent's ability to kill the microorganism in question, but not always. Environmental factors such as pH, viscosity, and concentration of organic matter can also influence the effectiveness of a particular antimicrobial agent.

Although there are numerous chemical sterilants and disinfectants, not all of them are practical for mortuary purposes. For example, heavy metals such as silver, mercury, and copper are germicidal, but they are potentially hazardous to embalmers. However, not all heavy metals are hazardous; zinc-chloride contains a heavy metal and is found in mouthwash. The disinfectants suitable for mortuary procedures include halogens, alcohols, aldehydes, phenolic compounds, and quaternary ammonium compounds. Table 23-1 lists some chemical disinfectants used in healthcare settings, their uses, and the strengths at which they are used.

Halogens

Halogens are widely used disinfectants that work by oxidizing the components of microbial cells. Some halogens also react with cellular proteins. Halogens are the six elements found in the next to the last column on the far right side of the periodic table. The halogens share some commonalities, with the exclusion of hydrogen because it has its own unique properties, and astatine because it is radioactive. The remaining four halogens are fluorine, chlorine, bromine, and iodine. Each of these elements is extremely caustic and aggressive because each requires only one electron to reach stability. Both chlorine and iodine are used extensively as disinfectants.

Chlorine. Chlorine is used to treat municipal drinking water and for the maintenance of swimming pools. Chlorine is actually a gas, so it is often combined with water to form sodium hypochlorite. Household bleach contains about 5 percent sodium hypochlorite solution, which is several hundred times stronger than is needed to kill most disease-causing microorganisms. Chlorine is irritating to

Table 23-1 Chemical Disinfectants used in Health Care Settings and Their Recommended Strengths

Chemical	Uses	Common Recommended Strength
Phenol (carbolic acid)	Disinfects instruments, utensils, clothing, linen, sinks, toilets, excreta, floors; protective handwash for health care personnel	5% standard disinfectant
Lysol	Disinfects excreta, sinks, toilets, utensils; effective as a general disinfectant	2%–5%
Bichloride of mercury	Disinfects instruments, glassware, rubber articles; used in antiseptic ointments	0.1% (1 to 1000)
Formaldehyde	Disinfects excreta, linen, dishes, instruments, rubber gloves; tissue preservation and fumigation	1.5%–10%
Chlorine	Disinfects water supply, sewage, pools, bedpans, toilets, floors	Varies with amount of organic matter present
Ethyl or isopropyl alcohol	Preparation of skin prior to an injection or operation (scrubbing up); disinfects thermometers	70%
Hydrogen peroxide	Cleanses skin wounds, irrigates wounds; mouthwash, gargle	3%–20%
Iodine	Treats parasitic skin diseases, disinfects water, air (iodine vapors), food, utensils	2%
Mercurochrome	Wounds, abrasions, cuts	1%–2.5%
Metaphen	Skin	2%–5%
Argyrol (silver compound)	Infection of mucous membranes of eye, nose, throat, bladder (mild antiseptic)	10%–25%
Hexylresorcinol	Wounds, mouthwash, gargle	33⅓%
Acidine dyes: acriflavine and proflavine	Burns, wounds, ophthalmic applications, bladder irrigation	2%–3%
Sodium hypochloride	Spills, equipment, work areas	0.5%
Household bleach	Spills, equipment work areas	10%
New products for hands:		
Alcare®	Hand cleansing	Lotion with alcohol and aloe
Ultra safe®	Hand cleansing	Gel with alcohol and aloe Waterproof skin protectant
Antec®	Spills, counters, work area, equipment; bactericidal	1/50–1/200

the skin and mucous membranes, and it may react with certain organic compounds to form trihalomethane, which is a possible carcinogen. Hypochlorites are corrosive, and they do not make good sterilants due to the long exposure time required for them to kill endospores.

Iodine. Iodine, which controls microbial growth by oxidizing certain molecules within the microbial cell, can be used in the form of either a tincture or an iodophore. A *tincture* is a solution of iodine and alcohol that is primarily used as an antiseptic. Simply applying tincture of iodine to the skin does not assure sterilization because it does not kill endospores. Iodine can stain skin, but the stain can be removed with rubbing alcohol. An *iodophore* is a compound of iodine and a surfactant such as a detergent that can slowly release the free iodine. A common iodophore is providone-iodine, or Betadine, which is a common antiseptic. The most likely hazard associated with the use of tincture of iodine or iodophores as disinfectants and antiseptics in the embalming room would occur if the embalmer were allergic to iodine.

Alcohols

Alcohols, including ethyl alcohol and isopropyl alcohol, are used to control microbial growth. Alcohols are widely used disinfectants that control microbial growth by denaturing proteins and by dissolving lipids in the cell membrane of microorganisms. They are most effective in aqueous solution because proteins are not soluble in high concentrations of alcohol.

Alcohols are often added to other disinfectants such as iodine, chlorhexidine, and quaternary ammonium compounds to enhance their germicidal power. Alcohols are volatile, and they may evaporate before their germicidal effect occurs. Isopropyl alcohol also lacks the ability to destroy hydrophilic viruses, and neither isopropyl or ethyl alcohol can be used to sterilize instruments because they do not kill bacterial endospores. Alcohols are classified as intermediate-level disinfectants

Aldehydes

Aldehydes are a group of organic compounds that control microbial growth by reacting with the proteins in microorganisms and altering their chemical structure. In the early days of the poliovirus vaccine, low concentrations of formaldehyde were used to prepare the vaccine causing many people to contract the disease because the concentration of formaldehyde was not sufficient to produce a safe vaccine.

Formalin is a concentrated, liquid form of formaldehyde used as a disinfectant in which formaldehyde gas is dissolved in water. Formalin is 37 percent formaldehyde by mass and 40 percent formaldehyde by volume, which is an extremely concentrated form of formaldehyde used in mortuary preparations. Formaldehyde can cause irritation of the skin, eyes, nose, and throat. Ingestion of formaldehyde can cause severe pain, vomiting, coma, and death. Formaldehyde is also a possible carcinogen, meaning that it is a potential cause of cancer.

Glutaraldehyde is an effective disinfectant and is actually a cold chemical sterilant when activated in a 2 percent solution, which is germicidal in 10 minutes and kills endospores in 3 to 12 hours. Glutaraldehyde inactivates the DNA and RNA of microorganisms. Cold chemical sterilants like glutaraldehyde are important because they can be used on heat-sensitive objects like plastics, which would melt under high heat. Glutaraldehyde can also be used to sterilize embalming instruments when an autoclave is not available. It is less toxic than formaldehyde, and it is a common ingredient in hospital disinfectants. Glutaraldehyde is pH sensitive, and is only active in an alkaline environment. The possible side effects of glutaraldehyde include throat and lung irritation, headaches, difficulty breathing, nosebleeds, burning eyes, skin rash, brownish staining of the hands, hives, or nausea.

Phenolic Compounds

The phenolic compounds include phenol (carbolic acid), cresols (lysol), and hexachlorophene. Phenolics control microbial growth by denaturing proteins and disrupting cell membranes. In most cases, phenolic compounds are not effective in killing bacterial endospores, so they do not make good sterilants.

Carbolic Acid. Joseph Lister (1827–1912) first used phenol as a disinfectant during surgery to disinfect wounds. At that time, the idea that germs caused infections was new to medicine. Patients commonly died due to wound infection, and repeated amputations were not uncommon in the control of postoperative gangrene. Lister knew that phenol had been used to deodorize cesspools and drains, so he tried it on an 11-year-old boy who had an exposed bone in his leg, resulting from an accident with a cart. The boy survived and did not develop an infection. Joseph Lister was a pioneer in the reduction of postoperative infections and their related deaths. The commercial antiseptic Listerine is named after this English surgeon.

Phenol is slightly acidic, and is also known as carbolic acid. It has a sickeningly sweet and tarry odor and is available commercially as a liquid. Phenol is flammable, and skin exposure to phenol has been shown to cause chemical burns, liver damage, diarrhea, dark urine, and hemolytic anemia. Phenol is also breathed into the lungs when smoking tobacco. Due to its toxic nature, phenolic derivatives have replaced phenol as a disinfectant and antiseptic.

Cresols. Cresols are phenolic compounds derived from a chemical known as toluene. There are three slightly different forms of cresols known as ortho-cresol, meta-cresol, and para-cresol. These three forms of cresols can appear individually or in combination with each other. Cresols are also used to produce the commercial product Lysol; additionally, cresols are used as deodorants and to produce insecticides.

Cresols are found in wood, tobacco, crude oil, and creosote, which is used in the manufacture of telephone poles and treated lumber. Effects observed in people who have been exposed to high levels of cresols include irritation and burning of skin, eyes, mouth, and throat; abdominal pain and vomiting; heart damage; anemia; liver and kidney damage; facial paralysis; coma; and death. Cresols are commonly used in mortuary disinfectants because they work well in the presence of other organic compounds.

Hexachlorophene. Hexachlorophene is about 450 times more effective as a germicide than phenol. It is such an effective antibacterial agent that it was commonly used in soaps, deodorants, toothpaste, talcum powder, mouthwash, and shaving cream. Newborns were once bathed in it, and it was an ingredient in surgical scrubs. In 1972, 35 babies died in a Paris hospital due to hexachlorophene in their talcum powder. Chlorhexidine is less toxic than hexachlorophene, and it is effective in the control of a wider array of bacteria. It has replaced hexachlorophene in many surgical scrubs, in the disinfection of patient's skin prior to surgery, and as a wound cleanser. Hexachlorophene is now only available with a prescription, but it is an ingredient in several commercial embalming chemicals.

Quaternary Ammonium Compounds

Quaternary ammonium compounds, which are also known as quats, are chemical disinfectants and antiseptics that damage cellular membranes and denature microbial proteins. These surface active agents, or surfactants, are capable of altering the surface tension of cell membranes causing their cellular contents to leak out, thus destroying the cell. Quaternary ammonium compounds are deactivated in the presence of soap and other organic matter found in items like gauze.

Benzalkonium chloride is a topical antiseptic used on the skin before surgery, in nasal sprays to reduce the airborne transmission of disease in hospitals, and as a preservative in eye drops. Another member of the quats is benzethonium chloride, which is a topical antiseptic. Ceepryn chloride, or Cepacol, another quaternary ammonium compound, is commonly found in mouthwashes and throat lozenges.

The primary drawback of all of the quaternary ammonium compounds is that they are deactivated in the presence of soaps and other organic matter or any alkaline substance. The hazards associated with the quats are skin and respiratory irritation, and they may also cause birth defects in pregnant women, who may be exposed through inhalation, ingestion, or skin absorption.

REVIEW QUESTIONS

Matching

1. _____ fungicides
2. _____ Joseph Lister
3. _____ quaternary ammonium compounds
4. _____ iodophore
5. _____ halogens

a. a group of disinfectants that are deactivated in the presence of soap
b. first to use phenol as a treatment for wound infections
c. kill both fungi and their spores
d. a compound of iodine and a surfactant such as a detergent that can slowly release the free iodine
e. fluorine, chlorine, bromine, and iodine

Multiple Choice

1. Which of the following is the process of completely removing or destroying all life-forms, endospores, or their products on or in a substance?
   a. sterilization
   b. disinfection
   c. antisepsis
   d. scrubbing

2. Which of the following physical methods of sterilization incorporates both free-flowing steam and pressure?
   a. incineration
   b. cremation
   c. autoclaves
   d. boiling

3. Which of the following is a concentrated, liquid form of formaldehyde, which is 37 percent formaldehyde by mass and 40 percent by volume?
   a. Cepacol
   b. formalin
   c. glutaraldehyde
   d. tincture

4. Which of the following is an effective disinfectant and a cold chemical sterilant?
   a. iodine
   b. isopropyl alcohol
   c. halogens
   d. glutaraldehyde

5. Which of the following types of disinfectants includes benzalkonium chloride?
   a. quaternary ammonium compounds
   b. phenols
   c. halogens
   d. bleaches

Bibliography

Chamberlain, N. (2000a). *Introduction to microbiology*. Retrieved July 25, 2003, from the Kirksville College of Osteopathic Medicine at http://www.kcom.edu/faculty/chamberlain/Website/intmic.htm.

Chamberlain, N. (2000b). *Rickettsia, chlamydia, mycoplasma*. Retrieved July 15, 2003, from Kirksville College of Osteopathic Medicine at http://www.kcom.edu/faculty/chamberlain/Website/Lects/RICKETT.HTM#ri.

Control of microbial growth. (2003). Retrieved July 15, 2003, from the Department of Biology, City College of San Francisco at http://www.ccsf.edu/Departments/Biology/control.htm.

Decontamination. (2002). Retrieved July 15, 2003, from the University of Arizona Institutional Biosafety Committee at http://www.ibc.arizona.edu/WebBiosafetyman/ManCh14.html.

Edmonds, P. (1978). *Microbiology: An environmental perspective*. Basingstoke Hampshire, England: Macmillan Publishing.

Formaldehyde, Appendix A. (n.d.). Retrieved July 15, 2003, from the California Code of Regulations, Title 8, Division 1, Chapter 4, Subchapter 7, Group 16, Article 110, California Department of Industrial Relations at http://www.dir.ca.gov/title8/5217a.html.

Frobisher, M., Hinsdill, R., Crabtree, K., & Goodheart, C. (1974). *Fundamentals of microbiology*. Philadelphia: Saunders.

Gale, J. (2003). Bacteria. In *Watersheds*. Retrieved June 30, 2003, from the North Carolina State University Water Quality Group at http://h2osparc.wq.ncsu.edu/info/bacteria.html.

Gaudy, A., & Gaudy, E. (1980). *Microbiology for environmental scientists and engineers*. New York: McGraw-Hill.

Glutaraldehyde: Occupational hazards in hospitals. (2001). Retrieved July 15, 2003, from the National Institute of Occupational Safety and Health, Centers for Disease Control and Prevention at http://www.cdc.gov/niosh/2001-115.html.

Grover-Lakomia, L., & Fong, E. (1999). *Microbiology for health careers* (6th ed.). Clifton Park, NY: Thomson-Delmar Learning.

Hexachlorophene. (2003). Retrieved July 15, 2003, from the Integrated Risk Information System, U.S. Environmental Protection Agency at http://www.epa.gov/iriswebp/iris/subst/0338.htm.

Infectious waste management. (2002). In *Biological safety manual*. Retrieved July 15, 2003, from the Department of Environmental Health and Safety, University of Texas at El Paso at http://www.utep.edu/eh&s/ppm/biosafety/management.html

Issues in healthcare settings: Sterilization and disinfection. (n.d.). Retrieved July 25, 2003, from the Division of Healthcare Quality Promotion, Centers for Disease Control and Prevention at http://www.cdc.gov/ncidod/hip/Sterile/sterile.htm.

Krishna, G., Martin, S., & Brockmeir, B. (2002). *Physical and chemical control*. Retrieved July 15, 2003, from the Department of Biology, Moberly Area Community College at http://www.macc.cc.mo.us/~biology/Phys_Chem_Control.html.

Levy, S. (2001). Antibacterial household products: Cause for concern. In *Emerging Infectious Diseases*. Retrieved July 15, 2003, from the Centers for Disease Control and Prevention at http://www.cdc.gov/ncidod/eid/vol7no3_supp/levy.htm.

Mahon, C., & Manuselis, G. (2000). *Textbook of diagnostic microbiology* (2nd ed.). Philadelphia: Saunders.

Mayer, R. (2000). *Embalming: History, theory, & practice* (3rd ed.). New York: McGraw-Hill.

Neighbors, M., & Tannehill-Jones, R. (2000). *Human diseases*. Clifton Park, NY: Thomson Delmar Learning.

Nester, E., Anderson, D., Roberts, C., Pearsall, N., & Nester, M. (2001). *Microbiology: A human perspective* (3rd ed.). Boston: McGraw-Hill.

Pathology for funeral service. (1999). Dallas, TX: Professional Training Schools.

Sepsis: What you should know. (2003). In *ICU Issues and Answers*. Retrieved July 26, 2003, from the Society of Critical Care Medicine at http://www.sccm.org/patient_family_resources/brochures/sepsis.asp.

Shafer, R. (1999). Sterilization, disinfection, and antisepsis. Retrieved July 15, 2003, from the Robert C. Byrd Health Sciences Center, West Virginia University: http://www.hsc.wvu.edu/som/micro/MB26VIEW/lecture6.

Shelton, H. (1992). *Boyd's introduction to the study of disease* (11th ed.). Philadelphia: Lea & Febiger.

Tortora, G., Funke, B., & Case, C. (1998). *Microbiology: An introduction* (6th ed.). Menlo Park, CA: Benjamin/Cummings Publishing.

Tox FAQs for cresols. (2001). Retrieved July 15, 2003, from the Agency for Toxic Substances and Disease Registry, Centers for Disease Control and Prevention at http://www.atsdr.cdc.gov/tfacts34.html.

Tox FAQs for phenol. (2001). Retrieved July 15, 2003, from the Agency for Toxic Substances and Disease Registry, Centers for Disease Control and Prevention at http://www.atsdr.cdc.gov/tfacts115.html.

Universal precautions. (2001). Retrieved July 26, 2003, from the National Institute of Environmental Health Sciences, National Institutes of Health at http://www.niehs.nih.gov/odhsb/biosafe/univers.htm.

Using alcohol as a disinfectant. (2001). Retrieved July 15, 2003, from the Association for Assessment and Accreditation of Laboratory Animal Care International at http://www.aaalac.org/index.html.

Venes, D. (Ed.). (2001). *Taber's cyclopedic medical dictionary* (19th ed.). Philadelphia: F. A. Davis.

What are universal precautions? (2002). Retrieved July 26, 2003, from the Canadian Centre for Occupational Health and Safety at http://www.ccohs.ca/oshanswers/prevention/ppe/universa.html.

Xintarus, C. (1995). *Formaldehyde*. Retrieved July 15, 2003, from the Agency for Toxic Substances and Disease Registry, Centers for Disease Control and Prevention at http://www.atsdr.cdc.gov/mmg9.html.

CHAPTER 24

Microbe Virulence and Human Resistance

Learning Objectives

Upon completion of the chapter and review questions, the reader should be able to:

- List and describe the four factors that influence the occurrence of disease.
- Differentiate between exogenous, endogenous, local, focal, general, primary, secondary, and mixed infections.
- Describe the roles of host, reservoir, vector, and pathogen in the spread of disease.
- Discuss both direct and indirect modes of the transmission of disease.
- List the body's defenses against infection, and describe the types of immunity discussed in this chapter.

Key Terms

antibodies
antigen
attenuation
biological vectors
contamination
drug-fast
host
mechanical vector
opportunists

pathogen
pathogenicity
reservoir
resistance
septicemia
toxemia
universal precautions
virulence

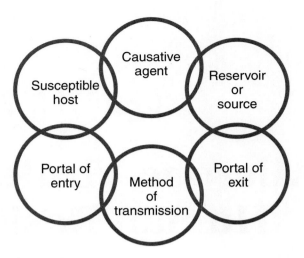

Figure 24-1 The chain of infection.

FACTORS INFLUENCING THE OCCURRENCE OF DISEASE

Infections occur when certain conditions are met. Figure 24-1 illustrates these conditions, which are referred to as the *chain of infection*. The chain begins with a causative agent, which can be any pathogenic microorganism. The pathogen must have a reservoir in which it can survive, such as the human body. **A reservoir** is the natural habitat of a disease-causing organism. The pathogen then exits the reservoir and is transmitted to a new host. The pathogen enters the new host through one of its portals of entry, such as the nose or mouth of a human. Finally, the new host becomes ill from the disease if the proper conditions are met.

Not every person who is infected with a pathogen will develop disease. Why is it that some individuals appear more prone to disease than others, and why do some diseases appear to occur more frequently? The answers to these questions lie in the relationship between the virulence of the microorganism and the resistance of the host. There are four factors that influence the occurrence of disease:

1. The virulence of the organisms
2. The portal of entry of the pathogen
3. The number of organisms present
4. The resistance of the host

VIRULENCE, RESISTANCE, AND INFECTION

The ability of the microorganism to survive is referred to as its virulence, while the ability of the human to defend against the pathogen is known as resistance. More specifically, **virulence** is the relative power and degree of pathogenicity possessed by organisms to produce disease, while **resistance** is the sum total of body mechanisms that interpose barriers to the progress of invasion, multiplication of infectious agents, or damage by their toxic products. The **host** is the organism from which a parasite obtains its nourishment, while a **pathogen** is an organism capable of producing disease. Stated differently, the host is the person who has the disease and the pathogen is the germ that causes the disease.

The act of introducing disease germs or infectious material into an area or substance is known as contamination. When disease-causing microorganisms are spread to humans, it is often the result of contact with contaminated surfaces. Being contaminated by the presence of microorganisms does not necessarily result in infection with disease. *Infection* is the state or condition in which the body, or part of the body, is invaded by a pathogenic agent that, under favorable conditions, multiplies and produces injurious effects. Pathogenicity is the ability to produce pathological changes and disease.

One reason why disease may not ensue after contact with a contaminated source is related to the microbe's virulence. Some microorganisms are real or genuine disease-producing organisms, and they are known as true pathogens. Other microorganisms, known as **opportunists**, exist as part of the normal microbial flora but can become pathogenic under certain conditions and result in disease. If a microorganism is virulent enough to resist pharmaceuticals designed to reduce disease, it is referred to as **drug-fast**. The reduction of a microorganism's virulence by diluting or weakening the microbe to reduce or abolish its pathogenicity is known as **attenuation**.

Exogenous and Endogenous Infections

Infection is the state or condition in which the body or a part of the body is invaded by a pathogenic agent that, under favorable conditions, multiplies and produces injurious effects. The source of the infection can be spread from the normal flora inside the human digestive tract, or it can arise from microorganisms transmitted from the outside of the body. Infections caused by bacteria that are normally nonpathogenic and that normally inhabit the digestive tract are known as endogenous infections, while infections caused by organisms not present in the body are called exogenous infections.

Communicable Diseases

Communicable diseases are those diseases that may be transmitted directly or indirectly from on individual to another. Endemic diseases occur continuously in a particular region but usually have a low mortality. Sporadic diseases occur occasionally or in scattered instances within a geographic region. Epidemic diseases are diseases that attack many people at the same time in the same geographic region, while pandemic diseases affect the majority of the population of a large region or are epidemic at the same time in many different parts of the world. Although some diseases are communicable, others do not spread from one person to another and these diseases are called noncommunicable diseases.

Local, Focal, and General Infections

Once an isolated area of the body becomes infected, the potential exists for the infection to spread throughout the body. A local infection is caused by microorganisms lodging and multiplying at one point in a tissue and remaining in that tissue. An abscess is a localized infection characterized by a collection of pus in any part of the body that results from disintegration or displacement of tissue. A focal infection is one in which the organisms are originally confined to one area but enter the blood or lymph vessels and spread to other parts of the body. Focal infections may arise from infections of the teeth, tonsils, or sinuses. If the infection becomes systemic, it is known as a general infection. Measles is an example of a systemic infection.

Primary, Secondary, and Mixed Infections

Some infections lead to more infections. An acute infection that causes the initial illness is known as a primary infection. Once the primary infection weakens the host, a secondary infection caused by a different organism can develop. Secondary infections of the skin and respiratory tract are common and may be more dangerous than the primary infection. Pneumocystis pneumonia is a secondary infection in cases of AIDS that is often fatal. Color Plate 37 is a photograph of lesions resulting from a secondary viral herpes simplex infection that occurred in a person who was under stress and already had a primary bacterial meningococcal infection.

A mixed infection is caused by two or more organisms. Infections that result from human bites frequently develop into mixed infections because the human mouth is a reservoir for a wide variety of microorganisms (Figure 24-2). These organisms typically do not result in infections in the mouth because they are not true pathogens. However, when these many different types of microorganisms are introduced deep into the tissues of the body by the crushing, penetrating action of the teeth, they can result in mixed infections in the injured tissue.

Blood Infections

There are many types of microorganisms that can infect the blood. The presence of viruses in the blood is known as *viremia*. The presence of bacteria in the blood is referred to as *bacteremia,* which can lead to death due to sepsis or toxic shock. **Septicemia**, which is commonly known as blood poisoning, occurs when the bacteria actually multiply in the blood. If the infection is allowed to progress, the bacteria can multiply and cause an overwhelming, fatal infection. The spread of bacteria through the blood in cases of septicemia sometimes causes a rash on the torso of the body, as indicated in Color Plate 38. Septicemia is also characterized by the following:

- Chills and fever
- Petechiae (pinpoint bleeding)
- Bleeding pustules

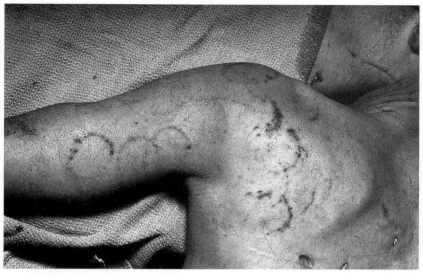

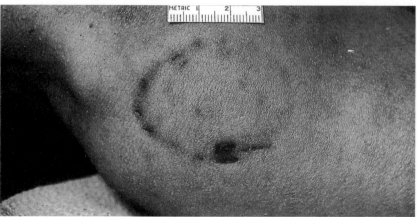

Figure 24-2 Bite marks. (Reprinted with permission from Vincent J. DiMaio and Dominick DiMaio, 2001, *Forensic pathology*, 2nd ed. Copyright CRC Press, Boca Raton, FL.)

- Abscesses
- Shock

Local or focal bacterial infections do not always develop into septicemia, but if the bacteria release poisonous toxins into the tissues, the toxin may spread throughout the body. **Toxemia** is the distribution throughout the body of poisonous products of bacteria growing in a focal or local site, thus producing generalized symptoms, which may include fever, diarrhea, vomiting, either an increase or decrease in pulse and respiration, and eventually shock and death. In cases of tetanus, the nervous system is especially affected, while in cases of diphtheria both nerves and muscles are involved. Table 24-1 lists examples of

Table 24-1 Examples of Bacteria That Produce Toxins, the Diseases They Cause, and Their Effects in the Body

Bacterium	Disease	Toxin's Effects
Bacillus anthracis	Anthrax	Swelling and bleeding in tissues; cardiovascular failure
Bordetella pertussis	Pertussis (whooping cough)	Damages cells of the respiratory tract by destroying cilia
Clostridium botulinum	Botulism	Causes paralysis by inhibiting the release of acetylcholine from nerve endings
C. tetani	Tetanus	Impairs the nervous system's ability to remove acetylcholine from nerves, which causes muscle spasms
Corynebacterium diphtheriae	Diphtheria	Blocks protein synthesis of cells in the nerves, heart, and kidney
Staphylococcus aureus	1. Scalded skin syndrome	1. Layers of skin separate, blister, and slough off
	2. Food Poisoning	2. Excessive secretion of intestinal fluids causes diarrhea
Vibrio cholerae	Cholera	Damages cells of the small intestine, causing extreme diarrhea

bacteria that produce toxins, the diseases they cause, and the effects of the toxin in the body.

Bacterial toxins may also have beneficial effects in humans. For example, *Clostridium botulinum* produces an extremely powerful poison. Although it can cause a type of food poisoning known as botulism, one type of toxin it produces is used in humans for both cosmetic treatments and to inhibit muscle spasms. Botox is a derivative of the botulin toxin produced by *C. botulinum*, which requires only a few milligrams to kill the entire population of a large city, but can also be used to remove facial lines. The Botox is extremely diluted and injected directly into facial lines, where it causes the muscles to relax. The treatment is temporary because the effects of the toxin wear off, and the procedure must be repeated within a few months. In diseases like cervical dystonia and Parkinson's disease, in which severe, involuntary muscle cramps occur, injections of diluted Botox directly into the muscles gives relief for months.

Factors Influencing the Virulence of Microorganisms

Microorganisms are more virulent, and thus more capable of producing disease in humans, if they contain or can produce toxins. Toxins are a poisonous substance of plant, animal, bacterial, or fungal origin. An *exotoxin* is a toxin, generally a protein, produced by a microorganism and excreted into its surrounding medium. In contrast, an *endotoxin* is a bacterial toxin confined within the body of a bacterium that is freed only when the bacterium is broken down. Endotoxins are found only in gram negative bacteria. Both *Staphylococcus aureus*, which causes toxic shock syndrome, and *C. tetani*, which causes tetanus, are virulent microorganisms because of their use of toxins. *S. aureus* contains an exotoxin that it releases into the tissues causing disease, while the endotoxin associated with *C. tetani* is released on the lysis of the bacterium by the immune system cells.

Some microorganisms are more virulent due to their ability to produce enzymes that damage human tissues. Hyaluronidase can cause blood to clot, resulting in the presence of fibrin threads in the blood. Another enzyme known as fibrinolysin is capable of digesting these fibrin threads. Coagulase is an enzyme that aids in the blood's ability to clot. These three enzymes can be used by certain bacteria to better use blood as a nutrient source, which results in disease in the infected human. *S. aureus* is a good example of a bacterium that uses enzymes to enhance its virulence.

There are three enzymes produced by *S. aureus* that add to its virulence: coagulase, hyaluronidase, and lipase. Coagulase causes blood to clot by converting fibrinogen into fibrin. Hyaluronidase allows *S. aureus* to penetrate the body's connective tissues, permitting it to spread throughout the body. Lipase acts with the oils and fats secreted by the sebaceous glands, allowing *Staphylococci* to colonize in the skin.

Microorganisms that contain a capsule or that can produce endospores are virulent. These microorganisms are capable of withstanding changes in the environment. The capsule helps protect the microorganism from antimicrobial agents, and the endospores allow the microorganism to assume a "dormant" form until a more suitable environment for survival is present. Both the capsule and the endospores help the microorganism survive changes in temperature, moisture, pH, light, and osmotic pressure that could otherwise be damaging to it. They also help the microorganism withstand periods in which a nutrient source is not readily available.

SOURCES OF THE SPREAD OF DISEASE

Diseases caused by infectious pathogens are spread through three sources of infection: (1) animals or persons ill of the infection; (2) chronic animal or human carriers; and, (3) the environment. The ability of a pathogen to spread depends on its specific reservoir. The natural habitat of a disease-causing organism is known as its reservoir.

The reservoir of a pathogen is important because it affects the extent and distribution of a disease. The disease coccidioidmycosis, for example, is endemic to the hot, dry, dusty areas of the Western Hemisphere because its causative agent, the fungus *Coccidioides immitis,* can only survive under these conditions. Table 24-2 lists examples of microorganisms, the diseases they cause, their reservoirs, and their mode of transmission.

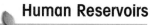

Human Reservoirs

One of the most important reservoir for disease transmission is infected humans. Diseases spread by human reservoirs are also often some of the easiest to control. In some cases, the pathogen in human reservoirs can also spread

Table 24–2 Examples of Microorganisms, Diseases, Reservoirs, and Methods of Transmission

Microorganism	Disease	Reservoir	Transmission
Bacillus anthracis	Anthrax	Livestock	Contact with contaminated air, food, or animal hides
Borrelia burgdorferi	Lyme disease	Field mice, deer	Tick bite
Chlamydia psittaci	Parrot fever	Birds	Direct contact
Coxiella burnetii	Q fever	Livestock	Inhalation, livestock hides, milk, etc.
Francisella tularensis	Tularemia	Wild rabbits	Deer-fly bites and contact with contaminated rabbits
Leptospira	Leptospirosis	Wild mammals, dogs, cats	Contact with urine, soil, or water
Rabies virus	Rabies	Bats, skunks, foxes, dogs, cats	Bite
Rickettsia rickettsii	Rocky Mountain spotted fever	Rodents	Tick bite
R. typhi	Typhus fever	Rodents	Flea bite
Salmonella species	Salmonellosis	Poultry, rats, turtles	Eating contaminated food or water
Trichophyton; microsporum; epidermophyton	Ringworm	Domestic mammals	Direct contact and nonliving objects
Yersinia pestis	Plague	Rodents	Flea bites

through animal reservoirs, or even the environment. When infected humans are the only reservoir, the disease can often be controlled through programs aimed at its elimination.

The eradication of smallpox is an example of a disease that virtually no longer exists but was once one of the largest killers in the world. The smallpox virus was eliminated by a global effort to vaccinate individuals before they became infected and to isolate those who were infected. By controlling the human reservoir that the smallpox virus needs to survive, scientists were able to virtually eradicate a deadly disease from the world. Although smallpox was officially eradicated in 1980, the CDC (*Smallpox emergency* 2002) now considers smallpox to be a potential bioterrorism threat and has prepared a smallpox response plan.

Universal Precautions.   It is not always possible to tell if someone is infected with a disease-causing pathogen. Take the case of the sexually transmitted disease gonorrhea as an example. Up to 50 percent of women infected with the bacterium *Neisseria gonorrhoeae* are asymptomatic, meaning they show no obvious signs or symptoms of the disease. Although gonorrheal infections can be treated with antibacterial drugs, isolating everyone who is infected is nearly impossible due to cost and difficulty.

A paramount assumption within the deathcare industry is that there is no 100 percent effective method of identifying a person who harbors a disease-causing pathogen. Since it is not possible to eliminate anyone from being suspect of being infected by a pathogenic microorganism, it is necessary to treat all human remains as though they are potential carriers of disease. **Universal precautions** are the guidelines designed to protect workers with occupational exposure to bloodborne pathogens. They were recommended initially in 1985 by the Centers for Disease Control and Prevention, and they became required by OSHA in 1991 for all healthcare workers. Protection of the funeral service practitioner begins by following these guidelines:

- All human remains are to be treated as though they are infectious.
- Always wear appropriate personal protective clothing, including gloves, face shield, mask, full-length gown, head cover, and shoe covers, as pictured in Figure 24-3.
- Topical disinfectants should be utilized to disinfect the deceased, the deceased's clothing, and the removal cot. Linen should always be laundered between removals.
- Always handle the deceased's clothing with care to inhibit the aerosolization of microorganisms.
- Avoid spattering body fluids by utilizing drain tubes and closed drainage systems, and cleaning up body fluids from contaminated surfaces immediately (Figure 24-4).

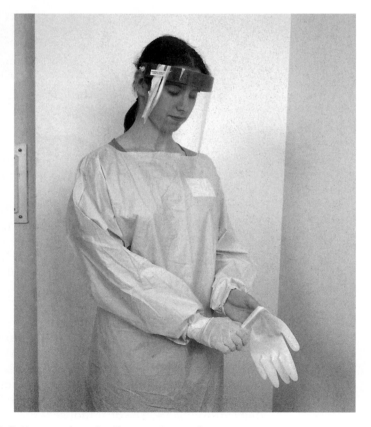

Figure 24–3 Personal protective equipment.

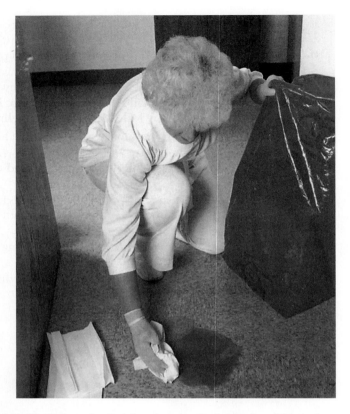

Figure 24-4 Spilled chemicals, blood, or body fluids should be cleaned up immediately.

- Always utilize approved sharps containers for the disposal of sharps such as needles, needle injector wires, and scalpel blades.
- Always utilize approved biohazardous waste containers and dispose of waste via an approved biohazardous waste handler.
- Always disinfect all work surfaces, instruments, equipment, and floors in the embalming facility after each embalming.
- Embalmers should always wash their hands on leaving the embalming facility and shower after embalming (Figure 24-5).

Nonhuman Animal Reservoirs

Some pathogens are harbored by nonhuman animal reservoirs. Both *Campylobacter* and *Salmonella* are bacteria found in infected poultry. Rabies, which is caused by a virus, is another disease that is found in wildlife such as foxes, raccoons, skunks, rabbits, bats, mice, chipmunks, squirrels, and even cattle. Even the innocent-looking prairie dog is host to the deadly bacterium *Yersinia pestis* that causes plague. The deer mouse is reservoir to hantavirus, which has become more significant since the late 1980s.

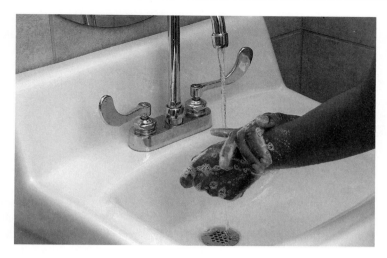

Figure 24–5 Hand washing is an essential component of limiting the spread of disease.

Environmental Reservoirs

Environmental reservoirs are largely found in water and soil. *Clostridium botulinum*, which causes botulism, and *C. tetani*, which causes tetanus, are both widespread in soils. A more recently discovered disease, Legionnaires' disease, is transmitted by contact with amebas in contaminated water found in air conditioning units on buildings. Contaminated items in the embalming room, such as sponges, may serve as a temporary reservoir long enough for the embalmer to become infected.

MODES OF TRANSMISSION OF DISEASE

For a disease to spread, the disease-causing pathogen must be able to move from its infected reservoir to its next potential host. There are two modes of transmitting infection: direct and indirect. The three mechanisms of direct transmission include physical contact, droplet infection, and congenital transmission. Some of the more common forms of indirect transmission of infection are food, milk, fomites, water, soil, and both biological vectors and mechanical vectors.

Direct Transmission of Infection

Direct transmission of infectious agents is usually associated with some form of contact, typically person-to-person contact through casual or intimate contact. Shaking hands is an example of casual contact, while sexual intercourse is an intimate form of contact. The type of direct contact required to allow transmission is determined largely by the virulence of the microorganism.

Although physical contact includes several mechanisms of direct contact between individuals that result in the spread of disease-causing pathogens, fecal-oral transmission and sexual transmission are two of the most common. In the course of shaking hands, for example, more virulent microorganisms, such as the intestinal pathogen *Shigella*, are capable of being spread from person to person.

Since it only takes about 10 to 100 *Shigella* organisms to induce infection in a new host, shaking hands is enough contact between individuals to result in the spread of disease. After the host's hand is contaminated, the bacteria can enter the body through a break in the skin or contact between the contaminated hand and the eyes, nose, or mouth. The transmission of *Shigella* is an example of the fecal-oral route of transmission. One of the easiest methods of diminishing the spread of disease is to combat the fecal-oral route of transmission through proper hand washing.

Sexually transmitted diseases are also spread through direct contact between individuals. Since many of the sexually transmitted diseases are caused by less virulent microorganisms, these fragile pathogens cannot withstand cold, dry environments and cannot be transmitted through casual contact like shaking hands. For example, *Treponema pallidum* and *Neisseria gonorrhoeae* cause syphilis and gonorrhea, respectively. These bacteria require the moist, warm environment of the host for survival. Sexually transmitted diseases may also be spread congenitally from mother to fetus. Additionally, any blood-to-blood contact can result in the spread of disease, so embalmers are at risk of acquiring sexually transmitted diseases through needle-stick injuries, contact with body fluids through open lesions, or any form of parenteral injury.

Indirect Contact

The transfer of disease-causing pathogens via indirect contact is typically the result of an individual coming in contact with inanimate objects. Fomites are any inanimate objects to which infectious material adheres and can be transmitted. The primary mechanisms of indirect contact are food, water, air, and zoonoses.

Food and Water. Many pathogens enter the human host through the ingestion of food or water. Food can harbor disease-causing microorganisms when it is prepared for cooking, cooked insufficiently, or handled improperly after cooking. When cattle are slaughtered to produce hamburger or steak, the normal flora within the animal's digestive tract may be spread to the meat if proper slaughter techniques are not followed. The spread of microbes from the digestive tract of poultry contaminates food resulting in salmonella poisoning.

If foods are not appropriately cooked, they may also harbor disease-causing microorganisms. Examples of diseases induced by undercooking foods include trichinosis resulting from undercooked pork, and salmonella poisoning from eating raw eggs in dishes like eggnog and salad dressings. Food may also become contaminated after being properly prepared and cooked when appropriate food-handling techniques are not followed. Placing cooked chicken back on the same cutting board that was used to prepare the raw chicken prior to cooking can lead to the spread of disease. Handling of properly prepared and cooked foods by carriers of hepatitis A who did not wash their hands after defecating can result in the spread of typhoid through the fecal-oral route of transmission.

Many diseases are spread through untreated water supplies that have become contaminated through overpopulation of a particular region. Throughout the developing world, refugees who are temporarily living in makeshift housing may, through necessity, be emptying sewage from human and nonhuman animals into the same water supply that they use for bathing, food preparation, and drinking water. Examples of diseases that can be spread through such incidences of untreated water include dysentery and cholera. Contaminated water supplies are not exclusive to refugee camps, however. There have been many outbreaks of diseases in the United States due to contaminated water supplies. Limiting the spread of disease through waterborne organisms requires water filtration, chlorination, and proper disposal and treatment of sewage.

More recently, the CDC (Evans et al. 2003) reports that both bottled water and vegetables on salad bars in restaurants are independently associated with campylobacter infection. According to the CDC, legislation in Europe prohibits water bottlers from chemically treating natural mineral water. Mineral water has been identified in the past as a vehicle of transmission during a cholera epidemic and as a potential source of typhoid fever in travelers. Drinking untreated, bottled natural mineral water may increase the risk of contracting certain diseases, while drinking treated tap water is less likely to result in disease transmission.

Air. Besides being ingested in food or water, some pathogens are spread through airborne transmission. The respiratory spread of infectious disease is commonly the result of the inhalation of aerosolized secretions from coughing, sneezing, and talking. These tiny pathogens are suspended in the air as the residue of the evaporation of larger droplets. The transmission of disease through airborne pathogens requires that the disease-causing organism be resistant to drying and inactivation by ultraviolet light.

Airborne microorganisms must defeat the body's defense mechanisms, penetrate the mucous layer of the respiratory tract, and embed within the epithelial tissues to cause disease. Although several diseases are transmitted through the air, (i.e., streptococcal sore throat, sinusitis, otitis media, diphtheria, and the common cold), *Mycobacterium tuberculosis* is an important example of an airborne pathogen. Tuberculosis is spread by this invasive, highly virulent, intracellular pathogen, which survives well and multiplies within the body's own immune system cells.

Zoonoses. In addition to diseases being spread through food, water, and air, some infectious diseases are spread through zoonoses. Diseases that are communicable from animals or animal products are zoonoses. Over 250 organisms are known to cause zoonotic infections, of which 20 to 40 spread from pets and animals used by the visually impaired and the hearing impaired. Individuals with suppressed immune systems and persons who work with animals are especially at risk of developing zoonoses.

Rabies is a fatal zoonotic disease spread by animal bites, especially from wild animals. Brucellosis is a zoonotic disease characterized by fever that may be contracted by farmers who handle the secretions of cattle, sheep, or hogs. Both tularemia and listeriosis are zoonotic diseases that can be transmitted to humans who handle the carcasses of infected animals. Although each of the previously mentioned zoonotic diseases can be spread through alternate routes, they are examples of diseases spread from animals to humans. A common route of zoonotic disease transmission is through one of the over 900,000 species of arthropods. Table 24-3 lists examples of arthropod vectors and the diseases they transmit.

Vectors. Arthropods are invertebrates with bilateral symmetry; a hard, jointed exoskeleton; segmented bodies; and jointed, paired appendages. Examples of arthropods include ticks, lice, fleas, and mites (Figure 24-6). A vector is a carrier, usually an insect or other arthropod, that transmits the causative organisms of disease from infected to noninfected individuals. Often the disease-causing organism goes through one or more stages in its life cycle on or inside the vector. Vectors can carry pathogens externally on their body or internally within their body.

Biological vectors are animal vectors in which the disease-causing organism multiplies or develops within the animal prior to becoming infective for a susceptible person. There are often several stages in the life cycle of microorganisms spread by biological vectors. Malaria is an example of a disease that is spread by a biological vector. *Plasmodium malariae* is the protozoa that causes malaria, and it undergoes several stages in its life cycle:

Stage 1: Malaria is a vector-borne disease that is spread when mosquito #1 bites a human, injecting *Plasmodium malariae* #1 under the skin.

Stage 2: The *P. malariae* then migrates to the human liver and reproduces.

Stage 3: From the liver, the *P. malariae* then develops in the human red blood cells.

Stage 4: Mosquito #2 then bites the infected human and becomes infected.

Stage 5: In the intestine of mosquito #2, the male and female reproductive cells of *P. malariae* unite to form *P. malariae* #2.

Stage 6: The *P. malariae* #2 then migrates to the salivary glands of mosquito #2, and the whole process is repeated when the mosquito bites and infects human #2.

Table 24-3 Examples of Arthropod Vectors and the Microorganisms and Diseases They Transmit

Arthropod Vector	Microorganism	Disease
Anopheles mosquito	*Plasmodium malariae*	Malaria
Tsetse fly	*Trypanosoma brucei gambiense* and *Trypanosoma brucei rhodesiense*	African sleeping disease
Mosquito	Encephalitis virus	Encephalitis
Body louse	*Rickettsia prowazekii*	Epidemic typhus
Rat flea	*Rickettsia typhi*	Endemic murine typhus
Ticks	*Rickettsia rickettsii*	Rocky Mountain spotted fever
Rat flea	*Yersinia pestis*	Plague
Ticks	*Borrelia burgdorferi*	Lyme disease

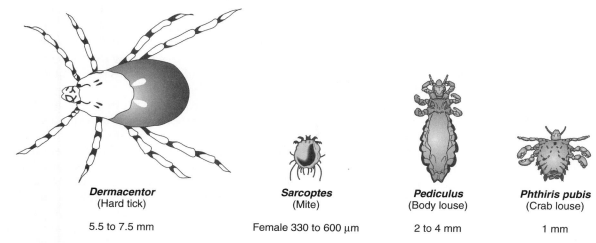

Dermacentor
(Hard tick)

5.5 to 7.5 mm

Sarcoptes
(Mite)

Female 330 to 600 µm

Pediculus
(Body louse)

2 to 4 mm

Phthiris pubis
(Crab louse)

1 mm

Figure 24–6 Significant arthropods.

P. malariae cannot grow without both the mosquito and the human. If the pathogen must grow within the vector's body, the vector is referred to as a biological vector. Vectors may also deposit pathogens on human skin when they defecate, which is then introduced into the bite when the human scratches.

A **mechanical vector** is a vector in or on which growth and development of the infective agent do not occur. Unlike biological vectors, pathogens spread by mechanical vectors may not reproduce in the vector's body. A fly acts as a mechanical vector when it lands on feces, picks up intestinal pathogens (i.e., *Escherichia coli* or *Shigella* sp.), and then transmits the pathogens to nearby food on its legs. The fly is a mechanical vector rather than a biological vector because the pathogen is carried on the outside of its body, and the microorganism does not grow inside the fly.

PORTALS OF ENTRY AND EXIT FOR PATHOGENS

Not every microorganism that enters the body will result in disease within the host. The route by which pathogens gain access to the body is specific to the properties of the disease-causing microorganism. For example, organisms that enter the respiratory system must be able to circumvent both the respiratory system's mechanical and chemical defenses. Additionally, microorganisms that cannot penetrate the thick, mucous secretions that cover the epithelial tissues of the respiratory system will not be able to survive and establish disease in the host. There are five portals of entry and exit by which pathogens may enter or exit the body: the skin and mucous membranes; the respiratory tract; the digestive tract; the genitourinary tract; and the placenta.

Skin and Mucous Membranes

Abrasions, lesions, and open wounds in the skin are an invitation to the introduction of disease-causing microorganisms. Pathogens that would otherwise not be able to establish injurious disease are able to bypass the open skin and enter the warm, moist, hospitable environment of the body's tissues. Insects may penetrate the tissues with their proboscises, resulting in the transmission of pathogens. Nonhuman animal bites are capable of tearing the tissues as well as forcing microorganisms and debris deep inside the tissues where bleeding may not flush the wound properly and infection may result.

Of all injuries to the skin, a human bite may result in the greatest inflammatory reactions. Although many of the microorganisms found in the mouths of nonhuman animals may not result in disease in humans, the majority of microorganisms in the human mouth are pathogenic when introduced under the skin. The mucous membranes of the eyes and ears may also become infected with pathogenic microorganisms, which is frequently the result of rubbing of the eyes and ears. Examples of diseases spread through the non-intact skin and mucous membranes include tetanus, malaria, yellow fever, African sleeping sickness, typhoid fever, tuberculosis, dysentery, rabies, typhus fever, and bubonic plague.

Respiratory Tract

The respiratory tract is often invaded by airborne pathogens capable of multiplying in its warm, moist environment. These pathogens may be spread through sneezing, coughing, touching contaminated surfaces and then touching the mouth or nose, and by dust particles that contain human or nonhuman wastes. Pathogenic bacterial spores may also be inhaled and enter or exit the body through the respiratory tract. Examples of diseases spread through the respiratory tract include the common cold, influenza, tuberculosis, histoplasmosis, and pneumonia.

Digestive Tract

Ingestion of infected or contaminated food and water is a frequent cause of the spread of disease. The possibility of contamination is especially significant at social functions where larger than normal quantities of food may be prepared in advance and stored without proper food-safety and food-handling education. Since children and the elderly—two groups that may not have fully functional immune systems—often attend large social functions, they are at a greater risk for the transmission of pathogens through the digestive tract. Examples of disease that spread through the digestive tract are typhoid fever, food poisoning, and undulant fever.

Genitourinary Tract

Both sexually transmitted diseases and diseases of the urinary system are spread between hosts through the genitourinary tract. Human sexual behavior can contribute to the spread of genitourinary tract infections. For example, anal intercourse increases the risk of introducing opportunistic pathogens into both the reproductive organs and the urinary tract in addition to increasing the risk of contracting numerous sexually transmitted diseases. The use of condoms can greatly reduce, but not eliminate, such risk. Examples of diseases spread through the genitourinary tract include bladder infections, syphilis, gonorrhea, and AIDS.

Placenta

Although the blood of the mother and the fetus do not mix, some pathogens are capable of spreading across the placenta into the fetus. One microorganism of great concern to pregnant embalmers is cytomegalovirus (CMV). Sixty percent of the population over 35 years of age are asymptomatic carries of CMV. Even though the virus usually does not cause symptoms in the adult, pregnant women may unknowingly pass the virus to the fetus through the placenta. CMV infection is especially prevalent among the poor and undereducated. Approximately 10 percent of infected infants develop CMV inclusion disease, which results in several blood disorders and liver problems, and 50 percent of these infants die.

Vehicles of Exit of Pathogens

Disease pathogens are spread through direct contact with body fluids, secretions, and blood, or contact with materials contaminated with body fluids, secretions, and blood. Items are considered contaminated if they potentially contain body fluids, secretions, or blood. Specifically, pathogens may be found in feces, urine, semen, vaginal secretions, sputum, saliva, blood, pus, and tears.

Feces, or excrement, is body waste containing food residue, bacteria, epithelium, and mucus discharged from the bowels by way of the anus. Semen is a thick, opaque secretion discharged from the ejaculatory duct of the penis during the male orgasm. Vaginal secretions include any fluids, including menstrual blood, that emanate from the vagina. Sputum is mucus expelled from the lung by coughing. Pus is a creamy-white mixture of cell fluid containing living and dead white blood cells, bacteria, and damaged body cells. However, pus need not be white. Pus resulting from the pathogen *Pseudomonas aeruginosa*, which is common in secondary infections of burns, is blue.

RESISTANCE OF THE HOST AGAINST INFECTION

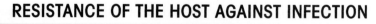

The relative ability of the body to defend itself against infection is known as resistance. Each of the body's defense mechanisms targets particular types of pathogens, and each is necessary to protect the body from the specialized features of pathogens that allow them to cause disease in the human host. The body is capable of limiting the occurrence of disease through its mechanical defenses, its physiological defenses, and, finally, its chemical defenses (Figure 24-7).

Mechanical Defenses Against Infection

One of the most important and effective barriers against infection is human skin. The outer surface of the skin, or epithelium, is a mechanical barrier that must be penetrated by potential pathogens. Most organisms capable of penetrating the

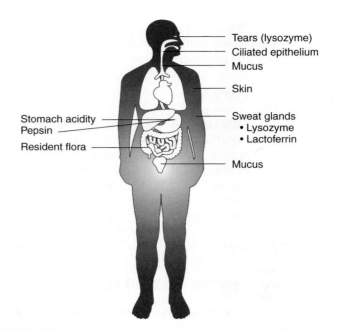

Figure 24-7 Defenses of the host.

mucous epithelium are not capable of penetrating unbroken, healthy skin. Although most organisms that penetrate the skin do so via animal or insect bites, some are capable of penetrating the unbroken skin. The skin is also host to numerous organisms that are not pathogens. The normal flora of the skin contributes to a low pH, competition for nutrients, and the production of by-products that are deadly to some pathogenic bacteria. The specialized oils in the skin produced by sebaceous glands add to the acidic environment, ensuring that few pathogenic organisms survive.

The body also has several mechanical defenses that function through cleansing processes. The skin has a mechanical defense system known as *necrobiosis,* which is the process by which the epithelial layer of the skin continuously dies, sloughs off, and is replaced with new cells. When the dead skin falls away, bacterial colonies are removed along with it. The eyes possess a mechanical barrier to pathogens in the form of tears. Since the eyes are continuously exposed to the environment, the process of blinking traps airborne particles, which are then washed away by tears. Tears also contain chemicals (i.e., immunoglobulin A and lysozyme) that are chemical defenses against infection.

The respiratory tract is lined by hairs in the nasal passage, ciliated epithelium, and mucous membranes, which trap debris and sweep them toward the esophagus, where they are swallowed. Even the urinary tract is cleansed by the flushing action of urine. These mechanical barriers to infection all function by reducing the number of organisms that enter the body through physical means.

Physiological Defenses Against Infection

The body is also capable of defending itself against foreign matter that enters the body through trauma. For example, stepping on a dirty, rusty, nail embeds the penetrated tissue with microorganisms and debris. Not only must the debris be removed, the body must defend itself against any pathogenic microorganisms that were introduced to the deep tissues during the trauma. To remove the foreign debris, the body initiates a physiological response known as inflammation.

During the process of inflammation, immune system cells are drawn toward the site of injury. The area swells with these cells that break down the foreign material. Pus may also be formed, which creates enough pressure to rupture the tissue and expel the foreign debris. After the debris is removed, the process of inflammation repairs the tissues to their normal, healthy state. The cardinal signs and symptoms of inflammation are:

- Heat
- Swelling
- Pain
- Redness
- Loss of function

In addition to the physiological defense mechanism of inflammation, which rids the body of foreign materials, the body also has a physiological defense mechanism known as fever. When fevers are caused by infections, certain white blood cells in the body, especially macrophages, release chemicals that increase the body's internal temperature. The temperature is raised by diverting blood from the superficial blood vessels of the body into the body's core. Diverting the blood into the body's core increases the core temperature and results in fever. The physical effect on pathogens is that at the temperature of 102°–104°F (39°–40°C), few human pathogens can survive. Fever may also affect the rate at which antibiotics function in the body, and fever can regulate access to chemicals like iron during infectious periods. Improved function of antibiotics kills more microorganisms, and restricting the available amount of necessary chemicals starves microorganisms of a viable nutrient source.

Besides the physiological defenses of inflammation and fever, the body possesses a physiological defense known as *phagocytosis*. A group of specialized cells known as phagocytes are produced in the body's bone marrow. These phagocytes contain chemicals capable of breaking down foreign cells and debris. The process of phagocytosis is quite complex, and it is illustrated in Figure 24-8.

Phagocytosis begins when a phagocyte encounters a foreign cell or particle. The phagocyte engulfs the foreign body and begins to break down the material through special chemicals produced by lysosomes. The phagocyte, which contains the ingested material, then moves to a part of the body where it can deposit the material for excretion from the body.

Chemical Defenses Against Infection

In addition to the mechanical and physiological defenses of the body, there are chemical defenses against infection. One of the body's lines of chemical defense

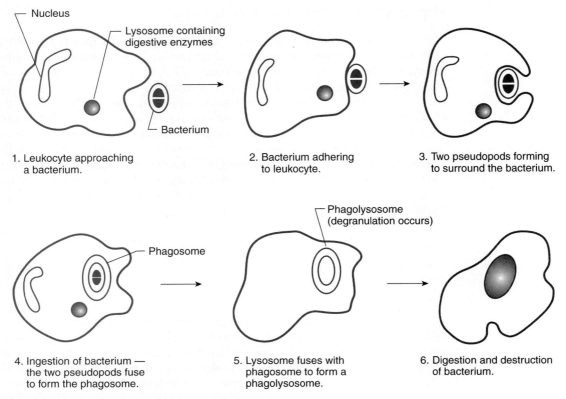

1. Leukocyte approaching a bacterium.

2. Bacterium adhering to leukocyte.

3. Two pseudopods forming to surround the bacterium.

4. Ingestion of bacterium — the two pseudopods fuse to form the phagosome.

5. Lysosome fuses with phagosome to form a phagolysosome.

6. Digestion and destruction of bacterium.

Figure 24-8 Phagocytosis.

is body secretions. Many body fluids and mucus contain chemicals that are antimicrobial. Additionally, phagocytes contain chemicals that defend the body against infection.

Lysozyme. Prokaryotes contain a peptidoglycan layer in their cell walls. Peptidoglycan is composed of amino acids and sugars. One method of killing prokaryotes is to destroy their cell wall. Lysozyme is a chemical enzyme in the body that uses water to break down the peptidoglycan layer in prokaryotic pathogens. Lysozyme is in many body fluids such as tears, breast milk, saliva, and sweat. Since many microorganisms are prokaryotic cells, lysozyme is an effective antimicrobial agent in the body.

Gastric Juice. Since one of the most common routes of disease transmission is through ingestion of infected or contaminated food and water, and the digestive tract is a portal of entry for many pathogens, the digestive system has many lines of chemical defense. The low pH of the stomach easily destroys most pathogens that enter the body through the nose and mouth. The low pH levels of the stomach are the result of the secretion of gastric juices that contain hydrochloric acid.

Interferon. To inhibit the spread of viruses in the body, a special group of cellular proteins are produced in eukaryotic cells in response to viruses. Interferon works to reduce the spread of viruses when a host cell infected with a virus produces interferon, which binds to the surface receptors of uninfected cells. The presence of the interferon on the uninfected cell causes the uninfected cell to synthesize enzymes that resist the viruse's ability to reproduce during the uninfected cell's next reproduction cycle. Although some interferon is antiviral, other forms of interferon stimulate the immune system in a more general way to enhance the effectiveness of phagocytes, natural killer cells, and cytotoxic T cells.

HUMAN IMMUNE SYSTEM

This chapter describes the relationship between a pathogen's ability to cause disease (virulence) and a host's ability to defend itself against that particular pathogen (resistance). So why is it that some people tend to be sick more often than others? Why can two people eat the same infected chicken and only one person contracts food poisoning? The answer lies in a healthy immune system. Three classes of people are more prone to contracting illness: children, the elderly, and individuals who are immunocompromised.

There are several reasons why a person may have a compromised immune system or low resistance to disease. Children are born with immature immune systems. If they are to develop a healthy, mature immune system, they must encounter pathogens so that their bodies can learn to defend themselves against specific pathogens. That is why children tend to contract numerous illnesses, but they tend to recover quickly; whereas an adult might contract the same illness and be symptomatic for a much longer period of time with a much slower recovery. The immune system also weakens with age. The elderly are typically prone to develop disease with greater frequency than younger, healthier individuals.

There are also numerous causes for immunosuppression in persons other than children and the elderly. For example, to reduce possible rejection of transplanted organs and tissues, recipients are often given pharmaceutical agents that reduce their immune system response. People with chronic inflammatory diseases frequently take nonsteroidal anti-inflammatory drugs (NSAIDS) to reduce the effects of the inflammation. NSAIDS function by suppressing the immune system. There are also a number of autoimmune diseases as well as pathogens that attack the immune system. AIDS is an example of a disease in which the infected host has a severely weakened immune system. Even people who are otherwise completely healthy may become immunocompromised through overexposure to cold or heat, and especially through sleep deprivation.

Antigens and Antibodies

In addition to the chemical defenses of the body found in body secretions, the human immune system produces a myriad of antimicrobial chemicals. **Antibodies**, which are also known as immunoglobulins, are glycoprotein substances produced by the body in response to specific antigens. The body recognizes cells by certain characteristics of the cell known as antigens. An **antigen** is a foreign substance that stimulates the formation of antibodies, which interact specifically with the antigen.

An antigen is a marker on every cell, including invading pathogens, by which the body recognizes unknown cells or disease-causing organisms. Antibodies are found in mucous secretions of the respiratory, genital, and digestive tracts. Antibodies neutralize or destroy antigens on disease-causing organisms in several ways. They can destroy pathogens by neutralizing the toxins the pathogen produces, by coating the pathogen with a substance that attracts phagocytes, by forming a substance that clumps the antigens together in a process known as agglutination, or by preventing the pathogen from adhering to the body's cells.

Types of Immunity

The classic method of describing different forms of immunity is to characterize them as either specific or nonspecific. Nonspecific immunity does not identify specific pathogens, and it can be further divided into physical barriers and the body's inflammatory processes. Specific immunity identifies a specific pathogen and can be divided into innate and acquired types, as well as active and passive forms.

Innate Immunity. Innate immunity, which is also known as natural immunity, is a form of immunity due to physical characteristics that can be attributed to biological differences such as race or sex. Certain groups of people are simply immune to certain diseases because they are born with a natural (innate) immunity. For example, some people are allergic to poison ivy, while others are not.

Acquired Immunity. Acquired immunity differs from innate immunity in that the individual must either form antibodies to a pathogen personally, or be given the antibodies from an alternate source. Natural active immunity is the result of developing a disease and recovering from it. For example, persons who contract mumps will be able to defend themselves against the mumps paramyxovirus in the future. Natural passive immunity is the result of placental transfer of antibodies in the uterus, or from the transfer of antibodies in the mother's first breast milk, which is known as colostrum. Artificial active immunity is the result of receiving a vaccination. As an example, children in the United States are routinely given the MMR vaccine against measles, mumps, and rubella.

Artificial passive immunity is the result of the injection of antibodies in the form of immune serums. Immune serums are the result of gathering antibodies from previously infected human and nonhuman animal hosts, and then introducing the antibodies into someone to reduce an existing disease or prevent disease from occurring. Immune serums are available against tetanus, rabies, and various forms of hepatitis, as well as other diseases.

REVIEW QUESTIONS

Matching

1. _____ antigen
2. _____ virulence
3. _____ host
4. _____ pathogen
5. _____ fomites

a. an organism capable of producing disease
b. any inanimate objects to which infectious material adheres and can be transmitted
c. relative power and degree of pathogenicity possessed by organisms to produce disease
d. a marker on every cell, including invading pathogens, by which the body recognizes unknown cells or disease-causing organisms
e. the organism from which a parasite obtains its nourishment

Multiple Choice

1. Which of the following is a chemical enzyme in the body that uses water to break down the peptidoglycan layer in prokaryotic pathogens?
   a. interferon
   b. antibody
   c. lysozyme
   d. immunoglobulin

2. Which of the following describes the state or condition in which the body, or part of the body, is invaded by a pathogenic agent that, under favorable conditions, multiplies and produces injurious effects?
   a. infection
   b. contamination
   c. aerosolization
   d. attenuation

3. Which of the following describes infection caused by bacteria that are normally nonpathogenic and that normally inhabit the digestive tract?
   a. endogenous infection
   b. mixed infection
   c. exogenous infection
   d. opportunistic infection

4. Which of the following is a carrier, usually an insect or other arthropod, that transmits the causative organisms of disease from infected to noninfected individuals?
   a. host
   b. vector
   c. reservoir
   d. pathogen

5. Which of the following portals of exit and entry allow the spread of pathogens causing tetanus, malaria, African sleeping sickness, typhoid fever, tuberculosis, dysentery, rabies, typhus fever, and bubonic plague?

   a. skin and mucous membranes

   b. respiratory tract

   c. digestive tract

   d. genitourinary tract

Bibliography

Abedon, S. (1998). *Acquisition of disease.* Retrieved July 26, 2003, from supplemental lecture notes for Micro 509 at the Ohio State University at http://www.mansfield.ohio-state.edu/~sabedon/biol2050.htm.

Abedon, S. (2003). *Arthropod vectors.* Retrieved July 26, 2003, from supplemental lecture notes for Micro 509 at the Ohio State University at http://www.mansfield.ohio-state.edu/~sabedon/biol3055.htm.

Chamberlain, N. (2000a). *Introduction to microbiology.* Retrieved July 25, 2003, from the Kirksville College of Osteopathic Medicine at http://www.kcom.edu/faculty/chamberlain/Website/intmic.htm.

Chamberlain, N. (2000b). *Rickettsia, chlamydia, mycoplasma.* Retrieved July 15, 2003, from Kirksville College of Osteopathic Medicine at http://www.kcom.edu/faculty/chamberlain/Website/Lects/RICKETT.HTM#ri.

Edmonds, P. (1978). *Microbiology: An environmental perspective.* Basingstoke Hampshire, England: Macmillan Publishing.

Evans, M. R., Ribeiro, C. D., & Salmon, R. L. (2003). Hazards of healthy living: Bottled water and salad vegetables as risk factors for campylobacter infection. *Emerging Infectious Diseases, 9*(10), 1219–1225.

Frobisher, M., Hinsdill, R., Crabtree, K., & Goodheart, C. (1974). *Fundamentals of microbiology.* Philadelphia: Saunders.

Gale, J. (2003). Bacteria. In *Watersheds.* Retrieved June 30, 2003, from the North Carolina State University Water Quality Group at http://h2osparc.wq.ncsu.edu/info/bacteria.html.

Gaudy, A., & Gaudy, E. (1980). *Microbiology for environmental scientists and engineers.* New York: McGraw-Hill.

Grover-Lakomia, L., & Fong, E. (1999). *Microbiology for Health Careers* (6th ed.). Clifton Park, NY: Thomson Delmar Learning.

The immune system. (1999). Retrieved July 26, 2003, from the National Institute of Allergy and Infectious Diseases, National Institutes of Health at http://www.niaid.nih.gov/final/immun/immun.htm.

Kennedy, V. (2001). Antigen. In *Medical Encyclopedia.* Retrieved July 26, 2003, from MedlinePlus, the U.S. National Library of Medicine and the National Institutes of Health at http://www.nlm.nih.gov/medlineplus/ency/article/002224.htm.

Kimball, J. (2003). *Antigen presentation.* Retrieved July 26, 2003, from Kimball's Biology Pages at http://users.rcn.com/jkimball.ma.ultranet/BiologyPages/A/AntigenPresentation.html.

Mahon, C., & Manuselis, G. (2000). *Textbook of diagnostic microbiology* (2nd ed.). Philadelphia: Saunders.

Mayer, R. (2000). *Embalming: History, theory, & practice* (3rd ed.). New York: McGraw-Hill.

Mosquito-borne diseases. (2001). Retrieved July 26, 2003, from the National Center for Infectious Diseases, Centers for Disease Control and Prevention at http://www.cdc.gov/ncidod/diseases/list_mosquitoborne.htm.

Neighbors, M., & Tannehill-Jones, R. (2000). *Human diseases.* Clifton Park, NY: Thomson Delmar Learning.

Nester, E., Anderson, D., Roberts, C., Pearsall, N., & Nester, M. (2001). *Microbiology: A human perspective* (3rd ed.). Boston: McGraw-Hill.

Pathology for funeral service. (1999). Dallas, TX: Professional Training Schools.

Rollins, D. (2000). *Nonspecific defenses of the host*. Retrieved July 26, 2003, from the University of Maryland at http://www.life.umd.edu/classroom/bsci424/BSCI223WebSiteFiles/Chapter16.htm.

Scott, P., & Pierce, J. (1996). *Edward Jenner and the discovery of vaccination*. Retrieved June 26, 2003, from the Thomas Cooper Library, University of South Carolina at http://www.sc.edu/library/spcoll/nathist/jenner.html.

Sepsis: What you should know. (2003). In *ICU Issues and Answers*. Retrieved July 26, 2003, from the Society of Critical Care Medicine at http://www.sccm.org/patient_family_resources/brochures/sepsis.asp.

Shelton, H. (1992). *Boyd's introduction to the study of disease* (11th ed.). Philadelphia: Lea & Febiger.

Smallpox emergency preparedness and response. (2002). Retrieved April 10, 2004, from Centers for Disease Control and Prevention at http://www.bt.cdc.gov/agent/smallpox/prep/cdc-prep.asp.

Stephenson, J. (2003). *Defending against infection*. Retrieved July 26, 2003, from the University of Miami, Oxford, Ohio at http://www.cas.muohio.edu/~mbi-ws/Infection/DefendInfect.htm.

Tortora, G., Funke, B., & Case, C. (1998). *Microbiology: An introduction* (6th ed.). Menlo Park, CA: Benjamin/Cummings Publishing.

Venes, D. (Ed.). (2001). *Taber's cyclopedic medical dictionary* (19th ed.). Philadelphia: F. A. Davis.

CHAPTER 25

Diseases Caused by Bacteria

Learning Objectives

Upon completion of the chapter, review questions, and case analysis, the reader should be able to:

- Match specific bacterial pathogens included in this chapter with the diseases they cause.
- Match the bacterial diseases described in this chapter with the genus of the bacterial pathogen.
- Identify the important disease conditions associated with the bacterial diseases described in this chapter.
- Identify the mode of transmission of the bacterial diseases described in this chapter.
- Identify lesions on human remains that suggest a potentially infectious bacterial disease.

Key Terms

buboes
coagulase
eschar

hyaluronidase
lipase

Historically, bacteria have caused some of the most deadly diseases and widespread epidemics in human society. Although diseases like malaria and smallpox, which are not caused by bacteria, may have killed more humans than bacteria, diseases like typhoid fever, bubonic plague, typhus, diphtheria, tuberculosis, and bacterial diarrhea have added significantly to human mortality. Table 25-1 lists significant pathogenic bacteria, the diseases they cause, their mode of transmission, and the signs and symptoms of the diseases they cause.

Table 25-1 Pathogenic Bacteria: Disease, Transmission, and Signs and Symptoms

Pathogen	Disease Name	Mode of Transmission	Signs and Symptoms
Bacillus anthracis	Cutaneous anthrax	Spore enters wound	Eschar (skin lesion)
	Inhalation anthrax (woolsorter's disease; pulmonary anthrax)	Inhalation of spores	Flulike symptoms, cyanosis, shock, disorientation, coma, respiratory failure
	Gastrointestinal anthrax	Ingestion of spores	Lesions in intestine, abdominal pain, nausea, anorexia, vomiting, bloody diarrhea
Bordetella pertussis	Whooping cough (pertussis)	Inhalation of respiratory droplets	A whooping sound between violent coughing spells, while gasping for air
Borrelia burgdorferi	Lyme disease (Lyme borreliosis)	Tick bite	Bull's-eye rash, polyarthritis, CNS infection, heart infection
Campylobacter jejuni	Intestinal ulcers	Ingestion of bacteria	Fever, chills, nausea, vomiting, bloody diarrhea
Clostridium botulinum	Botulism	Toxin	Paralysis, cardiac or respiratory failure, nausea, double vision, difficulty swallowing
	Food intoxication	Ingestion of spores	Abdominal pain and diarrhea
C. perfringens	Gas gangrene	Wound contamination	Necrosis of tissues
	Tissue gas (postmortem only)	Translocation from intestinal flora	Tissues swell with gas due to the bacteria's ability to ferment carbohydrates contributing to generalized decomposition
C. tetani	Tetanus (lockjaw)	Infection of wounds from contaminated soil	Contraction of muscles of the jaws and respiratory system leading to asphyxia
Corynebacterium diphtheriae	Diphtheria	Droplet or hand-to-mouth	Sore throat, fever, fatigue, swollen neck, pseudomembrane formation in pharynx, paralysis, demyelization of PNS
	Traveler's diarrhea	Ingestion of contaminated water or food	Fever, watery diarrhea, nausea, abdominal cramps
Escherichia coli	Enteroinvasive *E. coli* or enterohemorrhagic *E. coli*	Fecal-oral route	Fever, severe abdominal cramps, malaise, watery diarrhea with pus, mucus, and blood; low platelet count, hemolytic anemia, kidney failure

(continues)

Table 25-1 Continued

Pathogen	Disease Name	Mode of Transmission	Signs and Symptoms
Francisella tularensis	Tularemia (rabbit fever)	Inhalation, ingestion, bites, or skin breaks; also by the bite of deer flies, ticks, or rabbit lice	Local inflammation and small ulcer, enlargement of regional lymph nodes with pus, pneumonia and abscesses throughout the body
Haemophilus influenzae	Influenzal meningitis	Inhalation of respiratory droplets	Fever, headache, stiff neck, arthritis, bacterial pneumonia
Helicobacter pylori	Stomach ulcers (gastric ulcers; peptic ulcers)	Ingestion of bacteria	Nausea, vomiting, burning abdominal pain
Klebsiella pneumoniae	Nosocomial respiratory infections	Inhalation of respiratory droplets	Urinary, respiratory, and wound infections
Legionella pneumophilia	Legionnaires' disease (Legionellosis)	Possible airborne transmission	Fever, cough, and symptoms of pneumonia
Leptospira interrogans	Leptospirosis	Through the skin after contact with contaminated water, soil, or animal waste	Headache, muscle aches, chills, fever, renal and hepatic infection, CNS infection
Listeria monocytogenes	Listeriosis	Ingestion of contaminated food, soil, and water	Fever, muscle aches, nausea, diarrhea, stiff neck, confusion, convulsions
Mycobacterium avium	Mycobacterium avium complex (MAC)	Unknown but assumed to be environmentally acquired	Usually only found in persons with under 50 T4 cells; weight loss, fever, chills, night sweats, swollen glands, abdominal pain, diarrhea, weakness
M. tuberculosis	Tuberculosis	Inhalation of respiratory droplets	Coughing of blood or sputum, chest pain, weakness, weight loss, anorexia, chills, fever, night sweats
Neisseria gonorrhoeae	Gonorrhea	Direct sexual contact	Pustular discharge from genitalia, painful urination, sterility, rectal infections
	Ophthalmia neonatorum	Contact with the birth canal	Infant blindness
N. meningitidis	Meningococcal meningitis	Oral and respiratory droplets, or direct contact with infected sites on the body	Acute headache, stiff neck, fever, rash, spontaneous blood clotting, Waterhouse-Friderichsen syndrome
Proteus species	Infections in burns	Wound contamination	Infections in burns
Proteus vulgaris	Generalized decomposition	Bacterial translocation	Postmortem ptomaine formation from proteins
Salmonella enteritidis	Salmonella food poisoning (Salmonellosis)	Ingestion of contaminated food	Fever, chills, abdominal pain, watery diarrhea

Table 25-1 Continued

Pathogen	Disease Name	Mode of Transmission	Signs and Symptoms
S. typhi	Typhoid fever	Fecal-oral route	Fever, headache, abdominal pain, rose spots on abdomen, nosebleeds, whitish furlike growth on tongue
Shigella species	Bacillary dysentery (shigellosis; gay bowel syndrome)	Fecal-oral route by anal-oral sex, flies, fingers, and contaminated food or water	Severe diarrhea with blood and mucus, abdominal cramps, fever
	Food poisoning	Ingestion of contaminated food	Headache, vomiting, abdominal cramps, and diarrhea
Staphylococcus aureus	Skin and wound infections	Direct contact	Pimples, furuncles, carbuncles, septicemia
	Toxic shock syndrome	Tampons or surgical procedures	Fever, rash, dehydration, watery diarrhea, vomiting, hypotension, shock
Streptococcus agalactiae	Meningitis in newborns	Ingestion of raw milk	Lethargy, jaundice, respiratory distress, shock, pneumonia, anorexia
S. pneumoniae	Pneumococcal meningitis (bacterial meningitis)	Oral and respiratory droplets	Headache, stiff neck, fever
	Otitis media	Contaminated water, eardrum puncture, or skull fracture	Pus behind eardrum causes earache
S. pneumoniae	Pneumococcal pneumonia (lobar pneumonia; bacterial pneumonia)	Inhalation of respiratory droplets	Fluids are produced in the lungs accompanied by fever, chills, dyspnea, chest pain, bloody sputum
S. pneumoniae	Septic sore throat (strep throat)	Inhalation of respiratory droplets and close contact	Sore throat, malaise, fever, headache, nausea, vomiting, abdominal pain
S. pyogenes	Impetigo	Insect bite or skin abrasion	Small blisters that progress into weeping lesions; a crust forms when the lesions dry
S. pyogenes	Scarlet fever	Inhalation of respiratory droplets	Sore throat, red skin rash, high fever, spotted tongue with a "strawberry" appearance, loss of upper membrane of tongue, desquamation of skin lesions
S. pyogenes	Rheumatic fever	Inhalation of respiratory droplets	Polyarthritis, heart valve vegetation, St. Vitus' Dance

(continues)

Table 25-1 Continued

Pathogen	Disease Name	Mode of Transmission	Signs and Symptoms
S. pyogenes (cont.)	Childbirth fever (puerperal sepsis)	Contaminated instruments or hands of medical workers	Infection of uterus spreads to peritoneum, causing peritonitis (abdominal pain, vomiting, etc.)
Treponema pallidum	Syphilis	Direct sexual contact	Primary stage—chancre; secondary stage—rash; tertiary stage—gummas, blindness, and CNS infection
Vibrio cholerae	Asiatic cholera	Contaminated seafood	"Rice-water" stool, shock, increased blood viscosity
Yersinia pestis	Bubonic plague (black death; The Pest)	Flea bites, contact with infected animals, airborne transmission from infected persons	Dark hemorrhagic discolorations on the body, buboes on the lymph nodes

Table 25-2 Recently Discovered Bacteria and the Diseases They Cause

Year	Disease	Bacteria
1975	Lyme disease	*Borrelia burgdorferi*
1977	Legionnaires' disease	*Legionella pneumophilia*
1981	Toxic shock syndrome from tampon use	Toxin-producing *Staphylococcus aureus*
1983	Peptic ulcers	*Helicobacter pylori*

Although it is true that modern antibiotics, water purification, and immunization programs have drastically reduced the morbidity and mortality rates of many bacterial diseases, these changes have mostly benefited Western cultures. In the developing world, bacterial diseases remain significant contributors to both human morbidity and mortality. There are also new bacterial diseases discovered with regularity in the United States. Table 25-2 lists some of the significant bacterial diseases discovered in recent history.

STAPHYLOCOCCI

Staphylococci are spherical cells that may appear alone, in pairs, or in clusters that have been described as "bunches of grapes." These facultatively anaerobic microorganisms are nonmotile, and they do not form spores. *Staphylococci* are indigenous to the normal microbiota found on the skin and mucous membranes of both human and nonhuman animals. Staphylococcal infections are commonly spread through contact with contaminated fomites and close contact among humans in clinical settings.

Nosocomial infections are not unusual due to the close contact between patients and healthcare workers. *Staphylococci* are known to inhabit the nostrils of human carriers, so embalmers should be watchful for airborne transmission as well as direct contact with the nose. The proper and consistent use of topical disinfectants can help reduce the spread of *Staphylococcus*.

Staphylococcus aureus is a clinically significant species of *Staphylococci* with a unique virulence and pathogenicity due to the various poisons it produces in the human body. Even after the *S. aureus* cell is destroyed, the toxins it produced can result in injury in the human host. These toxins are capable of surviving in the gastric and digestive juices resulting in diarrhea and vomiting. Other toxins affect the cell membranes of both red and white blood cells leading to severe tissue damage. Toxins attacking platelets result in blood clotting failure in the human host. Another specialized toxin resists the human phagocytic cells.

Not only are *Staphylococci* virulent because of the toxins they produce, but the enzymes they produce—coagulase, hyaluronidase, and lipase—add to their virulence. The exact role of **coagulase** in the pathogenicity of *S. aureus* is unknown; however, its function is to cause blood to clot by converting fibrinogen into fibrin. The enzyme **hyaluronidase** allows *S. aureus* to penetrate the body's connective tissues, permitting the easy spread of infection throughout the body. **Lipase** acts with the oils and fats secreted by the sebaceous glands, allowing *Staphylococci* to colonize in the skin.

Staphylococci are becoming multidrug resistant. The antimicrobial agents used to control *Staphylococci* are less effective than they were previously because the bacteria are adapting. The emergence of highly resistant *S. aureus* strains is likely to present therapeutic challenges in the near future. The best method of controlling the spread of staphylococcal diseases is through proper hand washing and rigorous adherence to sanitization practices in the embalming room.

Certain species of *Staphylococci* have been known to cause diseases in humans, although their occurrence is relatively rare, while other species like *S. aureus* commonly cause disease in humans. The three most common Staphylococcal infections are food poisoning, skin and wound abscesses, and toxic shock syndrome.

Food Poisoning Caused by *Staphylococci*

Staphylococcal food intoxication is a gastrointestinal disorder caused by the enterotoxins produced by the *Staphylococcus aureus* bacterium. The normal processes through which food intoxication takes place are common at family reunions, major holidays, religious social functions, or service organization events. Many people have participated in such events without realizing the potential danger of improper food handling.

During the preparation of food, the *S. aureus* bacteria are usually killed through the process of cooking. However, after the food is cooked it is easily contaminated by food handlers who have bacteria on their hands as a part of their normal body microbiota. Food can also become contaminated by mechanical vectors like flies or ants, which can spread bacteria on their legs. If the food is then allowed to stand at room temperature to cool, or if it is cooked slowly in large masses, or if it is kept warm for any length of time at low temperatures, the bacteria have an opportunity to form enterotoxins. Reheating the food will kill the bacteria but not the toxin. Foods that contain mayonnaise or cream sauces may be infectious without any change in appearance, odor, or taste.

The signs of food poisoning typically occur one to six hours after ingesting contaminated food. Recovery is usually within 24 hours. Fever is not associated with food poisoning; however, the toxins may cause headaches, vomiting, abdominal cramps, and diarrhea. The mortality rate of staphylococcal food poisoning is quite low for healthy adults, but it is significant in weakened individuals, such as the elderly and children.

Skin and Wound Infections

Staphylococcus aureus is a bacterium associated with several toxic infections of the body. It begins on the surface of the skin where it penetrates the integumentary barrier through hair follicles causing a pimple. A more serious hair follicle infection is known as a furuncle, or boil. A furuncle is a superficial skin abscess, which is a localized area of pus surrounded by inflamed and necrotic tissue in which blood clots in the vessels and forms a "core." The core is either expelled or reabsorbed. If the body fails to contain the spread of an abscess, the surrounding tissue is invaded, forming a carbuncle, which is a hard, round, deep inflammation of the subcutaneous tissue under the skin. Carbuncles are common in cases of diabetes mellitus, requiring topical disinfection during embalming because the lesions contain numerous bacteria.

Toxic Shock Syndrome

Toxic shock syndrome (TSS) is caused by *Staphylococcus aureus* bacteria. Prior to the mid 1970s, TSS was not prevalent because tampons—which are inserted into the vagina with an applicator—were made of natural materials. These materials are less absorbent than newer superabsorbent tampons that contain synthetic materials, which swell with menstrual fluids and blood. These saturated tampons adhere to the vagina and can cause tears in the vaginal wall when removed. This trauma to the membranes of the vagina allows bacteria to enter the tissues, potentially resulting in septic infections. Half of the cases of TSS are associated with tampon use, while the other half are nosocomial infections. Nosocomial spread of TSS may result from surgical incisions, absorbent packing used after nasal surgery, and among women who have just given birth. TSS has also been found in males and premenstrual females.

Any wound caused by a strain of *S. aureus* that produces the TSS-1 toxin can cause TSS. The condition begins with a high fever, rash, and signs of dehydration due to watery diarrhea and vomiting for several days. Color Plate 39 is a photograph of the arm of a person exhibiting a rash due to TSS. Patients may also develop severe hypotension, causing shock. The rash is usually isolated to the trunk of the body although it may spread. Color Plate 40 is a photograph of a person with an eye infection due to TSS caused by *S. aureus*. TSS is best prevented by avoiding the use of tampons, using low absorbency tampons, and changing tampons frequently. Most persons with TSS recover; however, approximately 5 percent of the cases of TSS are fatal. Subsequent infection is also likely, with 60 percent of menstruating women experiencing recurrence of TSS.

Nosocomial Infections

Embalmers and other healthcare workers should also be aware of potential sources of staphylococcal infections associated with iatrogenic and nosocomial infections. Staphylococcal pneumonia may occur as a secondary infection associated with influenza. Intravenous drug abusers with fevers are suspect of staphylococcal bacteremia, and *S. aureus* can be present in their joint fluid, resulting in a septic arthritis. Localized inflammation in individuals with heart valve replacements, cerebrospinal fluid shunts, intravascular catheters, or other prosthetic devices may carry *S. epidermidis,* which is a common cause of urinary tract infection.

STREPTOCOCCUS

Species within the genus *Streptococcus* are gram-positive bacteria, which are virulent due to the toxins and enzymes they produce. Not only are some of the species of these bacteria among the most common and dangerous pathogens to humans, but many species are saprophytes that accelerate decomposition in the dead human body. There are three species of *Streptococcus* of clinical importance to embalmers: *S. agalactiae, S. pneumoniae,* and *S. pyogenes*.

Streptococcus agalactiae

The leading cause of bacterial sepsis and meningitis in newborns is *Streptococcus agalactiae*. This species of bacteria is common in raw milk, and it can present in newborns within the first five days of life. The infection is characterized by lethargy, jaundice, respiratory distress, shock, pneumonia, and anorexia. It is 50 percent fatal for low-weight neonates. *S. agalactiae* is also a primary cause of uterine infections accompanied by fever in postpartum women. As early as seven days, or as late as several months after delivery, symptoms of sepsis, meningitis, seizures, and psychomotor retardation may appear in mothers.

Pneumococcal Meningitis

The most common cause of bacterial meningitis in adults is *S. pneumoniae,* or pneumococcus, although half of the cases of pneumococcal meningitis occur in children under four. *S. pneumonia* is the causative agent of pneumococcal meningitis, which typically follows other infections with *S. pneumoniae* such as otitis media and pneumonia. *S. pneumoniae* is found in the nose and throat, and its capsule makes it highly virulent. Figure 25-1 depicts the capsule surrounding

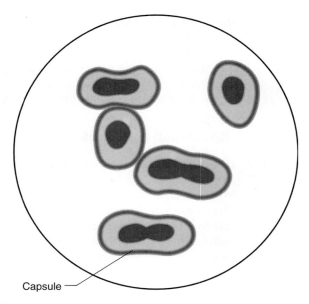

Capsule

Figure 25-1 *Streptococcus pneumoniae.*

S. pneumoniae, which explains its high virulence. The mortality rate of pneumococcal meningitis is high (40 percent), and the course of the disease is rapid. A vaccine for pneumococcal meningitis is available, and the disease is treated with penicillin.

 ## Otitis Media

Otitis media is often caused by the bacterium *S. pneumoniae,* although other microorganisms such as *Haemophilus influenzae* and *Staphylococcus aureus* are also known causes. Otitis media is an infection of the fluids of the middle ear, and it is often a complication of the common cold and infections of the nose and throat.

S. *pneumoniae* may be spread through contact with contaminated water found in swimming pools, through eardrum puncture, and through skull fractures. This postulant infection causes pressure behind the eardrum resulting in earaches. As a result of the narrow diameter of a child's eustachian tubes, these passages become easily occluded by bacterial colonies. When blockage occurs frequently, surgical tubes may be implanted to help keep the eustachian tube open. Otitis media is treated with antibiotics such as penicillin.

 ## Lobar Pneumonia

The most common cause of bacterial pneumonia is *S. pneumoniae.* Lobar pneumonia is isolated to the individual lobe of the lung where the infection occurs, although it can become systemic. If two lobes are involved, the resultant infection is known as double pneumonia. Lobar pneumonia is not usually a primary

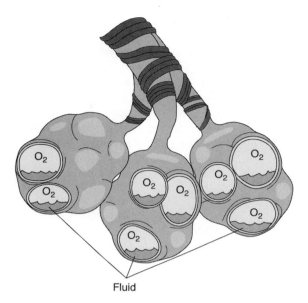

Figure 25-2 Pneumonia: alveolar filling with fluid.

infection; rather, it results from disturbance of the normal defense barriers of the body. Predisposing conditions include alcoholism, anesthesia, malnutrition, and viral infection of the respiratory system.

Lobar pneumonia involves the bronchi and the alveoli where edematous fluids are produced (Figure 25-2). The local production of fluid in the alveoli contributes to the infection's localization within the lobe of the lung. There is a vaccine available for pneumococcal pneumonia, used primary for the elderly. Lobar pneumonia is characterized by the following:

- Acute onset fever
- Chills
- Dyspnea (difficulty in breathing)
- Chest pain
- Bloody sputum

Strep Throat

Strep throat is caused by *S. pyogenes,* which is capable of producing injurious enzymes and toxins. Hyaluronidase, which is also known as spreading factor, is an enzyme produced by *S. pyogenes* that dissolves human connective tissues, allowing the organism to spread deep into the tissues.

Strep throat is common among children between 5 and 15. The symptoms appear within one to four days after exposure, including an acute onset of sore throat, malaise, fever, headache, nausea, vomiting, and abdominal pain. Color Plate 41 is a photograph of a person with strep throat. The disease is spread by droplets and close contact, and is treated with antibiotics.

Impetigo

S. pyogenes causes not only strep throat, but it is also the causative agent of impetigo. In addition, *Staphylococcus aureus* may also cause impetigo, which is a localized skin infection that begins with small vesicles that progress into weeping lesions (see Color Plate 42). After several days, a crust forms when the lesions dry. Children between two and five are most commonly infected. The disease spreads through insect bites, small abrasions in the skin, and contaminated hands on the face.

Scarlet Fever

Scarlet fever is a bacterial disease of the upper respiratory system caused by *S. pyogenes*. It is known as scarlet fever because of the reddening toxin produced by the bacteria, which results in inflammation of the throat. The toxin causes a pinkish-red skin rash (see Color Plate 43) and high fever. The tongue is spotted with a strawberry-like appearance (see Color Plate 44), after which it loses its upper membrane and becomes red and enlarged. The affected skin peels off of the body in a process known as *desquamation*. Scarlet fever is a communicable disease spread by inhalation of droplet spray. It does not have the high mortality rate that it once had in the United States due to the effectiveness of penicillin and other antibiotics in treating streptococcal infections.

Rheumatic Fever

Rheumatic fever is an autoimmune disease caused by a streptococcal infection. It occurs mainly between the ages of 4 and 18, where it develops as a type of arthritis noted by subcutaneous nodules at the joints. This septic infection may lead to inflammation of the heart valves, where it is known as rheumatic heart disease. Rheumatic heart disease is characterized by vegetative lesions of the heart valves, which prevent the valves from properly closing, allowing the blood flow to reverse. In the early 1980s, it was believed that rheumatic fever was being eradicated, but within a decade, cases began to appear with increasing regularity.

In approximately 10 percent of the cases of rheumatic fever, a condition known as Sydenham's chorea, or St. Vitus' dance, develops. St. Vitus' dance is characterized by purposeless, involuntary movements during waking hours. Self-injury may occur from flailing arms and legs. In many cases, the condition disappears in a few months without treatment.

In treating bacterial infections, it is important that antibiotics be continued even after the symptoms cease. It is possible for bacterial infections to remain dormant in the body for many years, only to surface at a later date causing severe disease. Failure to administer antibiotics to children until the antibiotics are depleted is more common among families of low economic and education levels. The remainder of the prescription should not be saved for recurrences of the symptoms or for other children who may potentially become ill. These practices can be detrimental to the afflicted child later in life.

Childbirth Fever

Puerperal sepsis, which was first known as childbed fever and is now also known as childbirth fever, is a septic disease mainly caused by *S. pyogenes,* although it may be caused by other bacteria. It is a nosocomial infection of the uterus resulting from childbirth or abortion. The *S. pyogenes* bacterium is spread to the uterus via contaminated surgical instruments or the hands of medical workers. The infection spreads from the uterus to the abdominal cavity, causing peritonitis. Modern disinfection techniques have reduced the occurrence of puerperal sepsis. The mortality rate associated with puerperal sepsis has also decreased due to the utilization of antibiotics such as penicillin in the treatment of streptococcal infections.

NEISSERIA GONORRHOEAE

Gonorrhea is a sexually transmitted disease caused by the *Neisseria gonorrhoeae* bacterium. It is spread through vaginal, oral, or anal sexual contact, including penis to vagina, penis to mouth, penis to anus, mouth to vagina, and mouth to anus contact. Ejaculation does not have to occur for gonorrhea to be transmitted or acquired. Humans are the only natural host for *N. gonorrhoea,* which is an aerobic, gram-negative diplococcus. *N. gonorrhoea* is uniquely virulent due to its capsule, pili, cell-wall proteins, endotoxin, and enzymes.

Gonorrhea is one of the most reported sexually transmitted bacterial disease in the United States. An ancient disease, it is most prevalent in young, sexually active teenagers and adults. Any sexually active person can be infected with gonorrhea. In the United States, the highest rates of infection are found in 15- to 19-year-old women and 20- to 24-year-old men. In 1999, 77 percent of the total number of cases of gonorrhea reported to the CDC occurred among African Americans (*Gonorrhea* 2001).

Gonococcus is extremely virulent in the body and attaches to tissues via its pili. Its most common symptom is a pustular discharge from the genitalia and painful urination (see Color Plate 45). Symptoms of rectal infection include discharge, anal itching, soreness, bleeding, and sometimes painful bowel movements. The symptoms appear a few days after infection. Sterility is a complication of gonorrhea due to infection of the testicles or scar tissue formation in the vas deferens, which is the tube that leads sperm from the testes to the ejaculatory duct.

Regardless of symptoms, once a person is infected with gonorrhea, he or she can spread the infection to others if condoms or other protective barriers are not used during sex. Both men and women often do not present signs of the disease and may be entirely unaware that they are spreading gonorrhea to their partners. Gonorrheal infections may also be transferred from the hands to the eyes, leading to possible blindness (see Color Plate 46). The heart, joints, meninges, and pharynx may also become involved in the infection. Color Plate 47 is a photograph of the feet of a person exhibiting gonococcal lesions. Gonococcus is not virulent outside of the body and dies readily in adverse environmental conditions.

Other areas of the body may also become infected with *N. gonorrhoea* through anorectal and oropharyngeal transmission. Although they may occur in females, infections in these sites are more common among homosexual males, resulting from the sexual practices of anal intercourse and oral sex, respectively. Approximately 30 percent to 60 percent of women with genital gonorrhea have concurrent rectal infections.

Antibiotics can successfully cure gonorrhea in adolescents and adults. Penicillin is no longer used to treat gonorrhea because many strains of the gonorrhea bacterium have become resistant to penicillin. Because many people with gonorrhea also have chlamydia, antibiotics for both infections are usually given together. Persons who have had gonorrhea and recovered can still contract the disease if they have sexual contact with another infected person.

In women, gonorrhea is a common cause of pelvic inflammatory disease. Of the 1 million women in the United States with pelvic inflammatory disease, many do not have symptoms or signs. If present, the signs and symptoms may include severe abdominal pain and fever, internal pus pockets that are hard to cure, long-lasting pelvic pain, and infertility. In men, gonorrhea can cause epididymitis, which is a painful condition of the testicles that can lead to infertility. Gonorrhea can also damage the prostate and lead to scarring of the urethra, making urination difficult. It can be fatal if it spreads to the blood or joints. Also, persons with gonorrhea can more easily contract HIV, the virus that causes AIDS.

The risk of contracting gonorrhea can be reduced through the proper use of latex condoms every time a person has sex. A condom put on the penis before starting sex and worn until the penis is withdrawn can help protect both partners from gonorrhea. However, condoms do not provide complete protection from sexually transmitted diseases because bacteria and lesions may be present in areas not covered by the condom, resulting in transmission of infection to another person.

A condition known as ophthalmia neonatorum is also caused by *N. gonorrhea*. During vaginal delivery, the infant's eyes may become infected from the presence of the bacteria in an infected mother's birth canal. The resultant infection can cause lesions on the eye and eventual blindness (see Color Plate 48). It can also cause joint infection or a life-threatening blood infection in the baby. Treatment of gonorrhea as soon as it is detected in pregnant women can lessen the risk of these complications. Ophthalmia neonatorum is rare in the United States because antimicrobial eye drops or silver nitrate are placed in newborns' eyes on delivery. Pregnant women should consult a healthcare provider for appropriate medications.

NEISSERIA MENINGITIDIS

Neisseria meningitidis, or meningococcus, is found in the nose and throat of up to 30 percent of asymptomatic individuals. It is an agent of endemic and epidemic meningitis, meningococcemia, pneumonia, purulent arthritis, eye infections, urogenital tract infections, and rectal infections. The virulence of *N. meningitidis* is due to the presence of a capsule and pili, and to the production of endotoxins. It can be spread through oral and respiratory droplets, or direct contact with infected sites on the body. Individuals living in close contact (i.e., college dorms and military barracks) are at an increased risk of contracting epidemic meningitis.

The carrier state may last several days to several months. Infection of the throat with *N. meningitidis* leads to bacteremia and meningitis. Meningococcal meningitis generally infects children under the age of two, although all age groups may be included. Its mortality rate is high (25 percent), and it is characterized by abrupt onset of headache, stiff neck, and sometimes fever. A rash may develop, and spontaneous blood clotting may also occur. Sometimes the disease is fulminant, resulting in a condition known as Waterhouse-Friderichsen syndrome. In these cases, death occurs within 12 to 48 hours from onset as a result of bleeding within the adrenal glands. *N. meningitidis* infections are treated with penicillin and other antibiotics.

CLOSTRIDIUM

All clostridia are spore-forming bacilli that are most frequently found in anaerobic infections or intoxications. Clostridia are spread by either ingestion or contamination of open wounds with soil. They are the causative agents of botulism, foodborne intoxication, gas gangrene, and tetanus. After death, *Clostridium perfringens* is also the cause of a postmortem condition known as tissue gas.

Botulism

Botulism is caused by an obligate anaerobic, gram-positive bacterial rod known as *Clostridium botulinum*. Botulin is the exotoxin produced by *C. botulinum* that causes food intoxication after ingesting the bacteria in contaminated foods such as home-canned vegetables, home-cured meats, and other preserved foods. The most common form of botulism in infants results from the ingestion of honey contaminated with *C. botulinum* spores. Only a small amount of botulin may block the release of acetylcholine from the synaptic end of nerves resulting in death. Botulism is characterized by the following:

- Paralysis
- Cardiac failure
- Respiratory failure
- Nausea
- Double vision
- Blurred vision
- Difficulty swallowing

Symptoms may appear as early as two hours or as late as three to eight days after ingestion of *C. botulinum*. Fever is not typically present in cases of botulism. *C. botulinum* is found in soil and water sediment, and wounds that become infected with the spores may develop into a systemic disease similar to foodborne intoxication.

Food Intoxication

Gastroenteritis is a form of food intoxication caused by improper handling of meat during the slaughtering of animals. Intestinal contents are allowed to contaminate meat as it is slaughtered. Cooking the meat lowers the oxygen level and provides obligate anaerobes like *C. perfringens* the opportunity to reproduce. Keeping foods warm for over 20 minutes and inadequate refrigeration are two main causes of the growth of *C. perfringens* colonies. These bacteria grow in the intestinal tract causing abdominal pain and diarrhea. Most cases of food poisoning are mild, with symptoms appearing 8 to 12 hours after ingestion of the bacteria.

Tetanus

Clostridium tetani is the causative agent of the bacterial infection that leads to tetanus, which is also known as lockjaw. *C. tetani* is an obligate anaerobic, endospore-forming, gram-positive rod. It is found in soil contaminated with animal feces. The symptoms of tetanus are caused by its neurotoxin, which is released on the death and lysis of the bacteria by phagocytes. The toxin moves toward the central nervous system via the peripheral nerves and blood.

The bacteria themselves cause no inflammation at the site of infection, and they do not generally move from the local site of infection. The tetanus neurotoxin tetanospasmin prevents muscle relaxation, causing opposing muscles to contract at the same time. The muscles of the jaw are affected first, spreading to the respiratory muscles where death occurs via asphyxia. Deep puncture wounds with little bleeding, similar to those caused by stepping on a nail, provide an excellent reservoir for *C. tetani*.

A serum is available that helps protect against tetanus; however, it requires a booster shot every 10 years and many Americans fail to receive their boosters. In certain parts of the world, tetanus is a common cause of death among infants who have had their umbilical cords treated with soil, clay, and manure as part of cultural practices. Worldwide, there are assumed to be several hundred thousand cases of tetanus from all causes each year. As a result of the widespread use of the diphtheria, tetanus, and acellular pertussis (DTaP) vaccine, tetanus is no longer common in the United States. Tetanus may also occur in newborns from the use of contaminated instruments during delivery, and it can occur in cases of septic abortions.

Gas Gangrene

Clostridium perfringens is a gram-positive, endospore-forming anaerobe that causes tissue gas in the postmortem state and gas gangrene, or myonecrosis, in the antemortem state. Gangrene is necrosis of tissue. *C. perfringens* is a saprophytic bacteria, meaning that it thrives on dead and decaying tissue. Gangrene is caused by a disruption in the flow of blood to tissues. It is often a complication of diabetes mellitus, especially of the feet and legs. When *C. perfringens* multiplies, it causes the fermentation of carbohydrates in the tissues, which releases carbon dioxide and hydrogen gases. The toxins move through the swollen tissue causing further necrosis of neighboring tissue. Gas gangrene is often fatal, spreading throughout the body via the blood. Embalming instruments exposed to *C. perfringens* must be disinfected, as the bacteria may spread on these fomites from one deceased person to another.

Tissue Gas

Clostridium perfringens is the causative agent of a postmortem condition known as tissue gas. *C. perfringens* is found in soil and water in the environment, and it is part of the normal intestinal flora of humans. Tissue gas may result from the presence of gas gangrene in the deceased before death, from bacterial translocation during the process of decomposition, or from the use of contaminated instruments during the embalming of the deceased. Even if appropriate embalming methods are followed, the quantity of microorganisms, the toxins they produce, and the organism's resistance to many disinfectants may collectively result in tissue gas formation.

Gases may form quite rapidly in the deceased, resulting in extreme disfigurement. Tissue damage is likely to occur in the soft tissues of the eyelids, neck, extremities, female breasts, and the male scrotum. Conditions that predispose the deceased to tissue gas formation include recent abdominal surgery; the presence of gangrene at the time of death; intestinal ulcerations or perforations; contaminated wounds of the skin; intestinal obstruction or hemorrhage; inadequate embalming; and contact with contaminated instruments.

CORYNEBACTERIA

Corynebacteria are a group of bacteria that are gram-positive, non-spore-forming rods that cause a wide range of infections. Many of the *Corynebacteria* are not well categorized, so there is a low rate of identification of these lesser-known species as pathogens of human disease. Bacteria of the genus *Corynebacterium* are facultative aerobic, free-living saprophytes, which can be found worldwide in fresh- and saltwater, soil, and the air. Mycobacteria are closely related to the *Corynebacteria*. The most widely studied and understood species in this genus is the diphtheria bacillus *Corynebacterium diphtheriae*. However, other species are becoming better understood as opportunistic human pathogens.

Each of the following microorganisms rarely occurs in humans, but they are becoming more prevalent—especially among immunosuppressed populations. *C. jeikeium* has been isolated as the cause of endocarditis after catheters or prosthetic valve replacement in the heart. *C. urealyticum* is the causative agent of urinary infections. *C. pseudotuberculosis* can cause respiratory illness in humans who have been in contact with infected sheep. *C. pseudodiphtheriticum*, *C. striatum*, and *Rothia dentocariosa* are all part of the normal flora of the human nose and throat, and they can all cause infections in humans.

Diphtheria

Diphtheria occurs in two forms, respiratory and cutaneous. The pathogen that causes diphtheria is *Corynebacterium diphtheriae*. Until 1935, diphtheria was the leading infectious killer of children in the United States. Now, however, it is considered uncommon in North America and Western Europe. Due to immunization programs in the United States, in particular the DTaP vaccine, the number of cases of diphtheria reported annually has fallen to five or fewer.

Although *C. diphtheriae* is readily killed by heat and most disinfectants, it is resistant to drying and remains viable in the environment for weeks. The diphtheria toxin is extremely potent and is lethal for humans in small amounts because it is able to block the production of proteins in human eukaryotic cells. Humans are the only natural host for *C. diphtheriae*.

C. diphtheriae is spread through airborne droplet transmission or hand to mouth contact. The following disease conditions occur within two to five days:

- Sore throat
- Red rash on the abdomen
- Fever
- Fatigue
- Swelling of the neck
- Bleeding in the throat
- Grayish-white pseudomembrane in the throat
- Paralysis

The most common site of infection is the tonsils or pharynx, which can bleed as a result. A tough, grayish-white pseudomembrane forms in the throat. The membrane is localized in the pharynx and contains dead tissue, fibrin, and bacterial cells. If the infection reaches the kidneys or heart, it can be acutely fatal. A red rash of the abdomen can also be present. Skin lesions are also possible in cases of diphtheria, as shown in Color Plate 49. Diphtheria can affect the nerves, causing partial paralysis due to the demylinating of peripheral neurons by the diphtheria toxin. Diphtheria is treated by the administration of antitoxins commercially produced in horses.

FRANCISELLA TULARENSIS

Tularemia is caused by the bacterium *Francisella tularensis*. This highly infectious, strictly aerobic, nonmotile, small, gram-negative bacillus is a facultatively intracellular parasite. Tularemia was discovered in Tulare County, California, and it is acquired in 90 percent of the cases in the United States by handling rabbits and then rubbing the eyes, hence its alternate name of rabbit fever. *F. tularensis* can enter the body through inhalation, ingestion, bites, or minor skin breaks.

The first sign of tularemia is a local inflammation and a small ulcer, as shown in Color Plate 50. About a week after infection, the regional lymph nodes enlarge and fill with pus. Septicemia, pneumonia, and abscesses throughout the body ensue. Ingestion of infected meat leads to infection in the mouth and throat. The bite of arthropods, such as deer flies, ticks, or rabbit lice may also be a mechanism of transmission of the disease.

MYCOBACTERIUM AVIUM

Organisms causing *Mycobacterium avium* complex (MAC), are commonly found in soil, water, and house dust. Coastal marshes have higher concentrations of the organisms than other areas. *M. avium* is a cause of disease in poultry and swine, but animal to human transmission has not been shown to be an important factor in human disease. However, the incidence of MAC has increased owing to the prevalence of AIDS.

MAC is a serious bacterial infection affecting persons with HIV. It is related to tuberculosis and is sometimes called *Mycobacterium avium* intracellulare. MAC infection is usually found only in people with under 50 T4 cells, meaning that healthy individuals would not usually contract this disease. MAC affects the intestines and inner organs first, and is noted by the following:

- Weight loss
- Fever
- Chills
- Night sweats
- Swollen glands
- Abdominal pains
- Diarrhea
- Fatigue

MYCOBACTERIUM TUBERCULOSIS

There are over 1 billion cases of tuberculosis infection worldwide, with 8 million to 10 million new cases and 3 million deaths each year. Although it was only first described by Robert Koch in 1882, tuberculosis is the oldest documented communicable disease. The incidence of tuberculosis in the United States was declining before 1985. The number of cases has risen since then, due to the prevalence of AIDS, increased IV drug use, and increased transmission within closed environments such as prisons and nursing homes.

Tuberculosis is caused by *Mycobacterium tuberculosis*, which is a highly resistant, rod-shaped bacterium with a high lipid content in its cell wall. Up to 60 percent of the dried mass of *M. tuberculosis* consists of fats, which is much higher than that of other bacteria. This high lipid content allows this bacterium to be resistant to desiccation and staining. *M. tuberculosis* can survive for weeks in dried sputum and is resistant to antiseptics and many disinfectants.

In healthy individuals, the tuberculosis bacterium is typically destroyed. However, in individuals with suppressed immune systems, this pathogen invades attacking macrophages. Once the macrophages engulf the microbe in the lungs, a tubercule forms (Figure 25-3). After a few weeks, the macrophages die, forming a caseous, or cheeselike, center in the tubercle. If the disease does not become dormant at this point, the caseous center enlarges in the process of liquefaction,

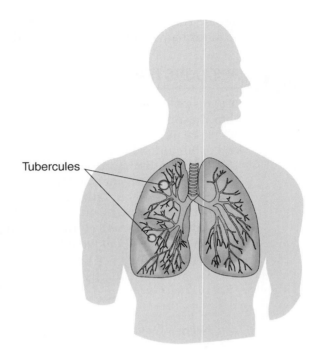

Figure 25-3 Tuberculosis.

allowing an air-filled tuberculosis cavity to form in which the bacteria grow. The formation of these cavities is known as cavitation. Liquefaction continues until the tubercle ruptures, allowing bacilli to invade the bronchiole and be disseminated throughout the respiratory system.

In 1991, 15 percent of the cases of tuberculosis were found to be resistant to a least one antituberculosis drug. The treatment of tuberculosis, therefore, often requires the use of more than one drug. Many strains of *M. tuberculosis* are drug-fast, meaning that they are multidrug resistant. The primary reason why treatment of tuberculosis fails is that patients do not comply with the drug therapy, which is associated with their socioeconomic status. In many places in the world, the expense of the necessary medications is a prohibitive factor in treatment programs (*Tuberculosis* 2002).

SPIROCHETES

Spirochetes have a flexible, helical shape. They are unicellular bacteria that are the causative agents of many important zoonotic diseases. Diseases that can be transmitted from animals to humans are known as zoonotic diseases. These bacteria differ from other bacteria because they have a flexible cell wall that is wound with several fibrils. These flagella-like fibrils allow a variety of motility in liquids. Spirochetes are free-living and may survive as either pathogens or as part of the normal microbiota of a host. They can utilize carbohydrates, amino acids, fatty acids, fatty alcohols, and carbon as energy sources. Depending on the species, they may be anaerobic, facultatively anaerobic, or aerobic. Spirochetes are gram-negative. Three common genera of spirochetes include *Borrelia*, *Leptospira*, and *Treponema*.

Leptospira interrogans

Leptospira interrogans is the spirochete that causes leptospirosis. Leptospirosis is primarily a disease of animals, although it can cause liver and kidney disease in humans. *L. interrogans* has a characteristically hooked end when viewed under a microscope. Humans become infected with the bacterium when they come in contact with the contaminated waste of infected animals or infected water or soil. Dogs, rats, and other rodents are the most common reservoirs for *L. interrogans* in the United States. The leptospires live in the lumen of renal tubules and are excreted in the urine of the host. Leptospires can survive in neutral waters for months.

According to the National Center for Infectious Diseases (*Leptospirosis* 2001), there are about 50 cases of leptospirosis reported each year in the United States. Symptoms begin about one week after infection. Leptospires are most likely to enter humans through nonintact skin or mucous membranes. The symptoms of leptospirosis, which typically subside within a few days, are headache, muscle ache, chills, and fever. A more severe, systemic infection known as Weil's disease, may also result from this spirochete. Weil's disease, which may be fatal, can include renal infection, hepatic infection, or central nervous system infection.

Borrelia burgdorferi

Lyme disease, or Lyme borreliosis, is caused by the gram-negative, highly flexible bacterial spirochete *Borrelia burgdorferi*. Lyme disease is named after Lyme, Connecticut, the geographic location in which it was first reported in the United States. Although the first reporting of Lyme disease in the United States occurred in 1975, a similar disease was described in Sweden in 1908. Dr. Willy Burgdorfer discovered the causative spirochetes in ticks during the 1975 outbreak of juvenile rheumatoid arthritis that is now known as Lyme borreliosis.

All *Borrelia* are arthropod-borne, and *B. burgdorferi* is transmitted by ticks, although other insects may also harbor the spirochete. Nymphs, which are young ticks, transmit the disease directly into human tissue by regurgitating during feeding. Lyme disease is the most common tick-borne disease in the United States, occurring most frequently between the months of June and September, when more people are outdoors. Although children were the first group to become infected, the disease affects people of all ages and both sexes.

Deer and field mice are the most common reservoirs from which ticks feed. Infection with *B. burgdorferi* causes a characteristic "bull's-eye" rash at the site of the bite (see Color Plate 51). About 60 percent of those infected exhibit this bull's-eye rash, which is technically known as erythema migrans (EM). As the rash fades, flu-like symptoms appear. *B. burgdorferi* has the ability to adhere to the endothelial cells of blood vessels, facilitating its growth.

If the disease enters a late stage, a pacemaker may be required to control damage caused to the heart by the spread of the bacteria. The nervous system may also become involved, leading to paralysis of the face, meningitis, and encephalitis. Arthritis often accompanies cases of Lyme disease due to the body's immune response to the pathogen. This arthritis may last for months or even years with relapsing episodes. Long-term Lyme disease cases resemble the later stages of syphilis, which is caused by a spirochete of the same family as *B. burgdorferi*.

To reduce the risk of contracting Lyme disease, individuals who participate in outdoor activities should utilize repellents and wear protective clothing. Attached ticks should be removed immediately because pathogen transmission is related to the length of attachment.

Treponema pallidum

Syphilis is a sexually transmitted disease caused by *Treponema pallidum*, which is an exclusively human pathogen. *T. pallidum* is a bacterial spirochete with three flagella inserted into each end of the cell, providing it a graceful motility in fluids. Because of its outer layer of lipids, *T. pallidum* causes little response from the body's immune system and has, therefore, become known as a Teflon® pathogen. Syphilis has often been called "the great imitator" because so many of its signs and symptoms are indistinguishable from those of other diseases.

The first cases of syphilis in Europe were reported at the end of the 15th century. Epidemiologists theorize that the disease was either brought back to Europe by Christopher Columbus's men from the West Indies, or it was endemic in Africa and transmitted by armies and civilians between continents. It was not until the 18th century that it was determined that syphilis is spread through venereal transmission. The causative agent for syphilis was discovered in 1908, and the name of the disease is attributed to a poem written in 1530, by Girolamo Fracastoro entitled, "Syphilis, or the French Disease." In the poem, the hero is a shepherd named Syphilus who was believed to be the first person to have the disease. He contracted the disease by cursing the gods, which reflects earlier humans beliefs in the origin of diseases.

Syphilis is spread through direct sexual contact with someone who has an active primary or secondary syphilitic lesion. These lesions are typically found on the genitals, which include the vagina and cervix in females and the penis in males. Nongenital contact with a lesion on the lips or anus may also spread the disease. Syphilis may also be transmitted from mother to fetus, resulting in congenital syphilis. It cannot be spread by toilet seats, door knobs, swimming pools, hot tubs, bath tubs, shared clothing, or eating utensils. While the health problems caused by syphilis in adults and newborns are serious in their own right, it is now known that the genital sores caused by syphilis in adults also make it easier to transmit and acquire HIV infection sexually.

Although there are no home remedies or over-the-counter drugs that will cure syphilis, penicillin and other antibiotics will kill the syphilis bacterium and prevent further damage. However, treatment will not repair any existing damage. Persons who receive syphilis treatment must abstain from sexual contact with new partners until the syphilis sores are completely healed. Persons with syphilis must notify their sex partners, so that they also can be tested and receive treatment. Having had syphilis does not protect a person from getting it again.

People who know that they are not infected, and who have sex only with each other, cannot contract syphilis. A good defense against becoming infected during sex is to use a latex condom before beginning sex and to keep it on until the penis is withdrawn. Condoms, however, do not provide complete protection because syphilis sores can be on areas not covered by a condom. Washing the genitals, urinating, or douching after sex does not prevent sexually transmitted diseases like syphilis. Any unusual discharge, sore, or rash, especially in the groin area, should be a signal to stop having sex and to see a doctor at once.

There are three stages of syphilis—primary, secondary, and tertiary—based on each stage's unique clinical manifestations.

Primary Stage. The primary stage of syphilis is noted by the appearance of a chancre, which is a small, hard ulcer (Figure 25-4) ulcer at the site of infection (e.g., penis, anus, vagina, cervix, or mouth) appearing approximately 10 to 90 days after contact. A serous exudate forms in the center of this painless lesion. Syphilitic chancres abound with treponemes, and they are extremely infectious. The chancre is frequently not visible in females because it appears on the cervix or the vaginal wall.

In both sexes, the chancre may be present in the anal canal without the knowledge of the infected individual. There are no systemic signs or symptoms of disease during the primary stage, despite the spread of bacteria throughout the blood and lymph systems during this stage of syphilis. In a few weeks, the

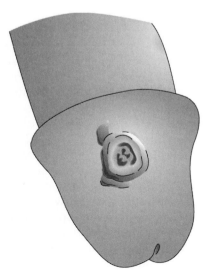

Figure 25-4 Syphilis chancre.

chancre disappears and infected individuals may, mistakenly, assume that they are no longer infected.

Secondary Stage. About 2 to 12 weeks after the chancre disappears, the secondary stage of the disease may begin in some individuals. The individual suffers from hair loss, swollen lymph nodes, sore throat, malaise, and low-grade fever. Infected individuals may also present with a rash that is unusual in that it can occur on the palms of the hands and the soles of the feet (see Color Plate 52). All secondary syphilitic lesions of the skin and mucous membranes are highly infectious. The secondary stage may either relapse for several weeks, or it may go entirely unnoticed by the infected individual. A person can easily pass the disease to sex partners when primary or secondary stage signs or symptoms are present.

Tertiary Stage. In about 25 percent of the cases of syphilis, the disease does not progress beyond the secondary stage, and another 25 percent of the cases become latent and no further symptoms are experienced by the infected individual, whether treated medically or not. The other 50 percent of cases of syphilis develop into a tertiary stage 2 to 20 years later. During the latent period, the individual may experience no symptoms of the disease.

During the tertiary stage of syphilis, a rubberlike lesion known as a gumma appears on the bone, viscera, and skin (see Color Plate 53). In the tertiary stage, syphilis may begin to damage the internal organs, including the brain, nerves, eyes, heart, blood vessels, liver, bones, and joints. The aorta can be affected, causing it to weaken. A loss of motor control can occur in cases of syphilis in which the central nervous system becomes infected. Syphilis can lead to seizures, blindness, and death. In the United States, the tertiary stage of syphilis is rarely seen due to medical intervention.

VIBRIO CHOLERAE

Asiatic cholera, which is also known as epidemic cholera, is caused by *Vibrio cholerae*, a gram-negative rod with a single, polar flagellum. *V. cholerae* is a bacterium found in contaminated seafood, usually from the Gulf coast of the United States. Cholera is more common in Asia and is endemic in India. According to the National Center for Infectious Diseases (*Cholera* 2001), in 1991–1992, 6,000 deaths occurred in a cholera epidemic in South America, and an eighth pandemic of epidemic cholera is spreading rapidly now. When untreated, cholera has a 50 percent mortality rate in comparison to treated cases in which the mortality is near 1 percent.

V. cholerae grows in the small intestine, producing an enterotoxin that results in the secretion of chlorides, bicarbonates, and water. These high levels of electrolytes and water cause "rice-water" stool (see Color Plate 54). The loss of between three and five gallons of fluid and electrolytes from the intestines each day causes fatal shock. The blood becomes extremely viscous due to the loss of fluids, causing failure of the organs. Fever is not a typical symptom of cholera.

BACILLUS ANTHRACIS

There are more than 50 species of *Bacillus* in the environment. Most of these rod-shaped microorganisms are commonly found in water and soil. *Bacillus* has been isolated from the subarctic to desert regions, from thermal springs and saltwater, and from various plants. These microorganisms are capable of survival in such diverse environments due to their ability to form endospores that can withstand temperatures ranging between 23°F and 167°F (–5°C and 75°C).

Bacillus anthracis is a gram-positive rod found singly or in chains; however, its gram staining changes with age or nutritional stress. It is an aerobic and facultative bacterium that forms spores aerobically. It is nonmotile, unlike other species of the genus *Bacillus*. The unique capsule on *B. anthracis* protects it from the body's phagocytic cells.

Anthrax is a disease common in livestock around the world. The animals do not spread the disease to one another; instead, they become infected by the spores found on plants they eat. The three forms of human anthrax include cutaneous, inhalation, and gastrointestinal anthrax. Each of these forms of anthrax results from wound contamination, the inhalation, or the ingestion of spores. In the United States, there are typically fewer than five anthrax cases per year reported. Worldwide, however, several thousand cases are reported annually.

The suspected use of anthrax as a biological weapon for terrorism in the United States requires a full understanding of the disease. Anthrax is typically treated with penicillin and a broad array of antibiotics. It is not a contagious disease. To become infected with any form of anthrax, the individual must be exposed to the spores of *B. anthracis*.

When embalming the deceased suspected of harboring anthrax, proper sanitization techniques and standard universal precaution procedures are sufficient to retard possible infection. As with all accidental exposures through needle sticks and other means, the embalmer should seek proper medical attention immediately. There is currently one vaccine for anthrax in the United States available to individuals, such as veterinarians, whose occupations require them to handle animals or animal products.

Cutaneous Anthrax

The overwhelming majority of anthrax cases in the world are cutaneous anthrax cases. When wounds such as skin cuts, abrasions, or insect bites become contaminated with anthrax spores, a small lesion appears about two to three days later. This lesion develops into a ring of small blisters surrounding a dark center that eventually ulcerates and dries. This area of dead tissue is known as an **eschar**, which does not form pus or cause pain (see Color Plate 55 and Color Plate 56). Within two to three weeks, the eschar dries, separates from the skin, and falls off, leaving a scar. Cutaneous anthrax lesions usually remain localized, but they may spread to the lymph glands. If a septic infection occurs, its symptoms are fever, malaise, and headache, although in normal cases of cutaneous anthrax septic infection does not develop.

Inhalation Anthrax

Woolsorter's disease, which is also called inhalation anthrax or pulmonary anthrax, is acquired when spores are inhaled into the lungs. Within two to five days of inhaling the *B. anthracis* spores, a mild respiratory infection occurs resembling a cold or flu. These cold- or flulike symptoms last about two to three days before a sudden phase of respiratory distress occurs. The ensuing respiratory failure occurs along with cyanosis, shock, disorientation, and coma. The severe phase of inhalation anthrax may only take 24 hours before death occurs.

Gastrointestinal Anthrax

The ingestion of *B. anthracis* spores may lead to an infection known as gastrointestinal anthrax, in which lesions form on the mucosal lining of the intestine. The characteristics of gastrointestinal anthrax are:

- Abdominal pain
- Nausea
- Anorexia
- Vomiting
- Bloody diarrhea

Gastrointestinal anthrax is the most difficult form to diagnose, and, therefore, has the highest fatality rate. Only 1 percent of all cases of anthrax in the world are gastrointestinal, and this form of anthrax has never been reported in the United States.

BORDETELLA

There are seven species of the genus *Bordetella*, which are small gram-negative bacilli that are all obligate aerobic bacteria. *Bordetella* infections are contracted through the inhalation of aerosolized particles into the respiratory tract. These microbes are uniquely adapted to reproduce on the ciliated cells of respiratory epithelium. Although the organism remains localized within the respiratory tract, the toxins it produces have systemic effects.

Whooping Cough

Whooping cough, which is also known as pertussis is caused by the bacterium *Bordetella pertussis*. It is one of the most highly communicable childhood diseases, infecting over 90 percent of susceptible households. Even in well-immunized populations like the United States, outbreaks of pertussis still occur every few years and isolated cases occur continuously. Adults appear to carry bacteria without symptoms, but they transmit the disease to children, especially when immunization rates decrease.

The initial infection takes about one to two weeks to develop into a mild respiratory infection resembling the common cold. At this stage, the disease is highly communicable due to the large number of microorganisms in the respiratory tract. Toxins released by *B. pertussis* inhibit the normal immune system response in the human host.

About one to two weeks after the initial stage of whooping cough, *B. pertussis* impedes the action of the tiny hairlike cilia of the respiratory tract, which help to expel mucus from the respiratory system. When the cilia are unable to perform this function due to a pertussis infection, the mucus accumulates in the respiratory system. The infected individual makes a whooping sound while gasping for air between violent coughs, which occurs with greater frequency at night. These spells of coughing can occur many times a day, followed by vomiting. The disease usually runs its course within about four weeks from initial infection, and it may take several weeks or months for complete recovery.

Less common but more severe complications related to pertussis are associated with its violent coughing episodes. These complications can include rupture of the alveoli in the lungs, which can permit inspired air to gain access to the subcutaneous tissues, resulting in a condition known as subcutaneous emphysema. Bleeding can also occur in the superficial blood vessels of the eyes and nose. Both umbilical and inguinal hernias can occur, as well as rupture of the diaphragm. In infants and young children, the rectum can prolapse, meaning that its mucosal lining protrudes through the anus.

DTaP Vaccine

The original vaccine against whooping cough was the diphtheria, tetanus, and pertussis (DTP) vaccine, which was developed in the 1930s. According to the United Stated Department of Health and Human Services National Immunization Program (*Diphtheria, tetanus, and pertussis vaccines* 2001), this vaccine is no longer used in the United States because it causes mild side effects in about 20 percent of immunized children. Currently, the DTaP vaccine is used to immunize children against these diseases. The vaccine is given to children at the ages of 2 months, 4 months, 6 months, 15–18 months, and 4–6 years old at the same time as several other vaccines. The Centers for Disease Control and Prevention's Vaccines for Children Program provides several vaccines for those children whose parents cannot afford the vaccine. The World Health Organization also supports vaccination programs throughout the world.

ENTERICS

Members of the family *Enterobacteriaceae* are also known as enterics, which include the genera *Escherichia, Klebsiella, Proteus, Salmonella,* and *Shigella.* Enterics are gram-negative, non-spore-forming, facultatively anaerobic bacilli.

Escherichia coli

The most significant opportunistic pathogen of all the enterics is *Escherichia coli.* This bacillus is common in human intestinal flora. Most strains of *E. coli* are motile and generally contain both pili and fimbriae. *E. coli* can cause several types of diarrheal illnesses, meningitis in newborns, urinary tract infections, and infections of wounds.

Traveler's diarrhea is caused by a strain of *E. coli* that is found in tropical and subtropical climates, especially in developing countries. When individuals travel from industrialized countries to developing countries, they may acquire this illness due to poor hygiene standards, inadequate sources of drinking water, and a lack of proper sanitation. Traveler's diarrhea is normally a self-limiting disease characterized by low-grade fever, nonbloody watery diarrhea, nausea, and abdominal cramps.

Two other strains of *E. coli* cause diarrheal illnesses that are much more severe than traveler's diarrhea. Enteroinvasive *E. coli* and enterohemorrhagic *E. coli* cause damage to the intestines that penetrates the intestinal wall. The former is transmitted from person to person through the fecal-oral route, and results in fever, severe abdominal cramps, malaise, and watery diarrhea with pus, mucus, and blood.

In cases of hemorrhagic diarrhea and colitis caused by *E. coli*, the classic progression is from watery diarrhea to a bloody diarrhea with cramps that may or may not present with a low-grade fever. The infection is fatal because it is accompanied by low platelet count, hemolytic anemia, and kidney failure. Children in daycare centers and schools, as well as the elderly in nursing homes, are especially at risk. The spread of the infection has been identified through processed meats, such as undercooked hamburgers from fast food restaurants, unpasteurized milk, and apple cider.

Klebsiella pneumoniae

Klebsiella pneumoniae is part of the normal gastrointestinal tracts of humans and animals, but it differs from other genera of enterics in that it is nonmotile. *K. pneumoniae* is unique because it possesses a polysaccharide capsule that resists human phagocytic cells, and it retards the absorption of antimicrobials. This gram-negative rod is a frequent cause of lower respiratory tract infections, especially in hospitals. Among immunosuppressed populations, *K. pneumoniae* has been known to cause urinary tract infections, wound infections, and outbreaks of nosocomial infections in newborn nurseries.

Proteus Species

Proteus is a genus of bacteria that is found in the human gastrointestinal tract. *Proteus mirabilis* and *Proteus vulgaris* are widely recognized human pathogens. Both species have been known to cause urinary tract infections, ear infections, and wound infections, particularly among burn patients. The colonies of these species have a unique odor that has been described as "burned chocolate." The primary importance of this gram-negative bacillus to the embalmer is its role in the decomposition of proteins. *P. vulgaris* is an obligate saprophyte that contributes to the decomposition of the body and the production of a ptomaine known as indole, which can inhibit proper cross-linking of proteins by the action of formaldehyde during the embalming process.

Food Infection

Salmonella gastroenteritis, or salmonellosis, is a type of food infection in which *Salmonella enteritidis* is ingested and grows by attaching to cells in the intestinal tract via fimbriae, approximately 8 to 36 hours after ingestion. Death associated with salmonellosis usually results from septicemia. Complications of salmonellosis include fever, chills, abdominal pain, and watery diarrhea.

Meat products, especially poultry, are commonly contaminated with *Salmonella* bacteria. To slow the transmission of *Salmonella* in the food preparation area, food handlers should thoroughly wash their hands after dealing with any meats or eggs. In addition, any items used in food preparation, such as cutting boards and mixing bowls, should be washed with soap and water after they have been in contact with raw meats or eggs.

Eggs cooked to allow the yolk to remain liquid may still be contaminated because the cooking time was not sufficient to kill the *Salmonella* bacteria. Foods containing raw eggs, such as hollandaise sauce, salad dressings, and eggnog, may also be contaminated. Salmonellosis is more likely to occur in children, the elderly, and individuals with sickle cell disease and other hemolytic disorders.

Typhoid Fever

Typhoid fever is an acute, contagious, bacterial infection of the digestive system. It is characterized by the presence of necrotic lesions in Peyer's patches, mesenteric glands, and the spleen. The incubation period for typhoid fever is about two weeks, and typhoid is caused by the *Salmonella typhi* bacterium, which is not found in animals. It is transmitted from one human to another through human feces. Although the incidence of typhoid has diminished in the United States in the last century, typhoid is still a frequent cause of death in countries with developing sanitation standards. Proper sewage disposal, water treatment, and food sanitation all help to reduce the incidence of typhoid. Currently, most cases of typhoid in the United States are acquired through foreign travel. Typhoid fever causes rose spots on the chest or abdomen, as pictured in Color Plate 57. Other complications of typhoid include:

- Prolonged fever
- Headache
- Abdominal pain
- Nosebleeds
- Whitish furlike material on the tongue
- Discoloration of the tongue

The most famous case of a typhoid carrier was Typhoid Mary. Mary Mallon became known as Typhoid Mary because she was a chronic carrier of *S. typhi* and allegedly spread the bacteria to several people as a cook in the early 1900s. *S. typhi* is carried in the gallbladder and found in the feces of the infected. Typhoid Mary worked in New York state and was assumed to be responsible for several outbreaks of typhoid fever and three deaths. The State of New York attempted several times to restrain her from working in food handling.

Shigella Species

Bacillary dysentery, which is also known as shigellosis, is caused by a group of anaerobic, gram-negative rods known as *Shigella* species. The *Shigella* bacteria are found only in the intestinal tracts of humans, apes, and monkeys. The disease is spread via the fecal-oral route by flies, fingers, and contaminated food or water. Young children in daycare centers; the impoverished who live in overcrowded, inadequate housing; and, people who participate in anal-oral sex are at a higher risk of contracting shigellosis.

In the United States, the most common species causing shigellosis are *S. sonnei* and *S. flexneri*. Although young children were once the most susceptible population for this disease, more recent demographic investigation indicates that young adults approximately 25 years old are most likely to contract shigellosis. This change is primarily a result of the occurrence of so-called gay bowel syndrome among homosexual men.

Dysentery is a severe form of diarrhea with blood and mucus in the stool. The blood and mucus result from damage to the colon by the *Shigella* toxin, although the bacteria remain in the small intestine. Symptoms and signs appear approximately 24 to 48 hours after ingestion of the microorganism. Sufferers may have up to 20 bowel movements per day, abdominal cramps, and fever. There are approximately 20,000–25,000 cases of dysentery in the United States reported each year. If untreated, the mortality rate of dysentery can be as high as 20 percent. Dysentery was one of the leading causes of death during the Civil War.

YERSINIA PESTIS

Over one-fourth of the population of Europe was killed in the Middle Ages due to the spread of *Yersinia pestis* from infected rats to fleas and then to humans. *Y. pestis* is the causative pathogen of bubonic plague. It is a gram-negative, short, plump rod that has a safety-pin appearance on staining. There are approximately 10 to 15 cases of plague in the United States each year (Plague 2001), and the World Health Organization reports 1,000–3,000 cases globally per year (Plague 2002). At the beginning of the 1900s, 10 million people were reported as having died due to the plague. Bubonic plague has a mortality rate of 50–75 percent. Also known as the black death, the plague receives this name from the dark hemorrhagenic areas present on the body.

Y. pestis has been isolated in rats, wild rodents, ground squirrels, prairie dogs, and chipmunks. Infection results from contact with infected animals, which can occur from scratches, skinning the animal, or similar contact. The disease spreads through the blood and lymph causing hyperplastic growths of the lymph nodes known as buboes (see Color Plate 58). Death occurs in untreated cases of plague in less than a week after the appearance of symptoms. There is also a pneumonic form of plague in which the infection is found in the respiratory system. Pneumonic plague can be transmitted from person to person, and it is often a result of bubonic plague.

HAEMOPHILUS INFLUENZAE

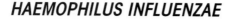

Haemophilus influenzae is the causative agent of influenzal meningitis. *H. influenzae* is a highly virulent gram-negative, nonmotile bacterium. Its high virulence is a function of its unique capsule and antigens on its outer membrane, which have been shown to paralyze the sweeping motion of ciliated respiratory epithelium. Influenzal meningitis is found in approximately 45 percent of the reported cases of meningitis in the United States each year. Influenzal meningitis is characterized by:

- Irritability
- Poor feeding in infants
- Fever
- Severe headache
- Nausea
- Vomiting
- Pain and stiffness in neck when flexed
- Pain in back when chin is flexed toward chest
- Unusual body posture
- Sensitivity to light

  H. influenzae received its name erroneously because it was thought to be the causative agent of the influenza pandemic of 1918. It is now understood that the presence of this bacterial rod in nasal and lung cultures taken from infected individuals was actually the result of a secondary infection. Influenza is actually caused by a virus and not the *Haemophilus influenzae* bacterium. Influenzal meningitis occurs mainly between the age of six months and six years, and it is the primary cause of childhood arthritis.

GASTROENTERITIS AND STOMACH ULCERS

The leading cause of gastroenteritis is *Campylobacter jejuni*, which is a gram-negative, non-spore-forming rod with an S-shaped, "seagull-wing" appearance. Figure 25-5 illustrates the infection with the stomach and small intestine. Individuals with gastroenteritis suffer from mild abdominal pain within 2 to 10 days after ingesting the organism. The bacteria are contracted through contact with infected pets (i.e., dogs, cats, birds), ingestion of contaminated water or dairy products, or ingestion of improperly cooked poultry. *C. jejuni* can also be transmitted through sexual contact. Bloody diarrhea may follow the initial signs of fever, chills, and, more rarely, nausea and vomiting. The disease usually resolves itself in two to six days, although untreated individuals may be carriers for several months.

  Another bacterium that is similar to *Campylobacter* bacteria has recently been determined to be the causative agent of upper gastrointestinal ulcers. Peptic ulcers may occur in the lower esophagus, the stomach, or the upper small intestine (Figure 25-6). Peptic ulcers are typically caused by the action of gastric

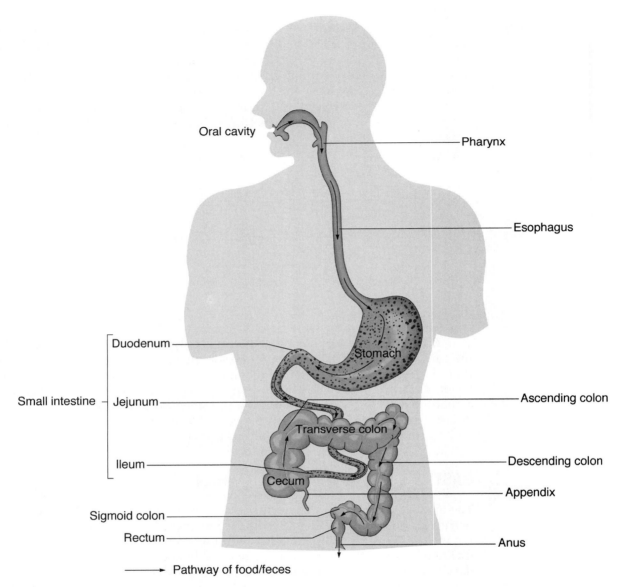

Figure 25-5 Gastroenteritis.

acid and the enzyme pepsin. These chemicals act on the mucosal layer of the digestive tract causing damage to the tissues.

The *Helicobacter pylori* bacterium is also associated with peptic and duodenal ulcers. The use of analgesics—which are medications to control pain—may also contribute to ulcer formation and aggravation. As more is understood about

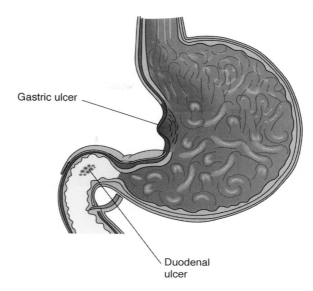

Gastric ulcer

Duodenal ulcer

Figure 25-6 Peptic ulcers.

H. pylori, researchers are beginning to hypothesize that long-term *H. pylori* infection can be an important risk factor for stomach cancer.

LEGIONELLA PNEUMOPHILIA

Legionellosis is a disease of the respiratory tract caused by a bacterial infection of *Legionella pneumophilia*. Legionellosis, or Legionnaires' disease, received its name from a group of men belonging to the American Legion who died after attending the same meeting in 1976. Symptoms of Legionnaires' disease are a high fever, cough, and symptoms of pneumonia. *L. pneumophilia* is found in the water of air-conditioning cooling towers, water faucets, shower heads, humidifiers, and contaminated respiratory therapy equipment, suggesting that it has an airborne transmission. The bacterium is resistant to chlorine for long periods. In cases of Legionnaire's disease, death may eventually result due to cardiovascular collapse.

LISTERIA MONOCYTOGENES

Listeria monocytogenes is a gram-positive, non-spore-forming bacillus, which is becoming recognized as a foodborne pathogen. Listeriosis is usually a mild, symptomless disease in healthy adults. However, among those with compromised immune system function it can be fatal. *L. monocytogenes* is capable of surviving within the white blood cells even after it has been engulfed by them. The bacillus can move from one macrophage to a neighboring macrophage, and infection frequently leads to fatal meningitis.

L. monocytogenes thrives at refrigerator temperatures and has been isolated from a variety of foods, including raw milk, cheese made from unpasteurized milk, hot dogs, and prepackaged meat products. Since *L. monocytogenes* is shed in the feces of infected animals, it is widely found in soil and water. Among infected pregnant women, there is a fetal mortality rate of 60 percent. Uterine infection may also result in a high rate of spontaneous abortion and stillbirths.

REVIEW QUESTIONS

Matching

1. _____ Asiatic cholera   a. *Clostridium perfringens*
2. _____ tissue gas   b. *Bordetella pertussis*
3. _____ rabbit fever   c. *Streptococcus pyogenes*
4. _____ whooping cough   d. *Vibrio cholerae*
5. _____ scarlet fever   e. *Francisella tularensis*

Multiple Choice

1. Which of the following is characteristic of the primary stage of syphilis?
   a. A chancre appears on the genitals.
   b. A rash is present on the palms of the hands and the soles of the feet.
   c. Cardiac failure and paralysis occur.
   d. Rubberlike lesions called gummas appear on the body.
2. Which of the following diseases is characterized by a bull's-eye rash?
   a. legionnaires' disease
   b. Lyme disease
   c. anthrax
   d. toxic shock syndrome
3. Which of the following diseases is caused by a spirochete?
   a. botulism
   b. leptospirosis
   c. gas gangrene
   d. food poisoning
4. Which of the following diseases is characterized by sore throat, fever, fatigue, swelling of the neck, and a tough grayish pseudomembrane in the throat?
   a. rheumatic fever
   b. shigellosis
   c. typhoid
   d. diphtheria

5. *Corynebacteria* have been shown to cause which of the following types of infections in humans?
   a. stomach ulcers, meningitis, and pneumonia
   b. paralysis, demyelization of peripheral neurons, colitis, and enteritis
   c. endocarditis, urinary infections, and respiratory illness after contact with infected sheep
   d. abdominal cramps, diarrhea with pus, rice-water stool, and bloody vomiting

Putting Learning to Work!

The purpose of the following case analysis is to allow you to apply the information you have learned in a real-world situation. Read the case carefully and try to answer the following questions:

What disease do you suspect the person had at the time of death?

How could the disease potentially spread to yourself or the public?

What precautions should you take as the embalmer to properly disinfect the body?

Case Analysis

A 63-year-old male died in the critical care unit of a local hospital. Both his groin and axillary spaces are swollen, and the skin in these areas appears red and bruised. There is also a localized enlargement in his left axillary space. The nurse at the hospital tells you that she has just started her shift, and that she is not aware of the cause of the man's death. One of the orderlies does mention that the deceased lived alone in a hunting cabin at a nearby lake, and that he was in a coma when he was admitted to the hospital. The deceased was also known to have eaten squirrel and rabbit, which he hunted and prepared himself.

Bibliography

Anthrax. (2002). Retrieved July 19, 2003, from the U.S. Food and Drug Administration at http://www.fda.gov/cber/vaccine/anthrax.htm.

Anthrax. (2003). Retrieved July 26, 2003, from the National Center for Infectious Diseases, Division of Bacterial and Mycotic Diseases, Centers for Disease Control and Prevention at http://www.cdc.gov/ncidod/dbmd/diseaseinfo/anthrax_g.htm.

Bahmanyar, M., & Cavanaugh, D. (1976). *Plague manual*. Geneva: World Health Organization.

Bloodborne pathogens and acute care facilities. (1992). OSHA 3128. Retrieved July 22, 2003, from the U.S. Department of Labor, Occupational Safety and Health Administration at http://www.osha.gov/Publications/OSHA3128/osha3128.html#Appendix.

Bordetella pertussis. (2001). Retrieved July 26, 2003, from the Office of Laboratory Safety, Health Canada at http://www.hc-sc.gc.ca/pphb-dgspsp/msds-ftss/msds20e.html.

Botulism. (2001). Retrieved July 26, 2003, from the National Center for Infectious Diseases, Division of Bacterial and Mycotic Diseases, Centers for Disease Control and Prevention: http://www.cdc.gov/ncidod/dbmd/diseaseinfo/botulism_g.htm.

Butler T. (1983). *Plague and other Yersinia infections.* New York: Plenum Press.

Chamberlain, N. (2000a). *Introduction to microbiology.* Retrieved July 25, 2003, from the Kirksville College of Osteopathic Medicine at http://www.kcom.edu/faculty/chamberlain/Website/intmic.htm.

Chamberlain, N. (2000b). *Rickettsia, chlamydia, mycoplasma.* Retrieved July 15, 2003, from Kirksville College of Osteopathic Medicine at http://www.kcom.edu/faculty/chamberlain/Website/Lects/RICKETT.HTM#ri.

Chlamydia in the United States. (2001). Retrieved July 20, 2003, from the Division of Sexually Transmitted Diseases Prevention, National Center for HIV, STD, and TB Prevention, Centers for Disease Control and Prevention at http://www.cdc.gov/nchstp/dstd/Fact_Sheets/chlamydia_facts.htm.

Chlamydia pneumoniae. (2002). Retrieved from the National Center for Infectious Diseases, Division of Bacterial and Mycotic Diseases, Centers for Disease Control and Prevention at http://www.cdc.gov/ncidod/dbmd/diseaseinfo/chlamydiapneumonia_t.htm.

Cholera. (2001). Retrieved July 26, 2003, from the National Center for Infectious Disease, Division of Bacterial and Mycotic Diseases, Centers for Disease Control and Prevention at http://www.cdc.gov/ncidod/dbmd/diseaseinfo/cholera_g.htm.

Cooper, D. (2002). Typhus. In *Medical Encyclopedia.* Retrieved July 26, 2003, from MedlinePlus, the U.S. National Library of Medicine and the National Institutes of Health at http://www.nlm.nih.gov/medlineplus/ency/article/001363.htm.

Diphtheria. (n.d.). Retrieved July 26, 2003, from the Centers for Disease Control and Prevention at http://www.cdc.gov/nip/publications/pink/dip.pdf.

Diphtheria, tetanus, and pertussis vaccines: What you should know. (2001). Retrieved July 19, 2003, from the U.S. Department of Health and Human Services National Immunization Program, Centers for Disease Control and Prevention at http://www.cdc.gov/nip/publications/VIS/vis-dtp.pdf.

Dixon, T. (1999). Anthrax. *New England Journal of Medicine, 341,* 815–826.

Edmonds, P. (1978). *Microbiology: An environmental perspective.* Basingstoke Hampshire, England: Macmillan Publishing.

Epidemic louse-borne typhus. (1998). Retrieved July 26, 2003, from the World Health Organization, Geneva at http://www.who.int/inf-fs/en/fact162.html.

Frobisher, M., Hinsdill, R., Crabtree, K., & Goodheart, C. (1974). *Fundamentals of microbiology.* Philadelphia: Saunders.

Gaudy, A., & Gaudy, E. (1980). *Microbiology for environmental scientists and engineers.* New York: McGraw-Hill.

Gonorrhea. (2001). Retrieved July 26, 2003, from the National Center for HIV, STD, and TB Prevention, Division of Sexually Transmitted Diseases, Centers for Disease Control and Prevention at http://www.cdc.gov/nchstp/dstd/Fact_Sheets/FactsGonorrhea.htm.

Grover-Lakomia, L., & Fong, E. (1999). *Microbiology for health careers* (6th ed.). Clifton Park, NY: Thomson Delmar Learning.

Haemophilus influenzae serotype b (Hib) disease. (2003). Retrieved July 19, 2003, from the Division of Bacterial and Mycotic Diseases, Centers for Disease Control and Prevention at http://www.cdc.gov/ncidod/dbmd/diseaseinfo/haeminfluserob_t.htm.

Legionellosis: Legionnaire's disease (LD) and Pontiac fever. (2001). Retrieved July 26, 2003, from the National Center for Infectious Disease, Division of Bacterial and Mycotic Diseases, Centers for Disease Control and Prevention at http://www.cdc.gov/ncidod/dbmd/diseaseinfo/legionellosis_g.htm.

Leptospirosis. (2001). Retrieved July 26, 2003, from the National Center for Infectious Disease, Division of Bacterial and Mycotic Diseases, Centers for Disease Control and Prevention at http://www.cdc.gov/ncidod/dbmd/diseaseinfo/leptospirosis_g.htm.

Listeriosis. (2003). Retrieved July 19, 2003, from the National Center for Infectious Disease, Division of Bacterial and Mycotic Diseases, Center for Disease Control and Prevention at http://www.cdc.gov/ncidod/dbmd/diseaseinfo/listeriosis_g.htm#symptom.

Lyme disease. (2001). Retrieved July 26, 2003, from the National Center for Infectious Diseases, Division of Vector-Borne Infectious Disease, Centers for Disease Control and Prevention at http://www.cdc.gov/ncidod/dvbid/lyme/index.htm.

Mahon, C., & Manuselis, G. (2000). *Textbook of diagnostic microbiology* (2nd ed.). Philadelphia: Saunders.

Maniloff, J., McElhaney, R., Finch, L., & Baseman, J. (Eds.). (1992). *Mycoplasmas: Molecular biology and pathogenesis*. Washington, D.C.: American Society for Microbiology.

Mayer, R. (2000). *Embalming: History, theory, & practice* (3rd ed.). New York: McGraw-Hill.

Mycobacterium avium complex. (2003). Retrieved from the National Center for Infectious Diseases, Division of Bacterial and Mycotic Diseases, Centers for Disease Control and Prevention at http://www.cdc.gov/ncidod/dbmd/diseaseinfo/mycobacteriumavium_t.htm.

Neighbors, M., & Tannehill-Jones, R. (2000). *Human diseases*. Clifton Park, NY: Thomson Delmar Learning.

Nester, E., Anderson, D., Roberts, C., Pearsall, N., & Nester, M. (2001). *Microbiology: A Human Perspective* (3rd ed.). Boston: McGraw-Hill.

Pathology for Funeral Service. (1999). Dallas, TX: Professional Training Schools.

Plague. (2001). Retrieved July 19, 2003, from the National Center for Infectious Diseases, Division of Vector-Borne Infectious Disease, Centers for Disease Control and Prevention at http://www.cdc.gov/ncidod/dvbid/plague/index.htm.

Plague. (2002). World Health Organization. Retrieved January 8, 2005, at http://www.who.int/mediacentre/factsheets/fs267/en/.

Shelton, H. (1992). *Boyd's introduction to the study of disease* (11th ed.). Philadelphia: Lea & Febiger.

Shigellosis. (2003). Retrieved July 26, 2003, from the National Center for Infectious Disease, Division of Bacterial and Mycotic Diseases, Centers for Disease Control and Prevention at http://www.cdc.gov/ncidod/dbmd/diseaseinfo/shigellosis_g.htm.

Sirisanthana, T., & Brown, A. (2002). Anthrax of the gastrointestinal tract. In *Emerging infectious diseases*. Retrieved July 19, 2003, from the Centers for Disease Control and Prevention at http://www.cdc.gov/ncidod/EID/vol8no7/02-0062.htm.

Stewart, K., & Stewart, D. (1998). *Bacteria and their characteristics*. Retrieved June 30, 2003, from the Food Safety Management Course, Stewart Enterprises at http://www.saturnnet.com/stewartent/webdoc201.htm.

Syphilis elimination: History in the making. (2001). Retrieved July 18, 2003, from the National Center for HIV, STD and TB Prevention, Division of Sexually Transmitted Diseases, Centers for Disease Control and Prevention at http://www.cdc.gov/nchstp/dstd/Fact_Sheets/Syphilis_Facts.htm.

Tetanus. (n.d.). Retrieved July 26, 2003, from the Centers for Disease Control and Prevention at http://www.cdc.gov/nip/publications/pink/tetanus.pdf.

Todar, K. (2002). Bacteria of medical importance. In *Todar's online textbook of bacteriology*. Retrieved July 18, 2003, from the Department of Bacteriology, University of Wisconsin-Madison at http://www.bact.wisc.edu/microtextbook/disease/overview.html.

Tortora, G., Funke, B., & Case, C. (1998). *Microbiology: An introduction* (6th ed.). Menlo Park, CA: Benjamin/Cummings Publishing.

Typhoid fever. (2001). Retrieved July 26, 2003, from the National Center for Infectious Disease, Division of Bacterial and Mycotic Diseases, Centers for Disease Control and Prevention at http://www.cdc.gov/ncidod/dbmd/diseaseinfo/typhoidfever_g.htm.

Tuberculosis. (2002). Retrieved March 16, 2004, from the World Health Organization at http://www.who.int/mediacentre/factsheets/fs104/en/.

Tularemia. (2002). Retrieved July 26, 2003, from the National Center for Infectious Diseases, Division of Vector-Borne Infectious Diseases, Centers for Disease Control and Prevention at http://www.cdc.gov/ncidod/dvbid/misc/tularemiaFAQ.htm.

Typhoid fever. (2001). Retrieved July 26, 2003, from the National Center for Infectious Disease, Division of Bacterial and Mycotic Diseases, Centers for Disease Control and Prevention at http://www.cdc.gov/ncidod/dbmd/diseaseinfo/typhoidfever_g.htm.

Venes, D. (Ed.). (2001). *Taber's cyclopedic medical dictionary* (19th ed.). Philadelphia: F. A. Davis.

CHAPTER 26

Diseases Caused by Mycoplasmas, Rickettsias, or Chlamydias

Learning Objectives

Upon completion of the chapter, review questions, and case analysis, the reader should be able to:

- Match specific pathogens included in this chapter with the diseases they cause.
- Match the diseases described in this chapter with the genus of the pathogen.
- Identify the important disease conditions associated with the diseases described in this chapter.
- Identify the mode of transmission of the diseases described in this chapter.
- Identify lesions on human remains that suggest a potentially infectious disease.

Key Terms

epidemic typhus   Rocky Mountain spotted fever
parrot fever   trachoma

This chapter covers bacterial diseases in the genera of rickettsia, chlamydia, and mycoplasma. Although each genus of microbe included in this chapter shares similarities with the bacteria discussed in Chapter 25, each causes diseases in humans that share similarities within the particular genus. Table 26-1 describes common pathogenic rickettsia, chlamydia, and mycoplasma diseases.

Table 26-1 Pathogenic Rickettsias, Chlamydias, and Mycoplasmas: Disease, Transmission, and Signs and Symptoms

Pathogen	Disease Name	Mode of Transmission	Signs and Symptoms
RICKETTSIA			
Coxiella burnetii	Q fever	Ingestion of raw milk, inhalation of airborne bacteria from animal products such as hides and placentas of goats, sheep, and cattle	Fever, headache, muscle pain, malaise, nausea, vomiting, chest pain
Rickettsia prowazekii	Epidemic typhus	Human body lice	Fatigue, headache, skin rash, stupor, CNS impairment, picking at bedclothes, black tongue with a white fur
Rickettsia rickettsii	Rocky Mountain spotted fever	Tick bite	Fever, headache, nausea, vomiting, muscle pain, rash, kidney and heart failure
Rickettsia typhi	Endemic murine typhus	Flea bite	Similar but less severe than epidemic typhus
CHLAMYDIA			
Chlamydia pneumoniae	Chlamydial pneumonia	Inhalation of respiratory droplets	90 percent are asymptomatic; otherwise, laryngitis, sinusitis, cough
Chlamydia psittaci	Parrot fever (psittacosis; ornithosis)	Inhalation of aerosolized bacteria from bird feces	Pneumonia, fever, headache, chills
	Trachoma of the eye	Person to person, fomite to person, fly to person	Loss of vision
Chlamydia trachomatis	Lymphogranuloma venereum	Sexual contact	75 percent of female and 50 percent of male cases are asymptomatic; blister appears on genitals, rupture and painlessly heal; enlargement of regional lymph nodes with pus
MYCOPLASMAS			
Mycoplasma pneumoniae	Primary atypical pneumonia (walking pneumonia)	Inhalation of respiratory droplets	Headache, fever, malaise, anorexia, sore throat, dry cough, earache

MYCOPLASMA PNEUMONIAE

Mycoplasmas were once thought to be viruses, but they are actually the smallest free-living organisms in nature. These microbes are resistant to penicillin and similar antibiotics because they do not posses a cell wall. *Mycoplasma pneumoniae* is a slowly growing, aerobic organism. Figure 26-1 illustrates the characteristic fried-egg appearances of *M. pneumoniae* colonies, which are capable of adhering to the epithelium of mucosal surfaces in the respiratory and urogenital tracts. *M. pneumoniae* are not removed by the passage of urine or mucous secretions. The microbes are spread through aerosol droplet spray produced by coughing.

M. pneumoniae can cause bronchitis, pharyngitis, or a common respiratory infection known as primary atypical pneumonia. The disease is best known by its common name: walking pneumonia. About half of the cases of pneumonia in the military and about 20 percent of the cases of pneumonia in the general population, especially among the young and the elderly, are caused by *M. pneumonia*. Other groups living in close contact, such as college students and prisoners, are also at a higher risk of contracting walking pneumonia. Walking pneumonia can include the following signs and symptoms:

- Headache
- Low-grade fever
- Malaise
- Anorexia
- Sore throat
- Dry cough
- Earache
- Cardiovascular complications
- Central nervous system involvement
- Gastrointestinal disorders

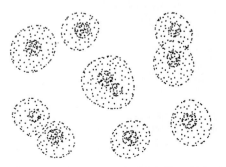

Figure 26-1 Fried-egg appearance of mycoplasmal colonies.

RICKETTSIA

The *Rickettsia* are short, nonmotile, gram-negative bacilli that are obligately intracellular pathogens. Most *Rickettsia* are transmitted to human hosts by arthropod vectors, where they infect the endothelial cells of the human vascular system and result in local blockages of small blood vessels.

Rickettsia are uniquely adapted to their arthropod hosts in that they typically cause no disease or only minimal disease in the arthropod. In some cases, when the arthropods bear young, the *Rickettsia* are passed along to the new generation of offspring. Arthropods, therefore, are not only vectors for *Rickettsia*, they are also reservoirs. However, this pattern does not hold true for *Rickettsia prowazekii*. This particular species causes the death of the arthropod vector, which is human body lice, and the human acts as a natural reservoir.

Rocky Mountain Spotted Fever

Rocky Mountain spotted fever is the most severe rickettsial infection, and it is caused by *Rickettsia rickettsii*. Rocky Mountain spotted fever is most prevalent in the southeastern United States and in Appalachia, although it was first reported in the Rocky Mountains. *Rickettsia rickettsii* is a parasite found in a variety of ticks. The pathogen is passed from one generation of ticks to another through their eggs. After being passed through the saliva of the tick to the human, the microbes multiply in the cytoplasm of the human cells. The microbes then pass directly through cellular membranes into adjacent cells without damaging the host cells.

A rash similar to measles is present in cases of Rocky Mountain spotted fever, with the exception that it is found on the soles of the feet and the palms of the hands. The rash begins on the extremities, usually around the ankles and wrists, and then spreads centripetally toward the trunk of the body (see Color Plate 59). The rash is not normally present on the neck or face. Other characteristics of Rocky Mountain spotted fever are:

- Headache
- Nausea
- Fever
- Vomiting
- Muscle pain

Death occurs in approximately 3 percent of the reported cases of Rocky Mountain spotted fever from kidney and heart failure, although the mortality rate can be as high as 20 percent in untreated cases.

Typhus

Epidemic typhus, which is also known as louse-borne typhus, is caused by *Rickettsia prowazekii*. This microbe grows in the intestinal tract of human body lice and is also found in flying squirrels located in the eastern United States.

The disease is transmitted when the human scratches the wound, rubbing fecal material into the bite left by the human body louse. The louse typically becomes infected with the disease and leaves when the human becomes febrile. Epidemic typhus is found primarily in crowded areas with poor sanitation, and it is still common in Africa, Central America, and South America. At one time, epidemic typhus was prevalent among sailors aboard ships and soldiers in military camps.

The tongue may be covered with a white fur or be black and rolled up in the back of the mouth. A measles-like rash is present on the body, which includes the palms of the hands and soles of the feet. The rash begins on the trunk of the body and spreads centrifugally away from the trunk. The neck and face are seldom involved. The mortality rate of epidemic typhus is high (40 percent) when not treated. Epidemic typhus can also cause the following:

- Extreme fatigue
- Headache
- Skin rash
- Stupor
- Neurological impairment
- Picking at the bedclothes

Endemic typhus, which is also known as either murine typhus or flea-borne typhus, is caused by *Rickettsia typhi*. This microbe is harbored in rats and is transmitted by the rat flea to humans, although the flea infests many domestic animals—which may explain the persistence of the disease in urban areas. Endemic typhus is usually self-resolving and complications are rare. Rat control decreases the occurrence of endemic typhus. Most cases contracted in the United States, which are usually fewer than 100 annually, are reported in the geographic regions of southern Texas and southern California.

Endemic typhus's symptoms are similar, yet less severe than epidemic typhus. Differing from both Rocky Mountain spotted fever or epidemic typhus, there is rarely a rash in cases of endemic typhus, and the rash is usually confined to the trunk and extremities if it is present. The rash is rarely found on the palms and soles.

Q Fever

Q fever is caused by the pathogen *Coxiella burnetii*. The cause of an outbreak of the disease in Queensland, Australia, during the 1930s was unknown so the disease was named Q fever, from the word "query," which refers to something that is unknown. *C. burnetii* is resistant enough to survive airborne transmission, although most *Rickettsia* are not. It is passed from animal to animal via tick bite after ticks feed on infected cattle. Humans, however, become infected by ingesting contaminated milk or inhaling aerosols of the microbe in dairy barns, especially from placental material at calving time. Handling infected animals such as goats, cattle, and sheep places workers at a higher risk of infection. Other sources of infection include meat- and hide-processing plants.

Unlike other rickettsial infections, no rash is present in cases of Q fever. The disease usually resolves without treatment in humans after about two weeks. A fatal endocarditis, which is an inflammation of the lining of the heart, can occur up to twenty years after infection in a small percentage of cases. In addition to the following characteristics of Q fever, about one-third of cases include chest pain:

- Fever
- Headache
- Muscle pain
- Malaise
- Nausea
- Vomiting

CHLAMYDIA

Three human pathogen species of *Chlamydia* are *Chlamydia trachomatis*, *Chlamydia psittaci*, and *Chlamydia pneumoniae*. These organisms are classified as bacteria due to the presence of certain structures in their cell walls and their ability to reproduce through binary fission, but they only grow intracellularly. *Chlamydia* have a unique growth cycle because they are incapable of producing enough energy by themselves, hence they are obligate intracellular parasites.

Chlamydia have two stages of growth, including both an infectious stage and a noninfectious stage. The first form of the organism is infectious and is referred to as an elementary body. The second form is noninfectious and is known as a reticulate body. The elementary body infects nonciliated, columnar, or transitional epithelial cells that line the conjunctiva, respiratory tract, or rectum. The elementary bodies utilize energy sources within the human cell and develop into reticulate bodies.

The mature reticulate bodies multiply within the cell through binary fission. The reticulate bodies then form new elementary bodies after dividing for about two days. When the human cell ruptures these infectious forms of *Chlamydia* infect adjacent cells, allowing the bacteria to spread within the host.

Chlamydial Pneumonia

The causative agent of chlamydial pneumonia is a recently recognized species of bacteria known as *Chlamydia pneumoniae*. This organism is an important respiratory pathogen, known to cause pneumonia, acute respiratory disease, and pharyngitis. Recently, *C. pneumoniae* has been believed to be a causative agent of otitis media, asthma, and cardiovascular disease. It is the third most common cause of infectious respiratory diseases, accounting for about 10 percent of outpatient and hospitalized cases of pneumonia. In addition, about 90 percent of the infections show no symptoms and, therefore, go undiagnosed. It is still unknown how *C. pneumonia* infections are spread.

Chlamydia trachomatis

Chlamydia trachomatis causes inflammation of the urinary tract and a sexually transmitted disease known as lymphogranuloma venereum. *C. trachomatis* is the most commonly spread sexually transmitted bacterial pathogen in the United States. There are between 4 million and 10 million new cases each year. In addition to sexually transmitted *Chlamydia,* a worldwide epidemic of blindness has been caused by *C. trachomatis.* When the bacteria is spread to the eye, a lesion known as a trachoma can develop. A **trachoma** is a chronic, contagious form of conjunctivitis that is one of the leading causes of blindness in the world. Conjunctivitis is an inflammatory condition of the membrane that surrounds the eye. The organism is spread from person to person, person to fomite, and fly to person. *C. trachomatis* is shed in the feces of infected persons. The urinary tract infection is known as either NGU (nongonococcal urethritis) or NSU (nonspecific urethritis).

Chlamydia is the most frequently reported infectious disease in the United States. The sexually transmitted disease, lymphogranuloma venereum, appears 7 to 12 days after exposure when a blister appears on the genitals. This vesicle ruptures and heals painlessly. In one to eight weeks, the regional lymph nodes enlarge and can become suppurative, which means they are infected with pus. Because approximately 75 percent of women and 50 percent of men have no symptoms, most people infected with chlamydia are not aware of their infections and, therefore, may not seek treatment. Initially symptomless diseases are not reported and treatment is not acquired. Lack of treatment allows the disease to spread, providing an opportunity for more severe symptoms to occur later in life.

Untreated, chlamydia causes pelvic inflammatory disease, which can result in infertility and birth defects. Chlamydial infections also increase the chance of becoming infected with HIV if exposed. When diagnosed, chlamydia can be easily treated and cured with antibiotics. Chlamydial infections can also cause severe reproductive and other health problems. Untreated chlamydia in men typically causes urethral infection, but can also result in complications such as swollen and tender testicles. Teenage girls have the highest rates of chlamydial infection, with 15- to 19-year-old girls representing 46 percent of infections and 20- to 24-year-old women representing another 33 percent.

Parrot Fever

Parrot fever, which is also known as psittacosis or as ornithosis, is a disease caused by *Chlamydia psittaci,* which is a gram-negative, obligate intracellular bacterium. The disease receives its name from its association with psittacine birds, such as parakeets and parrots. It can also be contracted from pigeons, chickens, ducks, and turkeys. Psittacosis is a form of pneumonia that causes fever, headache, and chills.

C. psittaci is spread to humans by inhaling the aerosolized microbes from bird droppings. People who work with birds are most at risk for this disorder, although those who work in buildings that provide nesting sites for birds may become infected from breathing the microbes. These bacteria enter buildings through ventilation systems, and courthouses and city buildings with ledges near the roof are excellent candidates for nesting.

REVIEW QUESTIONS

Matching

1. _____ murine typhus
2. _____ walking pneumonia
3. _____ parrot fever
4. _____ Rocky Mountain spotted fever
5. _____ Q fever

a. *Rickettsia rickettsii*
b. *Mycoplasma pneumoniae*
c. *Rickettsia typhi*
d. *Coxiella burnetii*
e. *Chlamydia psittaci*

Multiple Choice

1. Which of the following microorganisms has a characteristic fried-egg appearance?
   a. *Chlamydia pneumoniae*
   b. *Mycoplasma pneumoniae*
   c. *Coxiella burnetii*
   d. *Rickettsia Rickettsii*

2. Which of the following diseases is characterized by the presence of a measles-like rash on the palms of the hands and the soles of the feet?
   a. lymphogranuloma venereum
   b. Q fever
   c. tuberculosis
   d. Rocky Mountain spotted fever

3. In which of the following diseases might the tongue be covered with a white fur, or discolored black and rolled up in the back of the mouth?
   a. epidemic typhus
   b. endemic typhus
   c. Rocky Mountain spotted fever
   d. Q fever

4. Which of the following microorganisms undergoes both an infectious stage of growth and a noninfectious stage of growth?
   a. *Rickettsia*
   b. *Chlamydia*
   c. *Mycoplasmas*
   d. *Mycobacteria*

5. Which of the following microorganisms is the smallest free-living organism in nature?
   a. *Rickettsia*
   b. *Chlamydia*
   c. *Mycoplasmas*
   d. *Mycobacteria*

Putting Learning to Work!

The purpose of the following case analysis is to allow you to apply the information you have learned to a real-world situation. Read the case carefully and try to answer the following questions:

What disease do you suspect the person had at the time of death?

How could the disease potentially spread to yourself or the public?

What precautions should you take as the embalmer to properly disinfect the body?

Case Analysis

The deceased is a 57-year-old Chicano woman who died at her residence. She was employed as a janitor in a large, metropolitan school system in Texas. While at the home, her sister tells you that the deceased worked until about three weeks ago, despite her severe arthritis. You notice the numerous anti-inflammatory medications on the deceased's nightstand in her bedroom.

Her sister states that the deceased started "feeling bad" about three weeks ago, when she bent over in the boiler room at work to remove a dead rat. The deceased's sister states, "She just went downhill from there, and she said the doctor just gave her that cream for her rash, when she saw him two weeks ago. She lived alone, so I didn't know she was so sick." You notice a pair of sunglasses in the bed next to the deceased.

When you return to the funeral home, you notice that the deceased's nightgown is drenched in sweat. She has a mild rash on her trunk and extremities. She also has lesions on her ankles that look like insect bites.

Bibliography

Body lice. (2000). Retrieved July 26, 2003, from the National Center for Infectious Diseases, Division of Parasitic Infections, Centers for Disease Control and Prevention at http://www.cdc.gov/ncidod/dpd/parasites/lice/factsht_body_lice.htm.

Chamberlain, N. (2000a). *Introduction to microbiology*. Retrieved July 25, 2003, from the Kirksville College of Osteopathic Medicine at http://www.kcom.edu/faculty/chamberlain/Website/intmic.htm.

Chamberlain, N. (2000b). *Rickettsia, chlamydia, mycoplasma*. Retrieved July 15, 2003, from Kirksville College of Osteopathic Medicine at http://www.kcom.edu/faculty/chamberlain/Website/Lects/RICKETT.HTM#ri.

Chlamydia in the United States. (2001). Retrieved July 20, 2003, from the Division of Sexually Transmitted Diseases Prevention, National Center for HIV, STD, and TB Prevention, Centers for Disease Control and Prevention at http://www.cdc.gov/nchstp/dstd/Fact_Sheets/chlamydia_facts.htm.

Chlamydia pneumoniae. (2002). Retrieved from the National Center for Infectious Diseases, Division of Bacterial and Mycotic Diseases, Centers for Disease Control and Prevention at http://www.cdc.gov/ncidod/dbmd/diseaseinfo/chlamydiapneumonia_t.htm.

Cooper, D. (2002). Typhus. In *Medical Encyclopedia*. Retrieved July 26, 2003, from the U.S. National Library of Medicine and the National Institutes of Health at http://www.nlm.nih.gov/medlineplus/ency/article/001363.htm.

Edmonds, P. (1978). *Microbiology: An environmental perspective*. Basingstoke Hampshire, England: Macmillan Publishing.

Epidemic louse-borne typhus. (1998). Retrieved July 26, 2003, from the World Health Organization, Geneva at http://www.who.int/inf-fs/en/fact162.html.

Frobisher, M., Hinsdill, R., Crabtree, K., & Goodheart, C. (1974). *Fundamentals of Microbiology*. Philadelphia: Saunders.

Gaudy, A., & Gaudy, E. (1980). *Microbiology for environmental scientists and engineers*. New York: McGraw-Hill.

Grover-Lakomia, L., & Fong, E. (1999). *Microbiology for health careers* (6th ed.). Clifton Park, NY: Thomson Delmar Learning.

Mahon, C., & Manuselis, G. (2000). *Textbook of diagnostic microbiology* (2nd ed.). Philadelphia: Saunders.

Mayer, R. (2000). *Embalming: History, theory, & practice* (3rd ed.). New York: McGraw-Hill.

Mycobacterium avium complex. (2003). Retrieved from the National Center for Infectious Diseases, Division of Bacterial and Mycotic Diseases, Centers for Disease Control and Prevention at http://www.cdc.gov/ncidod/dbmd/diseaseinfo/mycobacteriumavium_t.htm.

Mycoplasma pneumoniae. (2002). Retrieved from the National Center for Infectious Diseases, Division of Bacterial and Mycotic Diseases, Centers for Disease Control and Prevention at http://www.cdc.gov/ncidod/dbmd/diseaseinfo/mycoplasmapneum_t.htm.

Neighbors, M., & Tannehill-Jones, R. (2000). *Human diseases*. Clifton Park, NY: Thomson Delmar Learning.

Nester, E., Anderson, D., Roberts, C., Pearsall, N., & Nester, M. (2001). *Microbiology: A Human Perspective* (3rd ed.). Boston: McGraw-Hill.

Pathology for funeral service. (1999). Dallas, TX: Professional Training Schools.

Psittacosis. (2003). Retrieved from the National Center for Infectious Diseases, Division of Bacterial and Mycotic Diseases, Centers for Disease Control and Prevention at http://www.cdc.gov/ncidod/dbmd/diseaseinfo/psittacosis_t.htm.

Q fever. (2003). Retrieved July 26, 2003, from the National Center for Infectious Diseases, Division of Viral and Rickettsial Diseases, Viral and Rickettsial Zoonoses Branch, Centers for Disease Control and Prevention at http://www.cdc.gov/ncidod/dvrd/qfever/index.htm.

Razin, S. (n.d.). Mycoplasmas. In *Medical Microbiology* (4th ed.). Retrieved July 15, 2003, from the University of Texas Medical Branch. At Galveston, TX at http://gsbs.utmb.edu/microbook/ch037.htm.

Razin, S., & Barile, M. (Eds.). (1985). *The Mycoplasmas*, Volume 4. Orlando, FL: Academic Press.

Rocky Mountain spotted fever. (2000). Retrieved July 26, 2003, from the National Center for Infectious Diseases, Division of Viral and Rickettsial Diseases, Viral and Rickettsial Zoonoses Branch, Centers for Disease Control and Prevention at http://www.cdc.gov/ncidod/dvrd/rmsf/index.htm.

Rottem, S., & Kahane, I. (Eds.). (1993). *Mycoplasma cell membranes*. New York: Plenum Press.

Shelton, H. (1992). *Boyd's introduction to the study of disease* (11th ed.). Philadelphia: Lea & Febiger.

Tortora, G., Funke, B., & Case, C. (1998). *Microbiology: An introduction* (6th ed.). Menlo Park, CA: Benjamin/Cummings Publishing.

Tuberculosis. (2003a). Retrieved July 26, 2003, from the National Center for HIV, STDs, and TB Prevention, Division of Tuberculosis Elimination, Centers for Disease Control and Prevention at http://www.cdc.gov/nchstp/tb/faqs/qa.htm.

Tuberculosis. (2003b). Retrieved July 26, 2003, from MedlinePlus, the U.S. National Library of Medicine and the National Institutes of Health at http://www.nlm.nih.gov/medlineplus/tuberculosis.html.

Tuberculosis resources. (n.d.). Retrieved July 26, 2003, from the Department of Biomedical Informatics at Columbia University at http://www.cpmc.columbia.edu/tbcpp/.

Venes, D. (Ed.). (2001). *Taber's cyclopedic medical dictionary* (19th ed.). Philadelphia: F. A. Davis.

CHAPTER 27

Diseases Caused by Prions or Viruses

Learning Objectives

Upon completion of the chapter, review questions, and case analysis, the reader should be able to:

- Match specific pathogens discussed in this chapter with the diseases they cause.
- Match the diseases described in this chapter with the genus of the pathogen.
- Identify the important disease conditions associated with the diseases described in this chapter.
- Identify the mode of transmission of the diseases described in this chapter.
- Identify lesions on human remains that suggest a potentially infectious disease.
- Categorize the viral diseases in this chapter as either dermatropic, pneumotropic, neurotropic, viscerotropic, or immunological.

Key Terms

Creutzfeldt-Jakob disease
hepatitis
mononucleosis

mumps
poliomyelitis
rabies

 ## PRIONS

Prions are small, proteinaceous, infectious particles that are resistant to most procedures that modify nucleic acids. Unlike viruses and viroids, prions do not contain either DNA or RNA, and they do not cause an immune system response in humans. Prions consist entirely of proteins that are produced by human genes and are, therefore, obligate intracellular parasites, just like viruses and viroids. Viruses, viroids, and prions are all nonliving agents, hence they can only replicate inside living cells. Prions are of particular concern to embalmers because they resist inactivation by both heat and formaldehyde and by ultraviolet and ionizing radiation as well. They are not destroyed by proteases or by nucleases, and they are much smaller than the smallest viruses.

Diseases caused by prions are collectively known as spongiform encephalopathies because they leave holes in the brain tissue that resemble a sponge. Prion-related diseases can be either inherited or develop sporadically and be transmitted through blood to blood contact. The common denominator of all prion disorders is the presence of amyloid deposits in the tissues.

Amyloid is a general term for any intracellular or intercellular starchlike protein deposit. These deposits stain easily with Congo red dye and appear homogenous, waxy, and translucent. Amyloid degeneration also occurs in non-prion-related pathological disorders such as tuberculosis, osteomyelitis, leprosy, Hodgkin's disease, and various cancers. Prion diseases like scrapie and mad cow disease are found in sheep and cows, respectively. Prions are suspected causes of human disease such as Creutzfeldt-Jakob disease, variant Creutzfeldt-Jakob disease, kuru, Gerstmann-Straussler-Scheinker syndrome, and fatal familial insomnia.

A disease known as kuru is also thought to be caused by a prion and has been linked to the former cannibalistic rituals of the Fore Highlanders in Papua New Guinea. As part of their mortuary rituals, the members of the tribe would smear the brains of the dead on their bodies, and eat the deceased.

Scrapie is a disease of sheep and goats that causes them to rub sores on their bodies. The sheep progressively lose muscle control and die. In cows, this disease is known as bovine spongiform encephalopathy, and the prion is believed to be spread to humans through the consumption of infected beef. Bovine spongiform encephalopathy is commonly referred to as mad cow disease.

Creutzfeldt-Jakob Disease

Creutzfeldt-Jakob disease (CJD) is thought to be caused by a prion. It is a progressive disease that causes spongiform—porous, like a sponge—degeneration of the brain. There is a long incubation period measuring between months, years, and decades associated with the disease. CJD has been transmitted to a pathologist via a scalpel nick during an autopsy, it has been experimentally transmitted to chimpanzees, it has been transmitted via cornea donation from an infected donor to a healthy recipient, and it is believed to be inherited. It is an extremely rare disease, with approximately one case appearing per million population worldwide. The symptoms of CJD are progressive dementia, loss of nervous system control, and blindness. In the majority of cases, CJD is fatal within approximately one year of the onset of symptoms.

There is no treatment for CJD. Embalmers must be certain to follow all universal precautions standards when dealing with all human remains. The prion that causes CJD is harbored in the central nervous system, so brain tissue contact should be avoided. During aspiration of the deceased, the trocar should be pointed away from the spinal column. Contact with the spleen should also be avoided as the prion is believed to be present in this organ as well as in the CNS.

Prion-Suspected Diseases

Recent research has tentatively identified the possible role of prions in certain nervous-system-related diseases besides the spongiform encephalopathies previously mentioned. The presence of prion proteins does not mean that the following diseases are transmittable. These diseases are inherited pathologies, indicating that some prions are infectious while others are not. Prions are poorly understood as microbial pathogens in humans, but recent work in mapping genes, gene therapy, and cloning is moving science into a new frontier and embalmers need to be aware of the potential role of prions in disease transmission.

Gerstmann-Straussler-Scheinker syndrome is a rare central nervous system disorder of families, which makes it fundamentally different from CJD. Since CJD is only present in families at the rate of 5 percent to 15 percent, it is not inherited at the rate of Gerstmann-Straussler-Scheinker syndrome. Normally occurring after 50, Gerstmann-Straussler-Scheinker syndrome is characterized by loss of reflexes in the legs and the development of dementia. The disease is noted for spongiform degeneration of the brain and spinal cord with the presence of amyloid plaque.

Fatal familial insomnia is a genetic disorder within families that results from a mutation of the normal prion protein in the brain. The specific portion of the brain affected in this disease is the thalamus, which is the sleep control center for the body. The presence of the waxlike buildup of amyloid tissues in the brain is a common aspect of fatal familial insomnia. As its name indicates, the disease ends in death, but first the following complications occur from sleep deprivation:

- Hallucinations
- Inefficient core body temperature regulation
- Blood pressure irregularities
- Abnormal heart rate
- Dementia
- Poor reflexes
- Inability to produce tears
- Failure to feel pain

VIRUSES

A virus is an intracellular, infectious parasite capable of living and replicating only in living cells. Viruses can infect almost any living cell including bacteria, fungi, parasites, plants, animals, and human cells. They are basically a piece of genetic material wrapped in protein, and they contain only one type of nucleic acid, either DNA or RNA. They replicate inside living cells by using the cell's own structures to reproduce more infected cells. Viruses are some of the smallest human pathogens (Figure 27-1).

Viruses lack enzymes such as ATP for producing energy, so they are dependent on their host cells. Some viruses are sensitive to disinfectants due to the presence of lipids in their coverings. For example, HIV, the virus that causes AIDS, can be inactivated by a solution of 10 percent household bleach in water. Both detergents and ether are capable of inactivating many viruses by dissolving their lipid coverings. Table 27-1 lists viral pathogens, the names of the diseases they cause, their modes of transmission, and the signs and symptoms of the diseases.

Dermatropic (Skin) Diseases

Smallpox. Variola is the poxvirus that causes smallpox. During the Middle Ages, much of Europe contracted smallpox. The disease ravaged Native Americans who had no previous exposure to it when it was brought to the Americas by European explorers. By the time the characteristic pox lesions form on the skin, many organs are already infected with the virus. The smallpox virus enters the body through the respiratory system. Smallpox has been eradicated through vaccination programs, although two samples of the virus have been stored in the former Soviet Union and the United States. Recent political developments have given rise to the speculation that the smallpox virus may be presently available for use as a biological weapon in certain countries. The first vaccine ever created was by Edward Jenner, and it was for smallpox.

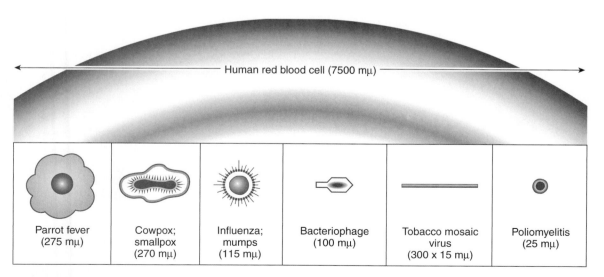

Figure 27-1 Relative size and shape of various viruses as compared with that of a human red blood cell. (Courtesy of the Centers for Disease Control and Prevention, Atlanta, GA.)

Table 27-1 Pathogenic Viruses: Disease, Transmission, and Signs and Symptoms

Viral Pathogen	Disease Name	Mode of Transmission	Signs and Symptoms
Cytomegalovirus (CMV)	Inclusion disease	Contact with body secretions such as saliva, urine, semen, vaginal secretions, and breast milk	Fetal birth defects; in adults symptoms sometimes include prolonged fever and mild hepatitis
Ebola virus	Ebola hemorrhagic fever	Body fluid contact	Acute fever, headache, arthritis, muscle pain, sore throat, weakness, diarrhea, vomiting, stomach pain, rash, red eyes, hiccups, internal and external bleeding
Encephalitis virus	Encephalitis	Mosquito bite	Chills, fever, headache, confusion, coma
Epstein-Barr virus	Mononucleosis (kissing disease; college disease)	Transfer of saliva	Infection of the parotid salivary glands, fever, sore throat, fatigue
Hantavirus	Hantavirus pulmonary syndrome	Inhalation of virus from infected rodents	Fatigue, fever, muscle aches, headache, dizziness, chills, nausea, vomiting, diarrhea, coughing, dyspnea
Hepatitis A virus	Infectious hepatitis	Fecal-oral route or ingestion of contaminated water or food	Anorexia, fatigue, nausea, diarrhea, fever, jaundice, chills
Hepatitis B virus	Serum hepatitis	Contaminated body fluids	Chronic or fatal, causing scarring and hardening of the liver, jaundice, liver cancer, or liver failure
Hepatitis C virus	Non-A, Non-B hepatitis (NANB)	Blood transfusion	Similar to hepatitis B
Herpes simplex 1 virus	Cold sore	Oral or respiratory route	Cold sore lesion on mouth
Herpes simplex 2 virus	Genital herpes	Sexually transmitted	Chronic painful blistering on genitals, flulike symptoms, fever, swollen glands
Human immunodeficiency virus (HIV)	Acquired immunodeficiency syndrome (AIDS)	Sexually transmitted, sharing IV drug needles	Failure of immune system
Influenza virus	Flu	Inhalation of respiratory droplets	Fever, chills, headache, cough, sore throat, extreme fatigue
Mumps virus	Epidemic parotitis	Inhalation of respiratory droplets	Swelling of parotid salivary glands, fever, painful swallowing, orchitis, meningitis, pancreatitis, inflammation of ovaries
Poliovirus	Poliomyelitis (polio)	Fecal-oral route, contaminated water	Sore throat, fever, nausea, vomiting, meningitis, paralysis

Table 27-1 Continued

Viral Pathogen	Disease Name	Mode of Transmission	Signs and Symptoms
Rabies virus	Rabies (hydrophobia)	Animal bite or inhalation of aerosolized virus	Encephalitis, inability to swallow, paralysis
Rubella virus	German measles	Inhalation of respiratory droplets	Red spots and fever that can lead to encephalitis
Rubeola virus	Measles	Inhalation of respiratory droplets	Red spots on face, trunk, and extremities that can lead to encephalitis; symptoms are more severe than in German measles
Varicella-zoster virus	Chicken pox (varicella virus)	Inhalation of respiratory droplets	Lesions of the face, throat, lower back, chest, and shoulders that fill with pus and dry, forming crusting
Varicella-zoster virus	Shingles (zoster virus)	Reactivation of varicella virus	Blistering of the waist, face, chest, and back that follows the sensory nerve paths and can lead to paralysis
Variola virus	Smallpox	Respiratory route	Characteristic pox lesions of the skin and organs
West Nile virus	West Nile encephalitis	Mosquito bite	Inflammation of nervous system

Monkeypox. Monkeypox is a viral disease with a clinical presentation in humans similar to that seen in the past in smallpox patients. Smallpox no longer occurs, following its worldwide eradication in 1980; however, the Centers for Disease Control (CDC) has current plans in place for response to an outbreak of smallpox as a result of potential bioterrorism. Monkeypox is still seen as a sporadic disease in parts of Africa. Most cases occur in remote villages of central and west Africa close to tropical rainforests where there is frequent contact with infected animals. It is usually transmitted to humans from squirrels and primates through contact with the animal's blood or through a bite.

The virus responsible for monkeypox is related to the virus that causes smallpox; both are orthopoxviruses. Vaccination against smallpox also gave protection against monkeypox. Before the eradication of smallpox, vaccination was widely practiced and protected against both diseases. Children born after 1980 have not been vaccinated against smallpox and are likely to be more susceptible to monkeypox than older members of the population. The death rate from monkeypox is highest in young children, reaching about 10 percent. The ending of vaccination programs against smallpox in the late 1970s has probably led to an increase in susceptibility to monkeypox.

The number of cases of monkeypox in the United States has recently increased, with 33 cases in the Midwestern states of Indiana, Illinois, and Wisconsin. These cases are believed to have stemmed from contact with pet prairie

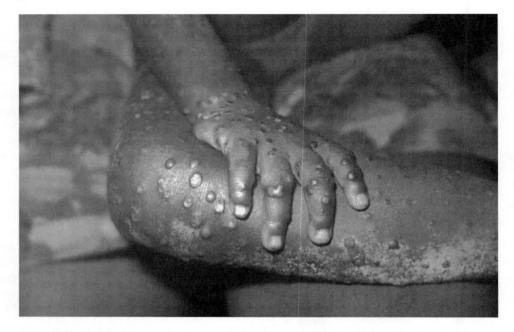

Figure 27-2 Monkeypox lesions on the arm and leg. (Courtesy of the Centers for Disease Control and Prevention, Atlanta, GA.)

dogs. The animals contracted the virus from an infected Gambian giant pouched rat, which came from central or west Africa. Although monkeypox does not spread readily among humans, it can be contracted though contact with contaminated animals. Figure 27-2 is a close-up of the monkeypox lesions on the arms and leg of an infected four-year-old.

Measles.   Rubeola virus is the cause of a dermatropic disease known as measles, and Figure 27-3 pictures its effect on normal cells. Measles is extremely contagious and is spread from person to person via the respiratory route. Humans are the only reservoir for the rubeola virus. Rubeola is similar to chickenpox and smallpox in its development. The infection spreads from the respiratory system after approximately 10 to 12 days, causing the same symptoms as the common cold. A rash appears on the face, which spreads to the trunk and then to the extremities (see Color Plate 60). Approximately one week after the rash appears, encephalitis can develop in some cases of measles.

German Measles.   German measles is caused by the rubella virus, which is pictured in Figure 27-4. It is a more mild form of measles than rubeola and often its symptoms are subclinical. German measles are characterized by a rash of red spots and fever (see Color Plate 61). Encephalitis can occur in adults who have contracted German measles. The incubation period of German measles is approximately two to three weeks. This disease is spread via the respiratory route.

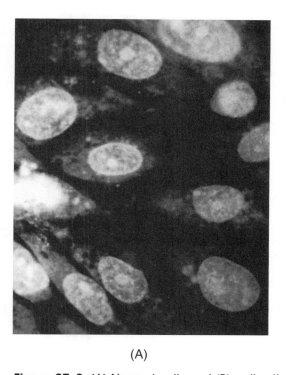

(A)

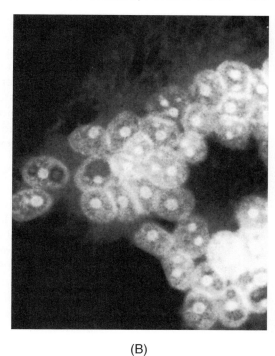

(B)

Figure 27-3 (A) Normal cells and (B) cells attacked by measles virus. The cells have clumped together into one giant cell. All the cytoplasm has fused into a single mass, and the nuclei have clustered together. (Courtesy of Pfizer, Inc.)

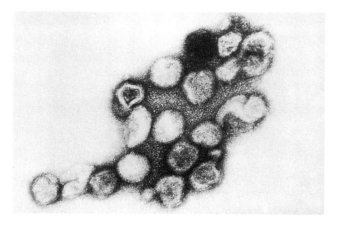

Figure 27-4 Cells infected with the rubella virus. (Courtesy of the Centers for Disease Control and Prevention, Atlanta, GA.)

Congenital rubella syndrome is a form of birth defect that occurs when the mother becomes infected with the rubella virus in her first trimester. In 1964 and 1965, a rubella epidemic in the United States caused thousands of infants to be born with congenital rubella syndrome. Fifteen percent of babies born with congenital rubella syndrome die within their first year. The others suffer from stunted growth, disfigurement of their bodies, deafness, cataracts, heart defects, and mental retardation. A vaccine has been developed to control the spread of rubella, and women who have been inoculated with the vaccine are protected 90 percent of the time for at least 15 years.

Chickenpox and Shingles. Chickenpox is an acute inflammatory disease caused by virus varicella-zoster, which also causes shingles. Chickenpox is an infectious disease spread by respiratory tract transmission. Its primary symptom is the development of lesions on the skin (see Color Plate 62). The blisters last three to four days and fill with pus, causing crusting. Lesions are typically found on the face, neck, and lower back but can occur on the chest and shoulders. Chickenpox can be fatal from related encephalitis and viral pneumonia. It is a childhood disease but can be contracted by adults. When chickenpox appears in adults, they are likely to develop more severe symptoms with a higher mortality rate than children who contract the disease.

Like all herpesviruses, the varicella-zoster virus can remain latent in the body. After recovery from chickenpox, the varicella-zoster virus remains indefinitely in the dorsal root ganglia of the spinal cord. Later, under periods of stress or compromised immunity, the virus is reactivated causing skin lesions in the form of shingles. The blisters are found around the waist, and on the face, chest, and back (see Color Plate 63). The vesicles follow the affected cutaneous sensory nerve and usually affect only one side of the body. Shingles is a painful disorder that can lead to nerve impairment and paralysis. It is fatal in approximately 17 percent of the reported cases in the United States.

Herpes. Herpes is both a sexually transmitted disease and an infectious disease of the integument. The herpes simplex 1 virus causes fever blisters and cold sores, and the herpes simplex 2 virus causes sexually transmitted herpes infections. Figure 27-5 pictures the herpes simplex virus.

Cold Sores. The herpes simplex 1 virus is transmitted by oral or respiratory routes. Almost everyone has been infected with the herpes simplex 1 virus during infancy. Cold sores, which are pictured in Color Plate 64, can appear due to excessive exposure to ultraviolet rays from the sun, emotional upsets, or hormonal changes during menstruation. In cases of herpetic keratitis, the herpes simplex 1 virus can lead to infection of the cornea of the eye. During latency, the herpes simplex 1 virus remains dormant in the trigeminal nerve ganglia of the brain.

Genital Herpes. Genital herpes, a sexually transmitted disease, is caused by the herpes simplex 2 virus. According to the National Center for HIV, STDs, and TB Prevention (*Genital herpes* 2001), nationwide, 45 million people ages 12 and older, or one out of five of the total adolescent and adult population, are infected

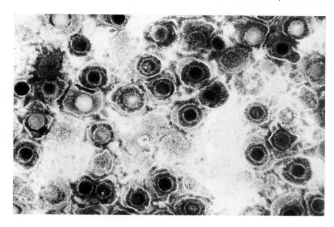

Figure 27-5 Cells infected with the herpes simplex virus. (Courtesy of the Centers for Disease Control and Prevention, Atlanta, GA.)

with herpes simplex 2 virus. Genital herpes is more common among African Americans (45.9 percent) than Caucasians (17.6 percent). The higher rate of genital herpes among minorities is due to other determinants of health such as poverty, access to good quality healthcare, behavior for seeking healthcare, illicit drug use, and living in communities with a high prevalence of sexually transmitted diseases. The largest increase in the rate of genital herpes is currently occurring among young Caucasian teens.

Most individuals have no signs or symptoms from herpes infection. When signs do occur, they typically appear as one or more blisters on or around the genitals or rectum (see Figure 27-6). The blisters break, leaving tender sores that

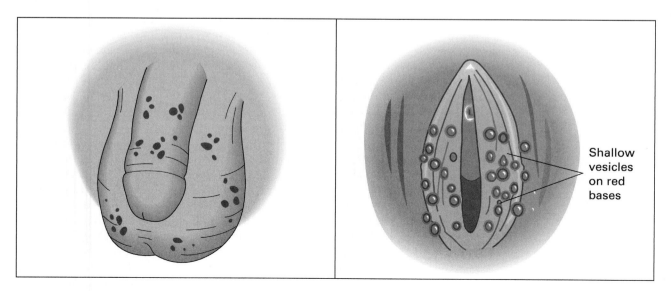

Shallow vesicles on red bases

Figure 27-6 Genital herpes.

may take two to four weeks to heal the first time they occur. Another outbreak can appear weeks or months after the first, but it almost always is less severe and shorter than the first episode.

The consistent and correct use of latex condoms can help protect against infection. However, condom use offers uncertain protection because the blisters appear on the external genitalia of women and at the base of the penis on men, which condoms do not cover. Herpes virus can be found and released from the sores that the viruses cause, but they also are released between episodes from skin that does not appear to be broken or to have a sore. There is no cure for genital herpes, although there are medications that can limit the number and severity of recurrences of the symptoms of the disease.

Pneumotropic (Respiratory Tract) Diseases

Influenza. The flu, or influenza, is an acute, viral, inflammatory disease of the respiratory system. The influenza virus consists of eight weakly linked RNA segments enclosed in a layer of protein and an outer bilayer of lipids. Because of the influenza virus's ability to recombine, it is able to spread through a variety of human and animal strains. Migratory birds are so-called mixing vessels that carry the virus over large geographic areas. Some of the more common types of influenza viruses are swine flu, Hong Kong flu, Asiatic flu, avian flu, and equine flu.

The symptoms of influenza are fever, chills, headache, cough, sore throat, and extreme fatigue. Diarrhea is not usually found in cases of influenza. Although Americans refer to stomach flu, this disorder is most likely a bacterial infection of the digestive tract and is not viral influenza at all.

Common Cold. According to the National Institute of Allergy and Diseases (The common cold 2001), over 1 billion colds occur in the United States each year. The signs and symptoms of the common cold are some of the most common of any illness known, since almost everyone has experienced them at some point in time. The common cold begins with sneezing, scratchy throat, and a runny nose. These symptoms and signs generally last only one to two weeks, but the common cold is one of the leading causes of healthcare visits and school or job absences. In 1996, colds caused 45 million days of restricted activity and 22 million days lost from school in the United States.

There are more than 200 different viruses known to cause the symptoms of the common cold. Rhinoviruses and coronaviruses are two of the most common causes of colds. The common cold is age dependent, with children having between six and ten colds per year due to their relative lack of resistance to infection, and people over 60 having one or no colds per year. Children in school or daycare, and adults who work with children are more likely to get a cold.

Symptoms of the common cold usually begin about two or three days after infection and often include nasal discharge, obstructed nasal breathing, swelling of the sinuses, sneezing, sore throat, cough, and headache. Occasionally, colds lead to secondary bacterial infections of the middle ear or sinuses. Since colds are spread through both direct and indirect contact, handwashing is one of the best ways to reduce the spread of the common cold.

Hantavirus Pulmonary Syndrome. Hantavirus belongs to the bunyavirus family, which contains five genera of viruses that are each made up of single-stranded RNA viruses. Hantavirus is the only virus in the bunyavirus family that is rodent-borne, all the others are arthropod-borne. Hantavirus causes a respiratory disease known as hantavirus pulmonary syndrome (HPS) or just hantavirus disease. Although HPS is spread through contact with rodents—especially mice—many infected people do not report contact with rodents.

According to the CDC's Special Pathogens Branch of the Division of Viral and Rickettsial Diseases (*All about hantavirus* 2003), in May of 1993, an outbreak of an unexplained illness occurred in the "Four Corners," an area of the Southwest United States shared by Utah, Nevada, Arizona, and New Mexico. Several previously healthy young adults developed a respiratory illness from which about half soon died. Researchers discovered that the disease was not being spread through person to person contact, but, rather, from contact with rodent droppings. Scientists also determined that the disease had existed since about 1959 in the area. To date, HPS has been identified in 31 states. The average age of infected persons is 37, and about 75 percent of the cases have been among Caucasians with 22 percent of the cases occurring among Native Americans. The mortality rate of HPS is 38 percent among reported cases. About 75 percent of all cases of HPS are contracted in rural areas.

The characteristics of hantavirus disease are:
* Shortness of breath
* Fever
* Muscle pain
* Headache
* Chills
* Dizziness
* Nonproductive cough
* Nausea and vomiting
* Diarrhea
* Joint, back, and abdominal pain
* Low blood pressure
* Irregular heart function

SARS. Severe acute respiratory syndrome (SARS) is a respiratory illness that has recently been reported in Asia, North America, and Europe. In general, SARS begins with a fever greater than 100.4°F (38.0°C). Other symptoms include headache, an overall feeling of discomfort, and body aches. Some people also experience mild respiratory symptoms. After two to seven days, a dry cough and trouble breathing may develop.

The primary way that SARS appears to spread is by close person to person contact and by respiratory droplet inhalation. Most cases of SARS have involved people who cared for or lived with someone with SARS, or had direct contact with infectious material (e.g., respiratory secretions) from a person who has SARS.

Most cases of SARS in the United States have occurred among travelers returning from other parts of the world where SARS is more prevalent. There have been a few cases resulting from close contact with family members and healthcare workers. Currently, there is no evidence that SARS is spreading in the United States. Scientists have detected a previously unrecognized coronavirus in patients with SARS. The new coronavirus is the leading hypothesis for the cause of SARS, although little is known about this new disease.

Neurotropic (Central Nervous System) Diseases

Rabies. **Rabies** is an acute, neurotropic, infectious disease caused by a rhabdovirus known as the rabies virus. The rabies virus is shaped like a bullet. Rabies can be spread to humans via the bite of infected animals or through aerosols of the virus entering the body. The rhabdovirus colonizes in skeletal muscle and connective tissue for a period of between a few days and several months. The rabies virus then travels along a peripheral nerve to the spinal cord and brain where it causes encephalitis.

Since lymph does not circulate in the brain and spinal cord, the immune system cannot suppress the infection once it reaches the central nervous system. Because of its relatively long incubation period, a vaccine can be given that is quite effective in controlling the spread of the virus to the central nervous system. The vaccine is administered in a series of five or six injections at intervals during a 28-day period. Unlike previous treatments that included injections in the abdomen, the current postexposure prophylaxis includes relatively painless injections in the arm similar to a flu or tetanus vaccine.

Rabies is characterized by alternating periods of calm and agitation. Infected persons present with spasms of the mouth and pharynx that cause the common sign of foaming at the mouth. The sight or thought of water can trigger these spasms. Because of this reaction to water, the disease was once well known as hydrophobia, which means fear of water. Death occurs within a few days after the final stage of the disease.

Polio. **Poliomyelitis**, or polio, is a neurotropic, viral infection caused by the poliovirus. Although the disease conjured images of paralyzed victims in the mid 1900s, less than 1 percent of those infected develop paralysis. Only about 10 percent of those infected with the virus even develop symptoms of sore throat, headache, fever, and nausea. Humans are the only known host for the poliovirus, and infected populations shed the virus in their feces. The virus is usually transmitted through contaminated water supplies.

The poliovirus multiples first in the throat and small intestine, and then it travels to the lymph nodes of the neck and ileum. The virus spreads to the blood causing viremia, at which point the infection has run its course in the vast majority of cases. If the disease spreads past this stage to the central nervous system, it migrates toward the anterior horn cells of the motor nerves of the spinal cord.

Color Plate 65 pictures a child displaying a deformity of her right lower extremity due to poliovirus infection.

There are two common vaccines for polio, the Salk vaccine and the Sabin vaccine. Dr. Jonas Salk's vaccine is administered in a series of injections, and Dr. Albert Sabin's vaccine is taken orally. Through the efforts of the World Health Organization, and service clubs like the Lions club, polio has been eradicated from most of the world.

Encephalitis. Viral encephalitis, which is an inflammation of the brain, is caused by an arthropod-borne arbovirus that has a variety of strains causing endemic outbreaks of encephalitis worldwide. Mosquitoes carry the virus from infected animals to humans. Viral encephalitis is fatal about 25 percent of the time, and is characterized by chills, headache, fever, confusion, and coma.

Other strains of viral encephalitis are more common and infection is asymptomatic. Some of the more commonly known strains of encephalitis are Eastern equine ("horse") encephalitis (EEE), Western equine encephalitis (WEE), St. Louis encephalitis (SLE), California encephalitis (CE), La Crosse encephalitis (LCE), and Japanese B encephalitis. The spread of encephalitis is best dealt with by controlling local populations of mosquitoes.

West Nile. West Nile virus is a flavivirus commonly found in Africa, West Asia, and the Middle East. It is closely related to the St. Louis encephalitis virus found in the United States. The virus can infect humans, birds, mosquitoes, horses, and some other mammals. West Nile virus usually causes mild disease in people, characterized by flulike symptoms lasting only a few days with no long-term health effects. The spread of disease is being limited through mosquito control.

More severe diseases due to this virus are West Nile encephalitis, West Nile meningitis, and West Nile meningoencephalitis. Encephalitis refers to an inflammation of the brain, meningitis is an inflammation of the membranes around the brain and the spinal cord, and meningoencephalitis refers to inflammation of the brain and the membrane surrounding it.

According to the Division of Parasitic Infections of the National Center for Infectious Diseases (*West Nile virus* 2003), West Nile virus has been found in humans, birds, and other vertebrates in Africa, Eastern Europe, West Asia, and the Middle East, but until 1999 it had not previously been documented in the Western Hemisphere. It is not known from where the United States virus originated, but it is most closely related genetically to strains found in the Middle East. It is also not known how long it has been in the United States, but CDC scientists believe the virus has probably been in the eastern United States since the early summer of 1999, and possibly longer. The continued expansion of West Nile virus in the United States indicates that it is now permanently established in the Western Hemisphere.

Viscerotropic (Visceral) Diseases

Hepatitis. **Hepatitis** is an inflammatory disorder of the liver. It is most commonly spread by five separate viruses. This chapter included the three most common viruses: hepatitis viruses A, B, and C.

Hepatitis A.　Hepatitis A, which is also known as infectious hepatitis, is spread via the fecal-oral route by the ingestion of contaminated water and food. The hepatitis A virus (HAV) contains single-stranded RNA. There are no animal reservoirs for HAV. The virus resides in the epithelial lining of the human intestinal tract. After sufficient growth in the intestine, the virus replicates in the blood, and the kidneys, liver, and spleen become infected.

The virus is believed to survive for days on countertops and other fomites. HAV is resistant to normal levels of chlorine in water. Mollusks, such as oysters, which live in contaminated water, may be a source of infection when eaten undercooked. The incubation period averages about four weeks, and there is no chronic form of HAV infection. By the time the symptoms of hepatitis A are observable, individuals are no longer infectious. Although most cases of hepatitis A are subclinical, the following disease conditions may be present:

- Anorexia
- Fatigue
- Nausea
- Diarrhea
- Fever
- Jaundice
- Chills

Hepatitis B.　Hepatitis B, or serum hepatitis, is spread through contaminated body fluids such as blood. The virus is pictured in Figure 27-7. HBV is a double-stranded DNA virus which is enveloped. Individuals who are most at risk of infection with HBV are healthcare professionals (i.e., embalmers, doctors, nurses). HBV has been isolated in numerous bodily fluids (i.e., blood, saliva, breast milk, semen, vaginal secretion).

According to the National Center for Infectious Diseases, Division of Hepatitis (*Viral hepatitis B* 2003), nearly 10,000 healthcare workers are infected

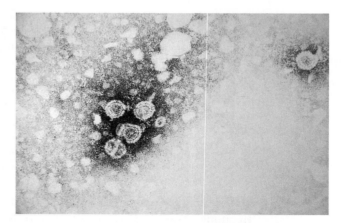

Figure 27-7　Cells infected with the hepatitis B virus. (Courtesy of the Centers for Disease Control and Prevention, Atlanta, GA.)

with HBV each year. Hepatitis B is a chronic, sometimes fulminant, disease, which means that it can rapidly lead to death, although 90 percent of acute hepatitis B infections end in complete recovery. The sharing of needles during intravenous drug abuse, contaminated tattoo needles, and unprotected sex all lead to higher incidences of HBV infection. Hepatitis B can cause any or all of the following:

- Jaundice
- Fatigue
- Abdominal pain
- Loss of appetite
- Nausea
- Vomiting
- Joint pain

According to the Occupational Safety and Health Administration's Blood-borne Pathogen Rule, all funeral home employees whose job description requires them to come in contact with body fluids or items soiled with body fluids are to be given the HBV vaccine at no cost to the employee. If the employee chooses not to receive the vaccination, the employee must sign a declination form, according to OSHA 3128 (Figure 27-8). The statement can only be signed by the employee following appropriate training regarding hepatitis B and the efficacy, safety, method of administration, and benefits of hepatitus B vaccination, and that the vaccine and vaccination are provided free of charge to the employee. The statement is not a waiver; employees can request and receive the hepatitis B vaccination at a later date if they remain occupationally at risk for hepatitis B.

Hepatitis C. Hepatitis C is caused by the hepatitis C virus (HCV), which is spread through direct contact with blood or other body fluids. Hepatitis C is subclinical in 80 percent of the suspected cases, with an incubation period of between 2 and 22 weeks. Half of the cases progress to chronic hepatitis. The characteristics of hepatitis C infection are similar to hepatitis B infection: jaundice, fatigue, dark urine, abdominal pain, loss of appetite, or nausea. Most cases of hepatitis C are transmitted through the use of illegal injected drugs. There is no vaccine for hepatitis C.

DECLINATION STATEMENT

I understand that due to my occupational exposure to blood or other potentially infectious materials I may be at risk of acquiring hepatitis B virus (HBV) infection. I have been given the opportunity to be vaccinated with hepatitis B vaccine, at no charge to me; however, I decline hepatitis B vaccination at this time. I understand that by declining this vaccine I continue to be at risk of acquiring hepatitis B, a serious disease. If in the future I continue to have occupational exposure to blood or other potentially infectious materials and I want to be vaccinated with hepatitis B vaccine, I can receive the vaccination series at no charge to me.

Figure 27-8 Declination statement for hepatitis B vaccination.

Mononucleosis. Infectious **mononucleosis**, which is also known as both kissing disease and college disease, is an infectious inflammatory disease caused by the Epstein-Barr virus (EBV). It affects young adults between the ages of 15 and 25. Outside the United States, the disease is asymptomatic for most children in less developed nations because they are exposed to EBV at an early age. The disease is generally self-limiting and few fatalities occur. When the disease is fatal, the cause of death is usually a ruptured spleen during vigorous activity.

EBV is spread by transfer of saliva by contacts such as kissing, sharing drinking glasses, or drinking from public fountains. The virus replicates in the parotid salivary glands until fever, sore throat, swollen lymph glands, and fatigue occurs. The incubation period for infectious mononucleosis is between four and seven weeks. EBV attacks the B memory cells within the immune system.

Inclusion Disease. Inclusion disease is a viral infection caused by the cytomegalovirus (CMV), a herpesvirus that causes cellular swelling resembling "owl's eyes." CMV infection is chronic. The virus is shed in body secretions such as saliva, urine, semen, vaginal secretions, and breast milk. It is estimated that 80 percent of the United States carries the cytomegalovirus. CMV is harbored in the parotid salivary glands and causes the following ailments:

- Fever
- Sore throat
- Swollen lymph glands
- Fatigue

CMV is important to embalmers due to the likelihood of transmission of the virus to children. According to the National Center for Infectious Diseases (*Cytomegalovirus* 2002), 4,000 children are born annually with cytomegalic inclusion disease, which is contracted in the womb or during infancy. Symptoms in infants are fever, enlargement of the liver and spleen, mental or motor retardation, and, possibly, death.

The virus may remain latent and exacerbate during pregnancy, immunosuppression therapy, or after multiple blood transfusions, causing deafness and neurological problems in the infant. Woman of childbearing age should be informed if they are nonimmune—some women have an innate immunity for CMV. CMV is a major cause of impaired vision in AIDS patients because the virus is reactivated during their illness. Both male and female embalmers can transmit the virus to the public.

Mumps. **Mumps**, which is also known as epidemic parotitis, is an infectious disease of the parotid salivary glands (Figure 27-9) caused by the mumps virus. The symptoms of mumps are swelling and pain in the parotid glands, fever, and painful swallowing (Figure 27-10). In males, four to seven days after the onset of symptoms, inflammation of the testicles can occur. Inflammation of the testicles is known as orchitis, a condition that can lead to sterility. A case of mumps can also lead to meningitis, inflammation of the ovaries (oophoritis), and pancreatitis.

The incubation period for epidemic parotitis is approximately 17 days. The mumps virus is spread via respiratory secretions and saliva. Children should be

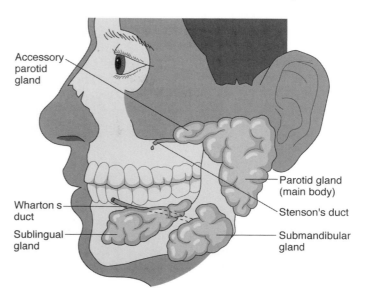

Figure 27-9 Salivary glands.

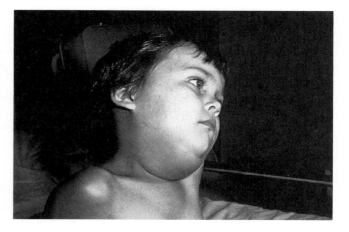

Figure 27-10 Mumps. (Courtesy of the Centers for Disease Control and Prevention, Atlanta, GA.)

vaccinated with the MMR vaccine, which provides children with immunity for measles, mumps, and rubella, to reduce the occurrence of mumps.

Ebola Hemorrhagic Fever. The Ebola virus causes a severe hemorrhagic fever with a high mortality rate (88 percent) that has appeared sporadically since it was initially discovered in Zaire, Africa, in 1976. Zaire is now known as the Democratic Republic of the Congo, and the Ebola virus is named after the river where it was first identified. The Ebola virus is an RNA virus that infects both human and nonhuman primates. Although the Ebola virus is believed to be harbored in certain animals in Africa, it was isolated from African imported monkeys in the United States. There have been no cases of Ebola hemorrhagic fever in the United States; however, several American research scientists were infected with the virus but did not become ill.

During outbreaks, it is assumed that the first infections occur due to contact with infected animals. The disease can then spread between people by way of nosocomial routes, needle-stick injury, or contact with infected bodily fluids. It is not known why some individuals recover from the disease and others do not, but Ebola hemorrhagic fever causes the following:

- Fever
- Headache
- Joint and muscle pain
- Sore throat
- Diarrhea
- Vomiting
- Rash
- Red eyes
- Hiccups
- Internal and external bleeding

Immunological Disease

AIDS. Acquired immunodeficiency syndrome (AIDS) is a contagious disease that compromises the immune system. It is caused by the human immunodeficiency virus (HIV), which is transmitted in body fluids. There is no cure for AIDS; however, a variety of chemotherapeutic agents are lengthening the lives of HIV-infected individuals. Like many microorganisms, however, HIV is capable of becoming multidrug-resistant. It is estimated that in 2000, 10 percent of newly HIV infected persons throughout Europe were infected with drug-resistant strains of the virus (McNeil 2003).

According to the National Center for HIV, STDs, and TB Prevention (*Human immunodeficiency virus type 2* 1998), in 1984, three years after the first reports of AIDS, researchers discovered the human immunodeficiency virus type 1 (HIV-1). In 1986, a second type of HIV, called HIV-2, was isolated from AIDS patients in West Africa. Both HIV-1 and HIV-2 have the same modes of transmission and are associated with similar opportunistic infections and AIDS. In persons infected with HIV-2, immunodeficiency seems to develop more slowly and to be milder than for HIV-1.

HIV is a retrovirus that affects T cells within the immune system. It attacks the RNA of the T cell causing the T cell to alter its DNA structure to that of HIV. The result is that when infected T cells replicate, the T cell creates more HIV. AIDS is the final stage of HIV infection. The average incubation period for AIDS development is 10 years from the point of initial infection.

HIV is spread by having unprotected sex with an infected partner. The virus can enter the body through the lining of the vagina, penis, rectum, or mouth during sex. HIV is also spread through contact with infected blood. Today, because of blood screening and heat treatment, the risk of getting HIV from blood transfusions is extremely small. HIV frequently is spread among IV drug abusers by the sharing of contaminated needles. Women can transmit HIV to their babies during pregnancy and birth, or through breast milk. If healthcare providers treat mothers with the drug AZT and deliver their babies by cesarean section, the chances of infecting the babies can be reduced to a rate of 1 percent.

According to the National Center for HIV, STDs, and TB Prevention (*HIV and its transmission* 2002) and the National Institute of Allergy and Infectious Diseases (*HIV infection and AIDS* 2003), more than 816,149 cases of AIDS have been reported in the United States since 1981. The AIDS epidemic is growing most rapidly among minority populations and is a leading killer of African-American males ages 25 to 44. AIDS affects nearly seven times more African Americans and three times more Hispanics than Caucasians.

People diagnosed with AIDS may get life-threatening diseases called *opportunistic infections,* which are caused by microbes such as viruses or bacteria that usually do not make healthy people sick. Some of the common diseases discussed in this text prove to be fatal for someone infected with HIV, and they are listed in Figure 27-11.

Pneumocystis carinii is a fungus that causes life-threatening pneumonia in AIDS patients but is rarely symptomatic in healthy individuals. *Toxoplasma gondii* is a protozoa that infects AIDS patients causing encephalitis. Cytomegalovirus causes fever, encephalitis, and blindness among individuals with AIDS. Herpes simplex viruses and the varicella-zoster virus, which causes chickenpox and shingles, can be fatal to AIDS patients as well. *Mycobacterium tuberculosis* can cause severe cases of tuberculosis. Kaposi's sarcoma is a common skin and blood vessel cancer found in cases of HIV infection (see Color Plate 66). Fungi such as *Histoplasma capsulatum,* which causes pulmonary infections; *Cryptococcus neoformans,* which causes meningitis; and *Candida albicans,* which causes overgrowths in the esophagus and respiratory tract, can all be fatal to those infected with HIV.

The increasing number of AIDS cases worldwide makes these otherwise benign infections even more hazardous to the embalmer. The threat to the embalmer is not AIDS itself, although the infection can be spread through needle-stick injuries. There are very few reported cases of healthcare workers becoming infected from accidental exposures. The threat to embalmers is the potential of spreading and contracting opportunistic infections from AIDS-related deaths.

Those individuals who have a T cell count in the teens—a normal count should be near 1,000—cannot defend themselves from infectious diseases. The sheer concentration of microbes in the deceased who has died of AIDS causes the embalmer to be at a higher risk of becoming contaminated with these microbes. Even if the embalmer does not develop symptoms of any diseases, it is possible to transmit the related microbes to the public.

The opportunistic pathogens associated with HIV infection can be found in the course of embalming anyone, regardless of their HIV status. Proper disinfection and preservation of the deceased is inherently hazardous to embalmers. The use of personal protective equipment and following universal precautions during all embalming operations reduces the likelihood of disease transmission. Utilization of personal protective equipment, proper biohazardous waste disposal, and thorough terminal disinfection of the embalmer, the embalming room, the removal vehicle and cot, and the deceased reduces the possible transmission of opportunistic pathogens.

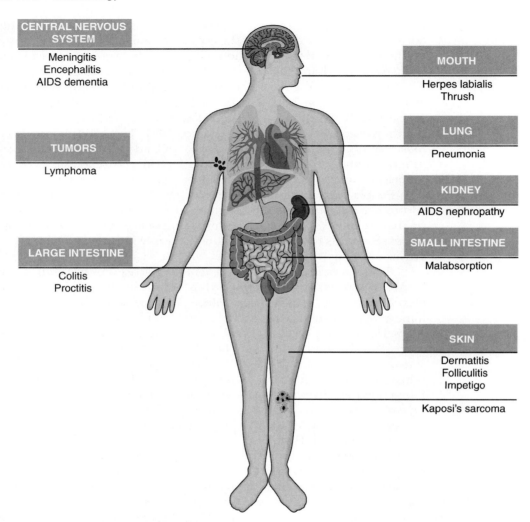

Figure 27-11 Pathologies associated with AIDS.

REVIEW QUESTIONS

Matching

1. _____ cold sores
2. _____ measles
3. _____ mononucleosis
4. _____ smallpox
5. _____ German measles

a. rubeola virus
b. variola virus
c. rubella virus
d. Epstein-Barr virus
e. herpes simplex 1 virus

Multiple Choice

1. Which of the following terms refers to viral infections that favor the body's abdominal organs?
   a. dermatropic
   b. pneumotropic
   c. neurotropic
   d. viscerotropic
2. Skin lesions caused by the herpes zoster virus are known as which of the following?
   a. ringworms
   b. trypanosomiasis
   c. dermatomycoses
   d. shingles
3. The first vaccine was developed by Edward Jenner, and it was a vaccine for which of the following?
   a. measles
   b. chickenpox
   c. smallpox
   d. West African sleeping disease
4. Orchitis and sterility can result from which of the following diseases?
   a. mumps
   b. rabies
   c. poliomyelitis
   d. mononucleosis
5. Which of the following types of hepatitis is spread through contact with blood and body fluids?
   a. hepatitis A
   b. hepatitis B
   c. hepatitis C
   d. hepatitis D

Putting Learning to Work!

The purpose of the following case analysis is to allow you to apply the information you have learned in a real-world situation. Read the case carefully and try to answer the following questions:

What disorder do you suspect the person had at the time of death?

What potential embalming complications do you anticipate?

What precautions should you take as the embalmer to limit the effects of these complications?

Case Analysis

The deceased is a 46-year-old male who died at an AIDS hospice center in Florida. His partner tells you that they have recently returned from a trip to Las Vegas and the Grand Canyon. He explains to you how difficult the trip was on his partner, especially due to the deceased's constant coughing and chest pain. He also tells you that he will have to purchase a new suit for his partner for the funeral because he has lost so much weight recently. When you see the deceased, you notice small cutaneous nodules on his face.

Bibliography

African trypanosomiasis. (1999). Retrieved July 26, 2003, from the National Center for Infectious Diseases, Division of Parasitic Diseases, Centers for Disease Control and Prevention at http://www.cdc.gov/ncidod/dpd/parasites/trypanosomiasis/default.htm.

All about hantavirus. (2003). Retrieved July 26, 2003, from the National Center for Infectious Diseases, Division of Viral and Rickettsial Diseases, Special Pathogens Branch, Centers for Disease Control and Prevention at http://www.cdc.gov/ncidod/diseases/hanta/hps/index.htm.

Basic information about SARS. (2003). Retrieved July 20, 2003, from the Centers for Disease Control and Prevention at http://www.cdc.gov/ncidod/sars/factsheet.htm.

Chamberlain, N. (2000a). *Introduction to microbiology*. Retrieved July 25, 2003, from the Kirksville College of Osteopathic Medicine at http://www.kcom.edu/faculty/chamberlain/Website/intmic.htm.

Chamberlain, N. (2000b). *Rickettsia, chlamydia, mycoplasma*. Retrieved July 15, 2003, from Kirksville College of Osteopathic Medicine at http://www.kcom.edu/faculty/chamberlain/Website/Lects/RICKETT.HTM#ri.

The common cold. (2001). In *Health matters*. Retrieved March 16, 2004, from the National Institute of Allergy and Infectious Diseases, National Institutes of Health, U.S. Department of Health and Human Services at http://www.niaid.nih.gov/factsheets/cold.htm.

Cytomegalovirus (CMV) infection. (2002). Retrieved July 26, 2003, from the National Center for Infectious Diseases, Centers for Disease Control and Prevention at http://www.cdc.gov/ncidod/diseases/cmv.htm.

Davey, M., & Altman, L. (2003). Suspected cases of monkeypox are rising. Retrieved June 10, 2003, from *New York Times*, electronic version, June 10, at http://www.nytimes.com/2003/06/10/national/10DOGS. html?th.

Ebola hemorrhagic fever. (2002). Retrieved July 26, 2003, from the National Center for Infectious Diseases, Division of Viral and Rickettsial Diseases, Special Pathogens Branch, Centers for Disease Control and Prevention at http://www.cdc.gov/ncidod/dvrd/spb/mnpages/dispages/ebola.htm.

Edmonds, P. (1978). *Microbiology: An environmental perspective.* Basingstoke Hampshire, England: Macmillan Publishing.

Epstein-Barr virus and infectious mononucleosis. (2002). Retrieved July 26, 2003, from the National Center for Infectious Diseases, Centers for Disease Control and Prevention at http://www.cdc.gov/ncidod/ diseases/ebv.htm.

Frobisher, M., Hinsdill, R., Crabtree, K., & Goodheart, C. (1974). *Fundamentals of microbiology.* Philadelphia: Saunders.

Gaudy, A., & Gaudy, E. (1980). *Microbiology for environmental scientists and engineers.* New York: McGraw-Hill.

Genital herpes. (2001). Retrieved July 26, 2003, from the National Center for HIV, STDs, and TB Prevention, Division of HIV/AIDS Prevention, Centers for Disease Control and Prevention at http://www.cdc.gov/ nchstp/dstd/Fact_Sheets/facts_Genital_Herpes.htm.

Grover-Lakomia, L., & Fong, E. (1999). *Microbiology for health careers* (6th ed.). Clifton Park, NY: Thomson Delmar Learning.

HIV and its transmission. (2002). Retrieved July 26, 2003, from the National Center for HIV, STDs, and TB Prevention, Division of HIV/AIDS Prevention, Centers for Disease Control and Prevention at http://www.cdc.gov/hiv/pubs/facts/transmission.htm.

HIV infection and AIDS: An overview. (2003). Retrieved July 22, 2003, from the National Institute of Allergy and Infectious Diseases, National Institutes of Health, U.S. Department of Health and Human Services at http://www.niaid.nih.gov/factsheets/hivinf.htm.

Human immunodeficiency virus Type 2. (1998). Retrieved July 22, 2003, from the National Center for HIV, STDs, and TB Prevention, Division of HIV/AIDS Prevention, Centers for Disease Control and Prevention at http://www.cdc.gov/hiv/pubs/facts/hiv2.htm.

Human papilloma virus. (1997). Retrieved May 29, 2003, from the Department of Gynecology and Obstetrics, University of Iowa at http://obgyn.uihc.uiowa.edu/Patinfo/Adhealth/hpv.htm.

Influenza (the flu). (2003). Retrieved July 26, 2003, from the National Center for Infectious Diseases, Division of Viral and Rickettsial Diseases, Special Pathogens Branch, Centers for Disease Control and Prevention at http://www.cdc.gov/ncidod/diseases/flu/fluinfo.htm.

Interferon. (2002). Retrieved July 26, 2003, from the British Association of Cancer United Patients at http://www.cancerbacup.org.uk/info/interferon.htm.

Mahon, C., & Manuselis, G. (2000). *Textbook of diagnostic microbiology* (2nd ed.). Philadelphia: Saunders.

Mayer, R. (2000). *Embalming: History, theory, & practice* (3rd ed.). New York: McGraw-Hill.

McNeil, D. Retrieved June 16, 2003 at http://nytimes.com/gst/health/article_page.html?nes=9807EEDD153 CC935A25754COA9659C8B63. Tenth of HIV cases in a study in Europe are resistant to drugs. *New York Times*.

Measles. (n.d.). Retrieved July 26, 2003, from the National Immunization Program, Centers for Disease Control and Prevention, http://www.cdc.gov/nip/publications/pink/meas.pdf.

Monkeypox fact sheet. (1998). Retrieved June 10, 2003, from the World Health Organization, Geneva at http://www.who.int/inf-fs/en/fact161.html.

Mumps. (n.d.). Retrieved July 26, 2003, from the National Immunization Program, Centers for Disease Control and Prevention at http://www.cdc.gov/nip/publications/pink/mumps.pdf.

Mycobacterium avium complex. (2003). Retrieved from the National Center for Infectious Diseases, Division of Bacterial and Mycotic Diseases, Centers for Disease Control and Prevention at http://www.cdc.gov/ ncidod/dbmd/diseaseinfo/mycobacteriumavium_t.htm.

Neighbors, M., & Tannehill-Jones, R. (2000). *Human diseases.* Clifton Park, NY: Thomas Delmar Learning.

Nester, E., Anderson, D., Roberts, C., Pearsall, N., & Nester, M. (2001). *Microbiology: A human perspective* (3rd ed.). Boston: McGraw Hill.

New variant CJD. (2003). Retrieved January 8, 2005, at http://www.cdc.gov/ncidod/diseases/cid/cjd_fact_sheet.htm.

Pathology for funeral service. (1999). Dallas, TX: Professional Training Schools.

Pneumocystis carinii pneumonia. (2003). Retrieved July 26, 2003, from the National Center for Infectious Diseases, Division of Parasitic Infections, Centers for Disease Control and Prevention at http://www.cdc.gov/ncidod/dpd/parasites/pneumocystis/default.htm.

Poliomyelitis. (n.d.). Retrieved July 26, 2003, from the National Immunization Program, Centers for Disease Control and Prevention at http://www.cdc.gov/nip/publications/pink/polio.pdf.

Rabies. (2001). Retrieved July 26, 2003, from the National Center for Infectious Disease, Division of Viral and Rickettsial Diseases, Viral and Rickettsial Zoonoses Branch, Centers for Disease Control and Prevention at http://www.cdc.gov/ncidod/dvrd/rabies/.

Shelton, H. (1992). *Boyd's introduction to the study of disease* (11th ed.). Philadelphia: Lea & Febiger.

Smallpox. (2002). Retrieved July 26, 2003, from Public Health Emergency Preparedness and Response, Centers for Disease Control and Prevention at http://www.bt.cdc.gov/agent/smallpox/overview/disease-facts.asp.

Tortora, G., Funke, B., & Case, C. (1998). *Microbiology: An introduction* (6th ed.). Menlo Park, CA: Benjamin/Cummings Publishing.

Update 2002: Bovine spongiform encephalopathy and variant Creutzfeldt-Jacob disease. (2003). Retrieved July 26, 2003, from the National Center for Infectious Diseases, Division of Viral and Rickettsial Diseases, Centers for Disease Control and Prevention at http://www.cdc.gov/ncidod/diseases/cjd/bse_cjd.htm.

Varicella disease (chickenpox). (2003). Retrieved July 26, 2003, from the National Immunization Program, Centers for Disease Control and Prevention at http://www.cdc.gov/nip/diseases/varicella/.

Venes, D. (Ed.). (2001). *Taber's cyclopedic medical dictionary* (19th ed.). Philadelphia: F. A. Davis.

Viral hepatitis A. (2003). Retrieved July 22, 2003, from the National Center for Infectious Diseases, Division of Hepatitis, Centers for Disease Control and Prevention at http://www.cdc.gov/ncidod/diseases/hepatitis/a/index.htm.

Viral hepatitis B. (2003). Retrieved July 22, 2003, from the National Center for Infectious Diseases, Division of Hepatitis, Centers for Disease Control and Prevention at http://www.cdc.gov/ncidod/diseases/hepatitis/b/index.htm.

Viral hepatitis C. (2003). Retrieved July 22, 2003, from the National Center for Infectious Diseases, Division of Hepatitis, Centers for Disease Control and Prevention at http://www.cdc.gov/ncidod/diseases/hepatitis/c/index.htm.

West Nile virus. (2003). Retrieved July 26, 2003, from the National Center for Infectious Diseases, Division of Parasitic Infections, Centers for Disease Control and Prevention at http://www.cdc.gov/ncidod/dvbid/westnile/wnv_factSheet.htm.

CHAPTER 28

Diseases of Fungi and Protozoa

Learning Objectives

Upon completion of the chapter, review questions, and case analysis, the reader should be able to:

- Match specific pathogens described in this chapter with the diseases they cause.
- Match the diseases described in this chapter with the genus of the pathogen.
- Identify the important disease conditions associated with the diseases described in this chapter.
- Identify the mode of transmission of the diseases described in this chapter.
- Identify lesions on human remains that suggest a potentially infectious disease.

Key Terms

dermatophytes
malaria

tsetse fly

FUNGI

Fungi are a group of often filamentous unicellular and multicellular organisms lacking chlorophyll and usually bearing spores. Fungi differ substantially from bacteria and viruses. Unlike bacterial cells, which are prokaryotic, fungal cells are eukaryotic cells containing a nucleus. Fungi are also different from plants because fungi do not contain chlorophyll.

Yeasts, molds, and dimorphic fungi are the three fundamental categories of fungi.

Yeasts are fungi that are typically encapsulated and are unicellular, while molds are fungi that are filamentous and multicellular. Dimorphic fungi alternate between unicellular and multicellular forms. Many fungi are saprophytes because they lack chlorophyll, and, therefore, grow on decomposing matter. Depending on the variety, fungi can reproduce either sexually or asexually through budding or reproductive spore formation (Figure 28-1). Some fungi produce toxins, which are harmful to humans. Table 28-1 lists some pathogenic fungi and the diseases they cause.

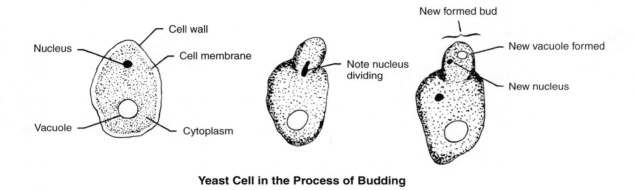

Yeast Cell in the Process of Budding

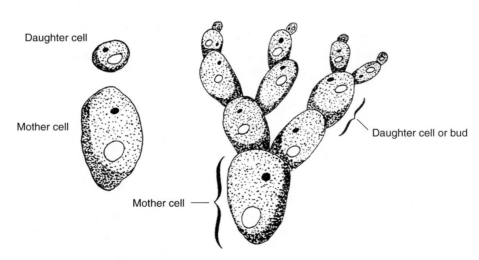

Chain of Yeast Cells as a Result of Budding

Figure 28-1 Budding yeast.

Table 28-1 Pathogenic Fungi: Disease, Transmission, and Signs and Symptoms

Pathogen	Disease Name	Mode of Transmission	Signs and Symptoms
Aspergillus fumigatus	Aspergillosis	Inhalation of fungus from manure or decaying vegetation	Lesions of the bronchi, lungs, aural canal, skin, eyes, nose, brain, bone, or urethra; nodules on kidneys, lungs, or liver; fever, cough, chest pain
Coccidioides immitis	Coccidioidomycosis (Posada-Wernicke disease; coccidioidal granuloma; valley fever/bumps; desert rheumatism; California disease)	Inhalation of fungal spores found in the dry, alkaline soils of the American Southwest, Mexico, and parts of South America	Angina, fever, coughing, anorexia, headache, weight loss, nodule formation, pulmonary disease, meningitis
Cryptococcus neoformans	Fungal meningitis	Inhalation of airborne yeast cells	Headache, fever, malaise, respiratory failure, deteriorating mental status, stiff neck
Histoplasma capsulatum	Histoplasmosis (cave disease; spelunker's disease; Darling's disease; reticuloendothelial Cytomycosis)	Inhalation of fungal spores from contact with bird feces	Lesions of the lungs or other organs, fatal chronic obstructive pulmonary disease (COPD)
Pneumocystis carinii (Pneumocystis jiroveci)	Pneumocystis pneumonia (PCP) (pneumocystosis)	Presumed to be through inhalation of fungus	Fever, cough, dyspnea, discolored skin and mucous membranes, respiratory failure
Trichophyton Microsporum Epidermophyton	*Tinea capitis* (scalp ringworm) *Tinea cruris* (jock itch) *Tinea pedis* (athlete's foot)	Person to person or fomite to person	Circular, raised lesions on the skin, discolorations of the nail beds, brittle nails, itching

Dermatomycoses

There are a wide variety of fungi that can infect the integumentary system. These infectious fungi are known as **dermatophytes**. The infections they cause are dermatomycoses. Dermatophytes grow in the keratin of the skin, hair, and nails causing infections called ringworms (tineas).

Ringworm of the scalp is known as *tinea capitis,* which begins as an infection of the hair follicle that spreads to the scalp (see Color Plate 67). *Tinea cruris* is a ringworm of the groin that is commonly referred to as jock itch. *Tinea pedis* is a fungal infection of the foot that is commonly known as athlete's foot (see Color Plate 68). These infections are caused by three genera of fungi: *Trichophyton, Microsporum,* and *Epidermophyton.* Recurrence of fungal infections of the integument are common, and many are chronic, especially those infecting the nails beds.

Coccidioidomycosis

Coccidioidomycosis is a respiratory disease caused by the fungus *Coccidioides immitis*. Other names for this disease include Posada-Wernicke disease, coccidioidal granuloma, valley fever, desert rheumatism, valley bumps, and California disease. *C. immitis* spores are found in dry, alkaline soils in the American Southwest, Mexico, and parts of South America. *C. immitis* is one of the most virulent mycotic pathogens in humans—inhaling only a few organisms results in infection. The wind carries the spores, transmitting the infection. Simply passing through endemic areas can lead to infection.

Most infections are subclinical, with less than 40 percent of those infected developing symptoms. However, coccidioidomycosis can be fatal, and Filipinos and African Americans run the highest risk of the disease becoming systemic. Among HIV-positive populations, a severe pulmonary disease can occur. Symptoms of the disease are angina (chest pain), fever, coughing, anorexia, headache, and weight loss for six weeks or longer. If the disease progresses to a secondary stage, it is accompanied by nodule formation, progressive pulmonary disease, and meningeal involvement. Men are nine times more likely to contract coccidioidomycosis than women.

Histoplasmosis

Histoplasmosis is a fungal infection of the respiratory system. Its other names include reticuloendothelial cytomycosis, cave disease, spelunker's disease, and Darling's disease. It is caused by the fungus *Histoplasma capsulatum*. In the United States, rates of histoplasmosis are highest in Ohio, Missouri, and the Mississippi Delta. *H. capsulatum* is found in the bodies of bats and in the fecal material of birds. The high nitrogen content of bird droppings makes a good breeding ground for this fungus. The disease is acquired from airborne spores, which may enter the ventilation systems of buildings where birds nest.

In most cases of the disease, the infected host is asymptomatic. This disease is not spread from contact with infected persons. In symptomatic cases, the fungus affects the lungs causing lesions, and any organ of the body can be affected as the disease progresses systemically. The clinical relevance of histoplasmosis is primarily of importance in immunocompromised cases. Once the disease reaches the systemic level, it causes fatal chronic obstructive pulmonary disease (COPD).

Candidiasis

Candidiasis is a disease caused by the fungus *Candida albicans*. The normal microbial flora of the body's mucous membranes is generally sufficient to prevent the growth of *C. albicans*. However, among infants who do not have a mature immune system and people with diseases that suppress the immune system, and when the normal microbiota are removed from mucous membranes the fungus is able to grow.

Infants often develop a white overgrowth of the tongue called thrush (see Color Plate 69). People with AIDS can develop a systemic infection caused by

C. albicans that can overgrow the esophagus or respiratory system and cause death. *C. albicans* can cause yeast infections in women due to frequent douching, which kills the normal bacteria of the vagina that would otherwise retard the growth of *C. albicans*. Diabetics and the obese may develop candidiasis of the moist skin. *C. albicans* is the fourth most common cause of nosocomial bloodstream infections in the United States, and it is 40 percent fatal once it reaches the systemic level.

Fungal Meningitis

Cryptococcus neoformans is the most common causative agent of a rare form of meningitis known as fungal meningitis, cryptococcal meningitis, or cryptococcosis. In cases of fungal meningitis caused by *C. neoformans*, a secondary fungal meningitis can also appear resulting from *Histoplasma capsulatum* infection, *Coccidioides immitis* infection, or *Aspergillus* species infection. Cryptococcosis may also infect the lung, as pictured in Figure 28-2. Even though fungi are widespread in the environment, fungal infections of the central nervous system in humans are rare.

Fungal meningitis is usually a chronic form of meningitis; however, it may appear acutely, mimicking bacterial meningitis. Individuals at risk of fungal meningitis include infants with histoplasmosis, IV drug abusers, and immunosuppressed populations including persons with cancer or AIDS. Fungal meningitis is noted by the following:

- Headache
- Low-grade fever
- Malaise
- Respiratory failure
- Deteriorating mental status
- Stiff neck

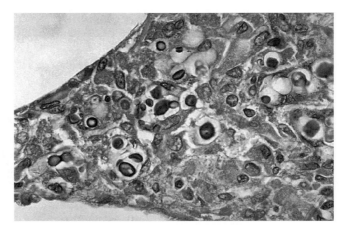

Figure 28-2 Cryptococcosis of the lung. (Courtesy of the Centers for Disease Control and Prevention, Atlanta, GA.)

C. neoformans is an encapsulate yeast cell present in the cerebrospinal fluid of infected persons. At autopsy, a mucus-like covering appears on the surface of the brain due to the capsule on these fungi. Microscopic flask-shaped cavities are also present in the brain tissue causing progressive dementia. All fungal infections of the CNS are difficult to treat, and fungal meningitis is fatal about 12 percent of the time.

Aspergillosis

Aspergillosis is a disease most commonly found among gardeners and farmers. It is caused by a fungus that is found in decaying vegetation and manure. *Aspergillus fumigatus* spores spread through ingestion or inhalation (Figure 28-3). The symptoms of aspergillosis are characterized by infection of the mucous membranes resulting in lesions that can be found in the bronchi, lungs, aural canal, skin, eyes, nose, or urethra. Nodules can form in the kidney, lungs, or liver. Other forms of aspergillosis can be caused by *A. flavus*, which is a mold found on corn, peanuts, and grains; *A. glaucus,* which is a bluish mold found on dried fruit; and *A. niger,* which forms black spores in the auditory meatus.

Persons with prolonged blood-related cancers, blood-related stem cell transplants, or organ transplants, and individuals receiving high-dose corticosteroids for chronic inflammatory diseases are most at risk for contracting aspergillosis. Those with HIV-positive infection may also contract this fungal disease of the lungs. Among immunosuppressed populations, aspergillosis begins as an invasive pulmonary infection, accompanied by fever, cough, and chest

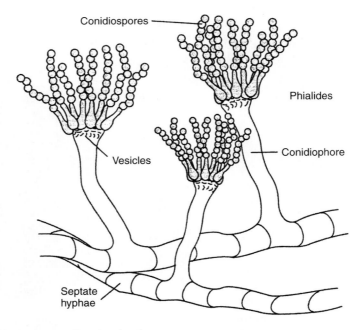

Figure 28-3 *Aspergillus fumigatus.*

pain. The fungi may then disseminate to other organs, including the skin, bones, and brain where the disease may cause fatal brain lesions.

Pneumocystis Pneumonia

At one time, *Pneumocystis carinii* was categorized as a yeast, then it was later believed to be a protozoan, and it is currently being reevaluated for classification as a fungus. The lifecycle of *P. carinii* is illustrated in Figure 28-4. *P. carinii*, which is now known as *P. jiroveci*, is a primary opportunistic pathogen in infections found among immunosuppressed populations (i.e., cancer patients, organ transplant recipients, AIDS patients). Pneumocystis pneumonia (PCP), which is also known as pneumocystosis, not only occurs in the immunosuppressed, but it was originally observed prior to and during World War II among malnourished infants and children in orphanages.

    P. carinii has a cell wall that increases its virulence against antimicrobial agents, which is why PCP is considered a multidrug-resistant disease. The fungus is widespread among animals, including dogs, cats, horses, and rodents, persisting in their lungs. It is unclear how the fungus is spread in humans, but most humans have become asymptomatic carriers of the infection by the time they are two or three years old. Scientists are uncertain if the disease is spread by

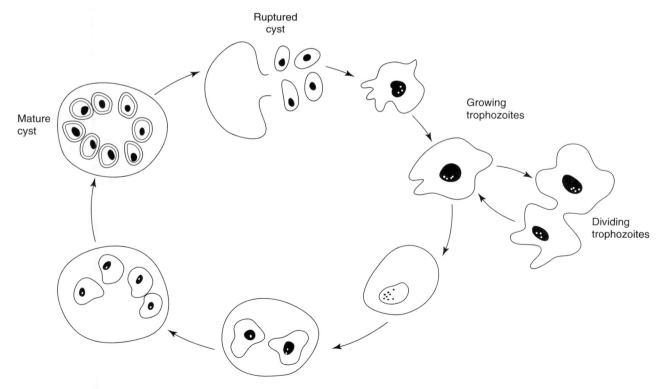

Figure 28-4 *Pneumocystis carinii* life cycle.

inhaling the fungus or if it is introduced into humans some other way. The fact that it has been isolated among hospitalized, malnourished infants, and elderly residents of nursing homes suggests that *P. carinii* is spread through airborne transmission.

Symptoms of *P. carinii* infection include fever, cough, and shortness of breath. As the disease progresses, a dusky discoloration appears on the skin and mucous membranes, which is due to the gradual loss of oxygen in the tissues. Respiratory failure is the result of the fungus entering the alveoli of the lungs, where they multiply until the alveoli fill with inflammatory fluid, macrophages, and the fungus. The progressive respiratory failure associated with PCP is ultimately fatal. Although PCP was once a leading cause of death among AIDS patients, early detection and treatment has resulted in the prevention of the disease before symptoms appear.

PROTOZOA

Protozoa are of the Kingdom Protista and are one-celled eukaryotes, although some may be colonial, with various mechanisms of motility. Even though protozoa lack a cell wall, they can have rigid forms that change based on their development through their life course. Although the majority of protozoa are free-living organisms with no disease-causing potential in humans, certain protozoa do cause serious diseases. There are more protozoa in the world than any other microorganism, and they play an important role in consuming both bacteria and multicellular organisms. Protozoa are responsible for such diseases as amebic dysentery, malaria, toxoplasmosis, African sleeping disease, giardiasis, and cryptosporidiosis. Table 28-2 lists some pathogenic protozoa and the diseases they cause.

Amebiasis

Amebic dysentery, which is also known as amebiasis, is caused by a protozoan named *Entamoeba histolytica*. The cyst form of *E. histolytica* is found in food and water, and is spread through the fecal-oral route to humans. Stomach acid destroys the vegetative cells but does not affect the cysts they form. The cysts enter the intestine, where the cyst's wall is digested and the vegetative form is released. The cells multiply in the epithelial cells of the colon. The typical mucous and bloody bowel movements indicate the protozoan's ability to feed on red blood cells and tissues of the gastrointestinal tract. *E. histolytica* can also infect tissues outside the digestive tract. Color Plate 70 is a photograph of the right flank of the torso of a person with an extraintestinal *E. histolytica* infection.

Amebiasis occurs in the United States primarily among male homosexuals who have many sexual partners, and among poor, migrant workers. Worldwide, there are approximately 30,000 deaths annually resulting from amebiasis. The symptoms of amebiasis are generally quite mild, but they may include chronic, mild diarrhea that lasts for months or years. In cases of ulcerative colitis associated with amebiasis, peritonitis may also occur. Amebiasis may also progress to an acute, fatal dysentery.

Table 28-2 Pathogenic Protozoa: Disease, Transmission, and Signs and Symptoms

Pathogen	Disease Name	Mode of Transmission	Signs and Symptoms
Cryptosporidium parvum	Cryptosporidiosis	Ingestion of contaminated food or water, fecal-oral route	Fever, anorexia, nausea, abdominal pain, profuse watery diarrhea
Entamoeba histolytica	Amebic dysentery (amebiasis)	Fecal-oral route	Chronic mild diarrhea that progresses to mucous bloody bowel movements
Giardia lamblia	Giardiasis	Ingestion of contaminated water, fecal-oral route, sexual transmission	Indigestion, gas, nausea, vomiting, explosive diarrhea, abdominal cramps, fatigue, weight loss
Plasmodium malariae	Malaria	Bite of the *Anopheles* mosquito	Chills, fever, anemia, hypertrophy of liver and spleen; symptoms alternate every 2–3 days with asymptomatic periods
Toxoplasma gondii	Toxoplasmosis	Ingestion of contaminated food or handling infected cat feces	Swollen lymph glands, muscle aches, fetal birth defects

Malaria

Malaria is a disease spread by the *Anopheles* mosquito, which is a biological vector. Malaria is caused by a protozoan of the genus *Plasmodium*. The most common forms of malaria are caused by *P. falciparum, P. vivax, P. ovale,* and *P. malariae*. The mosquito carries the pathogen in its saliva and transmits it to the human host through its bite.

Within 30 minutes of infection, the protozoan moves to the liver cells where it multiplies. Afterwards it reaches the red blood cells where it multiplies again. When the infected red blood cells burst, the symptoms of chills and fever appear. Other symptoms of malaria are anemia and hypertrophy of the liver and spleen. These symptoms alternate every two to three days with asymptomatic periods.

Mosquito control in the United States has decreased the number of cases of malaria. Nonetheless, malaria is still a serious disease in many parts of the world where mosquitoes breed uncontrollably. Malaria can be fatal. Quinine has been used with effectiveness in the treatment of malaria. According to the National Center for Infectious Diseases (*Malaria* 2002), there are 300 million to 500 million people worldwide infected annually with malaria, resulting in about 3 million deaths each year.

Toxoplasmosis

Toxoplasmosis is an infection caused by a single-celled protozoan named *Toxoplasma gondii*. It is found throughout the world. According to the National Center for Infectious Diseases (*Toxoplasmosis* 2003), more than 60 million people in the United States probably are infected with *T. gondii*, but the disease is usually asymptomatic. The lifecycle of *T. gondii* is presented in Figure 28-5.

Humans can contract toxoplasmosis by ingesting contaminated water or foods such as undercooked meats, although the most common form of transmission is through handling contaminated cat feces. Cats can only spread the protozoan for a few weeks after they become infected.

The mild flulike symptoms of toxoplasmosis are accompanied by swollen lymph glands, or muscle aches and pains that last for a few days to several weeks. *T. gondii* forms tissue cysts throughout the body, but especially in the skeletal muscle, myocardium, and brain. Persons with immune system problems, such as those with AIDS, those taking certain types of chemotherapy, persons who have recently received an organ transplant, or infants, may develop severe toxoplasmosis, which results in damage to the eye or the brain and is ultimately fatal. Infected infants can be born with severe mental retardation or with several

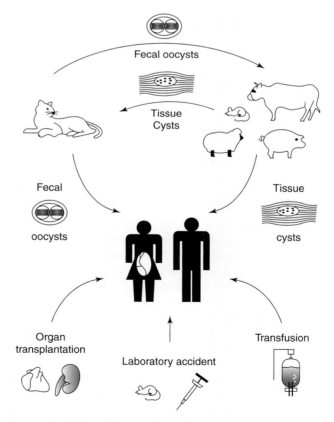

Figure 28-5 Life cycle of *Toxoplasma gondii*.

other serious mental or physical problems. The effects on the fetus range from convulsions to mental retardation, blindness, and death.

African Sleeping Sickness

There are two types of African trypanosomiasis, also called sleeping sickness, named for the areas in Africa in which they are found. According to the National Center for Infectious Diseases (1999), in the United States, 21 cases of East African trypanosomiasis have been reported since 1967 in travelers to Africa. There are approximately 20,000 cases of both East and West African sleeping disease reported each year worldwide. The disease is spread by the **tsetse fly**, which is a blood-sucking fly found only in Africa. The lifecycle of *Trypansoma* species is pictured in Figure 28-6.

East African Sleeping Disease.   East African trypanosomiasis is caused by a protozoan named *Trypanosoma brucei rhodesiense*, which is spread by the tsetse fly. A bite by the tsetse fly is often painful and can develop into a red sore. Fever, severe headaches, irritability, extreme fatigue, swollen lymph nodes, and aching muscles and joints are common symptoms of East African sleeping sickness. A skin rash can also be present. Progressive confusion, personality changes, slurred speech, seizures, and difficulty in walking and talking occur when the infection invades the central nervous system. If left untreated, death occurs within several weeks or months.

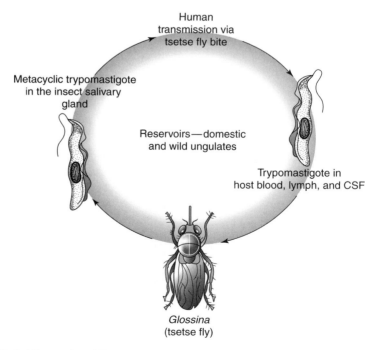

Figure 28-6 Life cycle of *Trypanosoma brucei gambiense* and *Trypanosoma brucei rhodesiense*.

West African Sleeping Disease. West African trypanosomiasis, also called Gambian sleeping sickness, is caused by a protozoan named *Trypanosoma brucei gambiense*. Symptoms include fever, rash, swelling around the eye and hands, severe headaches, extreme fatigue, and aching muscles and joints. Swelling of the lymph nodes on the back of the neck result in what is known as Winterbottom's sign. Weight loss occurs as the illness progresses.

Once the CNS becomes involved, personality changes, irritability, loss of concentration, progressive confusion, slurred speech, seizures, and difficulty in walking and talking occurs. Sleeping for long periods of the day and having insomnia at night is a common symptom of West African sleeping disease. If left untreated, death occurs within several months to years.

Giardiasis

The most commonly identified waterborne illness in the United States is called giardiasis. It is caused by the protozoan *Giardia lamblia,* which is found in both clear mountain streams and the chlorinated water supplies of the largest cities. The lifecycle of *G. lamblia* is illustrated in Figure 28-7. Although the main route of transmission of this disease is through contaminated water supplies, it can also be spread through the fecal-oral route. Contamination after diaper changing in daycare centers spreads the disease from the hands of the caregiver to the children. Giardiasis may also be spread sexually through anal intercourse.

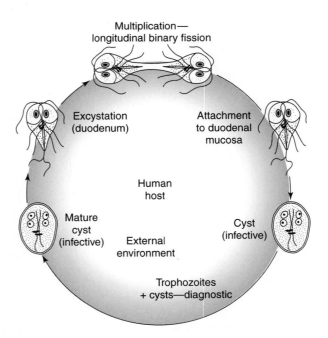

Figure 28-7 Life cycle of *Giardia lamblia.*

About two-thirds of exposed individuals develop the following symptoms approximately 6 to 20 days after infection:

- Indigestion
- Gas
- Nausea
- Vomiting
- Diarrhea
- Abdominal cramps
- Fatigue
- Weight loss

Even without treatment, the disease is normally self-resolving within about four weeks. Some cases, however, become chronic. Both symptomatic and asymptomatic persons may spread the infection unknowingly by excreting infectious cysts in their feces. A single human stool can contain 300 million *G. lamblia* cysts, and the establishment of infection requires only ten cysts. In cold water, the cysts can remain viable for up to two months, and chlorination of municipal water supplies is ineffective against these cysts.

Cryptosporidiosis

According to the Division of Bacterial and Mycotic Diseases of the National Center for Infectious Diseases (2003), over 403,000 people were involved in one waterborne outbreak of cryptosporidiosis, which is a protozoan disease caused by *Cryptosporidium parvum*. Many cases of traveler's diarrhea are caused by *C. parvum*, and it can be spread through contaminated food and water as well as the fecal-oral route. Epidemics have arisen from drinking water, swimming pools, a water slide, a zoo fountain, daycare centers, unpasteurized apple juice, and miscellaneous foods. The protozoan can be spread in the feces of infected humans and domestic animals such as dogs, pigs, and cattle. *C. parvum* is even more resistant to chlorine than *Giardia lamblia*.

The incubation period is approximately 4 to 12 days for this disease, with the symptoms lasting 10 to 14 days in most people. Cryptosporidiosis causes fever, loss of appetite, nausea, cramping abdominal pain, and profuse watery diarrhea. The disease is often fatal for individuals with suppressed immune systems, which include the elderly, children, cancer patients, organ transplant recipients, and persons with AIDS.

REVIEW QUESTIONS

Matching

1. _____ East African sleeping disease
2. _____ thrush
3. _____ PCP
4. _____ fungal meningitis
5. _____ amebic dysentery

a. *Candida albicans*
b. *Cryptococcus neoformans*
c. *Entamoeba histolytica*
d. *Trypanosoma brucei rhodesiense*
e. *Pneumocystis carinii*

Multiple Choice

1. Malaria is spread through which of the following vectors?
   a. ticks
   b. fleas
   c. mosquitoes
   d. human body lice
2. Which of the following refers to fungal infections of the skin, hair, and nails?
   a. tineas
   b. thrush
   c. owl's eyes
   d. kuru
3. Which of the following diseases is spread through handling contaminated cat feces?
   a. giardia
   b. toxoplasmosis
   c. histoplasmosis
   d. cryptosporidiosis
4. Which of the following microorganisms causes African trypanosomiasis and is spread by the tsetse fly?
   a. viruses
   b. bacteria
   c. fungi
   d. protozoa
5. Which of the following is the most commonly identified waterborne illness in the United States?
   a. giardiasis
   b. cryptosporidiosis
   c. toxoplasmosis
   d. amebiasis

Putting Learning to Work!

The purpose of the following case analysis is to allow you to apply the information you have learned in a real-world situation. Read the case carefully and try to answer the following questions:

What disorder do you suspect the person had at the time of death?

What potential embalming complications do you anticipate?

What precautions should you take as the embalmer to limit the effects of these complications?

Case Analysis

The deceased is a 42-year-old female who died on Halloween. Her 20-year-old son tells you that his mother was a single parent, and that she had a lumpectomy last Hanukah. Her breast cancer had been in remission until she found another lump Easter morning, while she was dressing. Since then, she had been undergoing chemotherapy and radiation therapy, but he says that she seemed to be doing well the last couple of weeks. "Mom is a veterinarian," her son states. "She worked until about two weeks ago. Then she got some kind of stomach flu. She had terrible diarrhea and stomach cramps, and I couldn't get her to eat anything. The doctors didn't know what was wrong with her."

Bibliography

African trypanosomiasis. (1999). Retrieved July 26, 2003, from the National Center for Infectious Diseases, Division of Parasitic Infections. Centers for Disease Control and Prevention at http://www.cdc.gov/ncidod/dpd/parasites/trypanosomiasis/default.htm.

Amebiasis. (2001). Retrieved July 26, 2003, from the National Center for Infectious Diseases, Division of Parasitic Infections, Centers for Disease Control and Prevention at http://www.cdc.gov/ncidod/dpd/parasites/amebiasis/factsht_amebiasis.htm.

Aspergillosis. (2002). Retrieved July 26, 2003, from the National Center for Infectious Diseases, Division of Bacterial and Mycotic Diseases, Centers for Disease Control and Prevention at http://www.cdc.gov/ncidod/dbmd/diseaseinfo/aspergillosis_t.htm.

Coccidioidomycosis. (2002). Retrieved July 26, 2003, from the National Center for Infectious Diseases, Division of Bacterial and Mycotic Diseases, Centers for Disease Control and Prevention at http://www.cdc.gov/ncidod/dbmd/diseaseinfo/coccidioidomycosis_t.htm.

Cryptosporidiosis. (2003). Retrieved July 26, 2003, from the National Center for Infectious Diseases, Bacterial and Mycotic Diseases, Centers for Disease Control and Prevention at http://www.cdc.gov/ncidod/dpd/parasites/cryptosporidiosis/default.htm.

Edmonds, P. (1978). *Microbiology: An environmental perspective*. Basingstoke Hampshire, England: Macmillan Publishing.

Frobisher, M., Hinsdill, R., Crabtree, K., & Goodheart, C. (1974). *Fundamentals of microbiology*. Philadelphia: Saunders.

Gaudy, A., & Gaudy, E. (1980). *Microbiology for environmental scientists and engineers*. New York: McGraw-Hill.

Giardiasis. (2001). Retrieved July 26, 2003, from the National Center for Infectious Diseases, Division of Parasitic Infections, Centers for Disease Control and Prevention at http://www.cdc.gov/ncidod/dpd/parasites/giardiasis/factsht_giardia.htm.

Grover-Lakomia, L., & Fong, E. (1999). *Microbiology for Health Careers* (6th ed.). Clifton Park, NY: Thomson Delmar Learning.

Histoplasmosis. (2003). Retrieved July 26, 2003, from the National Center for Infectious Diseases, Division of Bacterial and Mycotic Diseases, Centers for Disease Control and Prevention at http://www.cdc.gov/ncidod/dbmd/diseaseinfo/histoplasmosis_g.htm.

Mahon, C., & Manuselis, G. (2000). *Textbook of Diagnostic Microbiology* (2nd ed.). Philadelphia: Saunders.

Malaria. (2002). Retrieved July 26, 2003, from the National Center for Infectious Diseases, Division of Parasitic Infections, Centers for Disease Control and Prevention at http://www.cdc.gov/ncidod/dpd/parasites/malaria/default.htm.

Mayer, R. (2000). *Embalming: History, theory, & practice* (3rd ed.). New York: McGraw-Hill.

Meningococcal disease. (2003). Retrieved July 26, 2003, from the National Center for Infectious Diseases, Division of Bacterial and Mycotic Diseases, Centers for Disease Control and Prevention at http://www.cdc.gov/ncidod/dbmd/diseaseinfo/meningococcal_g.htm.

Neighbors, M., & Tannehill-Jones, R. (2000). *Human diseases*. Clifton Park, NY: Thomson Delmar Learning.

Nester, E., Anderson, D., Roberts, C., Pearsall, N., & Nester, M. (2001). *Microbiology: A human perspective* (3rd ed.). Boston: McGraw-Hill.

Pathology for funeral service. (1999). Dallas, TX: Professional Training Schools.

Pneumocystis carinii pneumonia. (2003). Retrieved July 26, 2003, from the National Center for Infectious Diseases, Division of Parasitic Infections, Centers for Disease Control and Prevention at http://www.cdc.gov/ncidod/dpd/parasites/pneumocystis/default.htm.

Shelton, H. (1992). *Boyd's Introduction to the Study of Disease* (11th ed.). Philadelphia: Lea & Febiger.

Taenia infection. (1999). Retrieved July 26, 2003, from the National Center for Infectious Diseases, Division of Parasitic Infections, Centers for Disease Control and Prevention at http://www.cdc.gov/ncidod/dpd/parasites/taenia/default.htm.

Tortora, G., Funke, B., & Case, C. (1998). *Microbiology: An introduction* (6th ed.). Menlo Park, CA: Benjamin/Cummings Publishing.

Toxoplasmosis. (2003). Retrieved July 26, 2003, from the National Center for Infectious Diseases, Division of Parasitic Infections, Centers for Disease Control and Prevention at http://www.cdc.gov/ncidod/dpd/parasites/toxoplasmosis/factsht_toxoplasmosis.htm.

Venes, D. (Ed.). (2001). *Taber's cyclopedic medical dictionary* (19th ed.). Philadelphia: F. A. Davis.

Wiser, M. (2000). *Free-living Protozoa and human disease*. Retrieved July 15, 2003, from Tulane University at http://www.tulane.edu/~wiser/protozoology/notes/free.html.

APPENDIX A

The Autopsy

THE AUTOPSY

An autopsy is performed by a forensic pathologist who has a degree from a medical school as well as specialized training in forensic medicine. Funeral directors and embalmers are not licensed forensic pathologists and do not perform autopsies. However, an understanding of the events that occur during the autopsy, and why they occur is necessary for the funeral service practitioner to better assist survivors and to prepare the deceased for funeralization.

Objectives of the Autopsy

According to Knight (1996:2), there are many facets of the autopsy that are common to every death investigation. The objectives of an autopsy are as follows:

1. To make a positive identification of the body and to assess size, physique, and nourishment.
2. To determine the cause of death.
3. To determine the mode of dying and time of death, where necessary and possible.
4. To demonstrate all external and internal abnormalities, malformations, and diseases.
5. To detect, describe, and measure any external and internal injuries.
6. To obtain samples for analysis and microbiological and histological examination, as well as other necessary investigations.
7. To retain relevant organs and tissues as evidence.
8. To offer an expert interpretation of those findings.

The External Examination

The autopsy begins with an external examination of the body, which is more important in forensic cases such as traumas than it is in autopsies related to natural diseases. In medicolegal cases, the description of the external attributes of the body is often the basis of inferences made about the nature of the weapon or the direction of attack. The routine for external examination of the deceased varies based on the nature of the case, but the procedure described here is typically followed by all forensic pathologists. Additionally, just as each embalmer prepares the deceased based on experience and personal preference, each autopsy differs according to the forensic pathologist and local custom.

After identification and removal of any clothing, the race and sex are noted. Other demographic characteristics such as age, eye color, and hair color are also noted. Conditions of the body associated with age (e.g., loss of hair, presence of age spots, loss of teeth) are also described. The body is measured for height and weight, and described in relation to general nutrition, physique, obesity, leanness, dehydration, and edema. Also of importance are any tattoos, congenital deformities, amputations, surgical scars, or other acquired external markings. The forensic pathologist also makes note of any external markings due to resuscitation attempts to distinguish them from original traumas. The body's limbs are flexed to note the degree of rigor mortis, and the degree of livor mortis is also noted. The forensic pathologist also examines each body orifice and collects samples where needed for the presence of vomit, blood, other body fluids, evidence of insect activity, or foreign matter.

The forensic pathologist then describes the condition of the body in relation to the presence of skin discolorations, such as cyanosis or congestion of the face, hands, or feet. Other discolorations may indicate specific diseases or forms of traumatic death. For example, localized discolorations of the limbs may indicate an arterial embolism, especially if the discoloration is only present in one limb. A brownish discoloration may indicate poisoning, and a bronze speckling of the skin may indicate blood poisoning due to a type of bacteria known as *Clostridium*. Pink or brownish pink patches over the large joints may indicate hypothermia, and a dark red discoloration may indicate cyanide poisoning deaths. Other common discolorations include cherry red associated with carbon monoxide poisoning, yellow associated with jaundice, and a bronze-copper discoloration associated with Addison's disease.

The Internal Examination

The internal investigation of the body begins with a Y-incision across the torso. The top of the Y is formed at each shoulder leading to the breast bone, and the lower half of the Y leads from the sternum to the pubic bone. The forensic pathologist makes a detour around the umbilicus. To access the brain, an incision is made across the scalp beginning behind one ear, following posterior to the crown of the head, and ending behind the opposite ear. The viscera are exposed by flaying the skin back from the Y-incision to expose the anterior rib cage. Similarly, the scalp is flayed back to allow access to the skull. With an autopsy saw, the anterior rib cage is removed, and the calvarium is removed from the superior portion of the skull. The viscera and the brain are examined, during which time they may be either partially or completely removed. The brain is almost always removed completely. Depending on the circumstances, the organs may be placed in a viscera bag and returned to the body cavity, or the forensic pathologist may keep them. In addition, portions of the organs may be returned to the body cavity, while other portions are kept by the forensic pathologist. Once the autopsy is complete, empty body cavities may be filled with absorbent materials.

Numerous aspects of the autopsy have not been included in this appendix. Only those aspects of the autopsy directly affecting the condition of the deceased, and specifically those that can potentially complicate the embalming process have been mentioned. The full investigation into the death often includes fingerprinting, toxicology, and radiological testing, as well as completing a full medical history of the deceased. The purpose of this appendix is merely to provide the reader with the most basic explanation of the events surrounding a postmortem examination.

Bibliography

Hill, Rolla B., & Anderson, Robert E. (1988). *The Autopsy—Medical practice and public policy*. Boston: Butterworths.

Knight, Bernard. (1996). *Forensic pathology* (2nd ed.). London and New York: Arnold and Oxford University Press.

Magath, Thomas B. (1934). *The Medicolegal necropsy*. Baltimore: Williams & Wilkins.

Spitz, Werner U., & Fisher, Russel S. (1980). *Medicolegal investigation of death: Guidelines for the application of pathology to crime investigation* (2nd ed.). Springfield, IL: Charles C Thomas.

Wetli, Charles V., Mittleman, Roger E., & Rao, Valerie J. (1988). *Practical forensic pathology*. New York: Igaku-Shoin.

APPENDIX B

Cellular Anatomy

THE CELL

Cells maintain their existence in the presence of internal and external fluids. The water inside the cell is known as intracellular fluid or cytosol. The body's cells are suspended in interstitial fluid, which is also referred to as extracellular fluid. Extracellular fluid contains 0.9 percent sodium chloride (NaCl, or salt), a similar salt concentration to that of sea water. All of the materials found in the cell are collectively known as *cytoplasm*, and both intracellular fluid and extracellular fluid contain many other dissolved substances in addition to water. Figure B-1 depicts the basic components of many human cells.

Nucleus

Most cells of the body contain at least one nucleus, but mature red blood cells have no nucleus, and muscle cells may have several nuclei. The nuclear envelope is not a solid structure; it contains many small openings that allow communication with the rest of the cell. These openings in the nuclear envelope are known as nuclear pores, and the collective substances within the nucleus are known as *nucleoplasm*.

Chromosomes and Genes

Chromosomes store genetic material in the human genes. There are 46 chromosomes in the healthy human. The sperm and egg each contribute 23 chromosomes to the cell. A chromosome is a long, coiled molecule of DNA (deoxyribonucleic acid) with a characteristic double-helix shape, as illustrated in Figure B-2. A double helix resembles a twisted ladder, with sides formed by alternating bands of sugar and phosphate. The rungs are formed by nitrogenous bases, which always pair in specific ways. Genes are segments of DNA that control the release

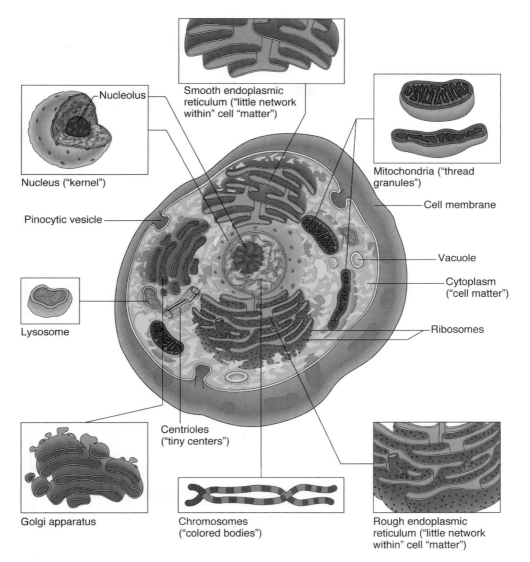

Figure B-1 Structure of a cell.

of proteins determining the cell's particular function. DNA also stores the genetic material allowing the cell to replicate and pass on its genetic material.

DNA is composed of nucleic acids, which are organic compounds containing carbon, oxygen, hydrogen, nitrogen, and phosphorus. Nucleic acids are formed from nucleotides, which are made of a sugar unit, a phosphate unit, and a nitrogenous base. In DNA, the nitrogenous bases are adenine (A), guanine (G), cytosine (C), and thymine (T). Nitrogenous bases always pair the same way in DNA, with thymine paring with adenine, and cytosine pairing with guanine.

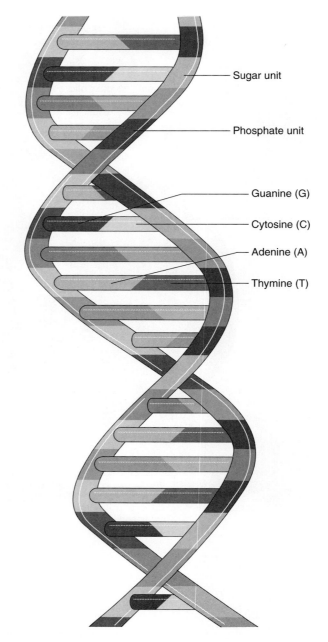

Sugar unit

Phosphate unit

Guanine (G)

Cytosine (C)

Adenine (A)

Thymine (T)

Figure B-2 DNA.

Ribosomes

The function of ribosomes is to synthesize proteins from amino acids. Ribosomes can be found attached to the endoplasmic reticulum, or they can be free in the cytosol. Ribosomes are small granules of protein and RNA (ribonucleic acid) that are integral in the process of combining amino acids into proteins.

Endoplasmic Reticulum

The endoplasmic reticulum (ER) is a series of intracellular membranes. The various shapes of the membranes of the ER allow it to synthesis proteins, carbohydrates, and lipids. In addition, the ER stores substances in the cell without affecting the other functions of the cell. Finally, the ER serves as an intracellular transport system allowing substances to travel from place to place within the cytosol.

Golgi Apparatus

The Golgi apparatus is found in cells that secrete chemical substances. The Golgi apparatus can modify the cell membrane because it is formed of layers of stacked membranes. Small fluid reservoirs in the Golgi apparatus store substances such as mucus and enzymes. This stored material is later secreted onto the surface of the cell in a process known as *exocytosis*.

Lysosomes

The digestive unit of the cell is the lysosome. Lysosomes contain a variety of digestive enzymes that aid in the cellular breakdown of proteins, nucleic acids, lipids, and carbohydrates. The constituent substances found in these materials are then released back into the cytoplasm, where they can be utilized to form new substances.

Lysosomes are of great importance to the embalmer due to their role in the decomposition of the dead and their activity in the immune system. During the process of decomposition, cells are unable to control the activity of lysosomes. As the lysosomes cross the cellular membrane, they enter the extracellular fluid where they begin to digest, or lyse, the body's own tissues. This process of self-digestion is known as *autolysis*. In addition, when invading microorganisms are destroyed by the immune system, lysosomes aid in the breakdown of the disease-causing microbes.

Mitochondria

Mitochondria are the energy production centers of the cell. The mitochondria produce most of the ATP (adenosine triphosphate) found in the cell, in a process requiring oxygen and generating carbon dioxide. Mitochondria contain their own DNA and ribosomes, so they are able to replicate within the cell. Muscle cells contain the most mitochondria due to their high demand for ATP production, which provides the cell with essential energy.

Cell Membrane

The cell membrane, which is also referred to as a *plasma membrane,* surrounds the entire cell, and it is composed of specialized fats called phospholipids. Although it is thin, the cell membrane is crucial in separating the cytoplasm from the extracellular fluid. The cell membrane contains channeled proteins that allow the cell to interact with extracellular fluid. The cell may also be coated with a thick fluid known as the glycocalyx that allows the cell to identify other cells.

Structures Providing Motility

Some specialized cells have attachments on their exterior. *Microvilli* are finger-like projections of the cell membrane allowing the absorption of materials from the extracellular fluid. Cells with microvilli are found in the digestive system, where nutrients are absorbed. *Cilia* are found on cells lining the respiratory tract. Cilia are hairlike structures that beat repeatedly, moving mucus and trapped particles toward the throat and away from the delicate tissues of the lungs. *Flagella* are whiplike structures on the surface of sperm that provide it with motion. A flagellum allows a sperm cell to travel within the female reproductive system once it becomes activated.

Bibliography

Saladin, K. (1998). *Anatomy & physiology: The unity of form and function.* New York: McGraw-Hill.

Scott, A., Fong, E., & Beebe, R. (2002). *Functional anatomy for emergency medical services.* Clifton Park, NY: Thomson Delmar Learning.

Van Wynseberghe, D., Noback, C., & Carola, R. (1995). *Human anatomy & physiology* (3rd ed.). New York: McGraw-Hill.

APPENDIX C

Blood

THE BLOOD: GENERAL CHARACTERISTICS

The pH level of blood is important because many enzymes within the body function best at the slightly alkaline pH of 7.35 to 7.45. The maintenance of the body's pH level is crucial for survival. If too many acids are released into the blood and tissue, as in the cases of renal acidosis and lactic acidosis, the death can result.

Blood is a relatively thick fluid with a viscosity of 3.3 to 5.5, meaning that blood is approximately three to five times thicker than water. The viscosity of blood may be higher in persons whose body has become dehydrated, in the presence of diseases that increase the production of certain blood components, or in cases of diseases that have altered blood clotting mechanisms. When blood flow slows, the blood begins to pool and thicken, or congeal, causing blood clots to form. Both chemotherapeutic agents and edema can lower the viscosity of blood, making it thinner.

In a living body, the temperature of blood is 100.4°F (37.8°C). This may sound odd at first because the body's temperature, as measured under the tongue, is 98.6°F (36.7°C). The reason for the apparent discrepancy is that the deep temperature of the body at its core is higher than more superficial surfaces. A condition known as hypothermia occurs when an individual's core temperature drops below normal, while an increase in core body temperature is known as hyperthermia.

PLASMA

Plasma contains 90 percent water and 7 percent blood proteins. The remainder of the plasma contains hormones, electrolytes, amino acids, waste products, enzymes, and nutrients such as glucose. One of the primary functions of plasma is to transport dissolved substances across the endothelium-lined walls of blood vessels. These dissolved substances can be exchanged with other substances in the interstitial fluid.

Interstitial fluid differs from plasma in two ways. First, there is a higher concentration of dissolved oxygen in plasma than there is in interstitial fluid, allowing the dissolved oxygen to diffuse from the bloodstream into the extravascular tissues. Second, the proteins found in plasma are larger than other blood proteins and remain in the blood vessels because they are unable to cross capillary walls into the lymph capillaries (Figure C-1).

There are three types of plasma proteins: albumins, globulins, and fibrinogen.

Albumins

Albumins are synthesized in the liver and maintain total blood volume by transporting water in the blood. They are the most abundant type of plasma protein, making up almost 60 percent of the plasma proteins. If the amount of albumins decreases, perhaps due to liver cancer or hepatitis, the fluid accumulates in the tissues, causing edema.

Globulins

There are three classes of globulins: alpha globulins, beta globulins, and gamma globulins. The liver produces alpha and beta globulins. They transport fats in the bloodstream. Low-density lipoproteins (LDL) transports cholesterol from the liver to body cells, while high-density lipoproteins (HDL) remove cholesterol from arteries. Gamma globulins function in the immune system as antibodies.

There are five categories of antibodies: IgA, IgD, IgE, IgG, and IgM. Each of these gamma globulin antibodies has a specific formula for defending the

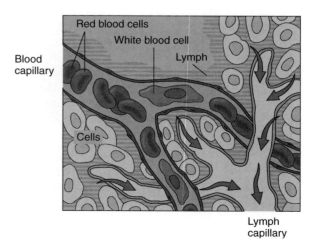

Figure C-1 Exchange of fluids between the lymph and blood vessels.

body against antigens present in disease-causing microorganisms. Gamma globulins are also known as immunoglobulins or antibodies, and some of the more important immunoglobulins are described in Table C-1.

Fibrinogen

Fibrinogen is a plasma protein that aids in blood clotting reactions. Given the appropriate conditions, fibrinogen molecules will interact to form fibrin. The insoluble strands that serve as the framework of blood clots are formed from fibrin. Fibrinogen is an exceptionally small protein. It would take more than 100 fibrinogen molecules lined up end-to-end to equal the diameter of one red blood cell, which is about the same size as the period at the end of this sentence.

Electrolytes

Electrolytes are inorganic compounds that separate into ions when dissolved in water. The presence of sodium ions in the plasma helps determine the amount of extracellular fluid by setting the osmotic pressure of the blood and controlling the direction of osmotic diffusion. Other ions in plasma are chloride, calcium, potassium, phosphate, magnesium, and bicarbonate.

ERYTHROCYTES

Erythrocytes, which are the red blood cells, transport oxygen and carbon dioxide in the blood. Figure C-2 includes both red blood cells and white blood cells. Erythrocytes are specialized cells that do not have a nucleus, ribosomes, or mitochondria, and must, therefore, be synthesized in the body. They circulate for approximately 80 to 120 days. Approximately 3 million new erythrocytes enter the circulation every second. They travel about 700 miles in their lifetime, and they make a single circuit of the circulatory system every 30 seconds.

Table C-1 Antibodies and Their Function

IgA	Found in exocrine excretions such as mother's milk, respiratory and intestinal mucus, saliva, and tears. IgA protects mucous surfaces from microbial infection. It also helps protect suckling newborns from infection.
IgD	Prepared from persons with high Rh antibody concentrations in their blood. It is administered to an Rh-negative mother after the birth or abortion of an Rh-positive fetus.
IgE	Attach to cells in the respiratory and intestinal tract. They are found in half of the patients with allergic diseases.
IgG	Moves across the placental barrier to provide immunity to the infant before birth.
IgM	Found in almost every immune response during the early period of the reaction. Its size prevents it from moving across the placental barrier to the fetus.

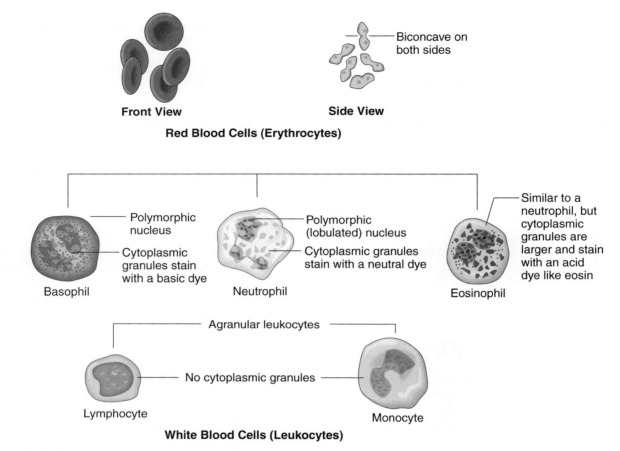

Figure C–2 Cellular components of blood.

Red blood cells have a characteristic biconcave-disc shape. They are shaped like a breath mint without the hole in the center. This biconcave shape gives the red blood cell a larger surface area, allowing it to exchange gases more easily. The total number of red blood cells in the body of an average size person is about 35 trillion. The surface area of these 35 trillion cells, when added together, is about 3,820 square meters. The total surface area of the entire human body is about 2,000 times less than that.

Oxygenated hemoglobin gives blood its red color. Deoxygenated hemoglobin has a bluish-purple color and gives the surface veins their characteristic blue color. In hemoglobin, oxygen binds to iron in a weak bond that is easily separated. Carbon dioxide can also bond to the hemoglobin, and the bond is similarly unstable. This instability allows the exchange of oxygen and carbon dioxide in the peripheral tissues of the body and in the lungs.

Interestingly, heme has over 200 times a greater affinity for carbon monoxide (CO) than it does for oxygen. The carbon monoxide–hemoglobin bond is stable. Over 20 percent of a tobacco smoker's hemoglobin is nonfunctional because it is bound to hemoglobin.

LEUKOCYTES

The body's primary defense against invading microorganisms is through the white blood cells, or leukocytes (Figure C-3). The white blood cells found in lymph are produced primarily by bone marrow. Leukocytes are found in the blood, the lymph nodes, and specialized lymphatic tissues of the body. Leukocytes can be divided into two categories: agranulocytes and granulocytes. Agranuloctyes are further divided into monocytes and lymphocytes, which can be further subdivided into T cells, B cells, and NK cells.

Monocytes

Monocytes are the largest blood cells, circulating in the blood for one to three days and then entering the peripheral tissues of the body. Once in the peripheral tissues, monocytes are known as free macrophages, which are the first cells to arrive at a site of injury, where they release chemicals that attract other phagocytic cells. A macrophage destroys invading microorganisms by engulfing the foreign cell and then releasing lysosomes that digest it.

Macrophages are found in lymph, in lymph nodes, and lining the walls of both blood vessels and lymphatic vessels. They are also found in the alveoli of the lungs, in Kupfer cells within the liver, and in the kidneys, spleen, and bone marrow. Groups of macrophages are able to encompass foreign bodies, walling off the microorganism and inhibiting its spread.

Lymphocytes

Although lymphocytes account for 20 percent to 30 percent of the white blood cell population, most are found in the body's lymphatic system. The function of lymph is to help cleanse the body tissues of disease-causing organisms as well as to remove decaying cells. Lymph is produced by lymph nodes and lymphatic tissues. The three types of lymphocytes are T cells, B cells, and NK cells.

T Cells.   T cells are actually a group of specialized lymphocytes within the body. There are many types of T cells. Although there are more than four types of T cells, this section describes only cytotoxic T cells, helper T cells, suppressor T cells, and memory T cells.

Cytotoxic T cells migrate from lymphoid tissue to the site of invasion, where they inject perforin into the invading microorganism. Perforin causes the invading cell to rupture within two hours. Cytotoxic T cells seem to have the ability to attach to another foreign cell and repeat this same process. The reaction is

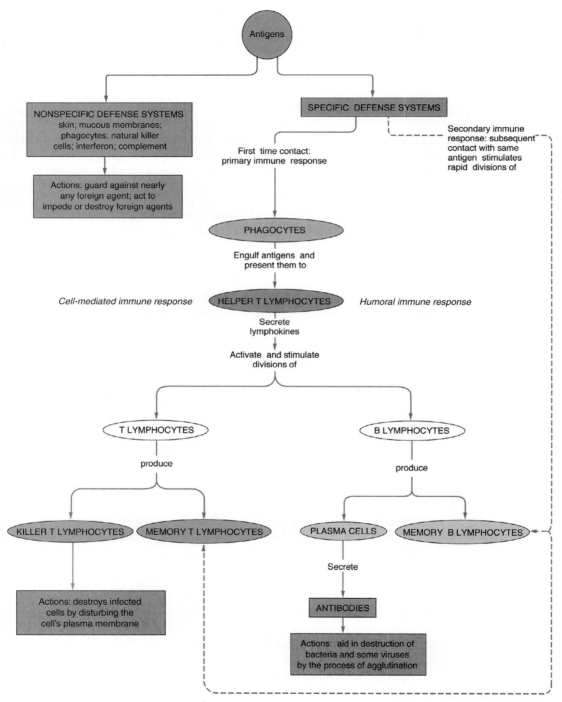

Figure C-3 Overview of the body's chemical defense mechanisms.

highly specific for certain types of invading cells. Cytotoxic T cells are the main cause of rejection of organ and tissue transplants, as well as acting against neoplasms.

The regulation of the immune response is aided by helper T cells, which work in direct association with B cells. The B cells produce antibodies that destroy invading microorganisms, and helper T cells activate B cells when contact is made with the specific antigen for that B cell. An antigen is a protein found on the surface of a cell that identifies it as a specific microorganism. Helper T cells also activate cytotoxic T cells to produce interferon that destroys viruses. Antibiotics do not destroy viruses.

Suppressor T cells help inhibit the immune system response. The action of lymphocytes is controlled by suppressor T cells, which can induce a negative feedback loop to inhibit the formation of helper T cells and B cells. The suppression of lymphocytes is necessary to reduce inflammation, allergic reactions, and autoimmune disorders.

Memory T cells are produced when activated T cells divide, which occurs when an individual is infected by a particular antigen. The memory T cells remain in reserve in the event that the same antigen presents itself again in the body.

B Cells. B cells can differentiate into plasma cells, which are then able to produce antibodies found in the blood plasma. Memory B cells hold the recipe for particular antigens and are able to stimulate the production of lymphatic reactions when the body is infected again with the same antigen.

NK Cells. Immunological surveillance is achieved by the presence of NK (natural killer) cells and activated macrophages in the peripheral tissues of the body. NK cells seek and destroy foreign cells, normal cells infected with viruses, and cancer cells.

Granulocytes

Granuloctyes are a category of white blood cell named according to the method utilized to stain them. Cells are frequently stained to observe their structures under the microscope. Neutrophils stain with neutral dye, eosinophils stain with an acid dye, and basophils stain with an alkaline dye.

Neutrophils contain lysosomal enzymes and bactericidal compounds that lyse, or digest, microorganisms. Dead microorganisms and neutrophils make up pus. Eosinophils are phagocytic cells that contain lysosomes that digest phagocytized materials. They are most likely to digest antibody-antigen complexes after the neutrophils lyse microorganisms. Eosinophils contain the protein plasminogen, which helps dissolve blood clots. Basophils are the least common of all the white blood cells. They have a life span of about 5 to 10 days and live for only a few hours once released in the blood stream. Once basophils enter the peripheral tissues, they release heparin and histamine. Heparin is an anticoagulant that prevents blood clotting, and histamine causes the blood vessels to dilate. The combination of histamine and heparin allows leukocytes to pass through blood vessel walls into the peripheral tissues.

THROMBOCYTES

Thrombocytes are not cells, as was once believed. The term *platelet* is a more accurate description of a thrombocyte. Platelets are flat, disc-shaped structures that act in blood clot formation. They are membrane-enclosed packets containing enzymes that initiate the blood clotting process. They also form temporary patches in the walls of damaged blood vessels by clumping together. Finally, platelets contain actin and myosin proteins that reduce the size of the clot and pull the cut edges of vessel walls back together, preventing further blood loss after blood clot formation. The constriction of broken or damaged blood vessels is further influenced by the presence of serotonin, which is released from platelets. Serotonin is a chemical that causes vasoconstriction.

PHARMACEUTICAL AGENTS AND BLOOD CLOTTING

Those who suffer from chronic inflammatory disorders will often follow a regimen of NSAIDs. Two over-the-counter medications classified as NSAIDs are Aleve (naproxen sodium) and aspirin (acetylsalicylic acid). One of the side effects of both of these drugs is that they inhibit proper blood clotting by preventing platelets from sticking together. This effect can lead to easy bruising and internal bleeding.

Streptokinase is a drug that digests fibrin threads. Certain streptococcal bacteria can release streptokinase into the blood in cases of bacteremia. Streptokinase activates plasminogen to speed up the digestion of fibrin. Tissue-plasminogen activator (tPA) is a genetically engineered medication. It is used to dissolve intravascular blood clots by delivering the tPA directly to a clotted area via a catheter. Dicumarol is often administered after surgery to prevent the formation of blood clots. It also prevents clots from forming during surgery. Dicumarol is commonly added to blood that will later be used for transfusion.

Bibliography

Saladin, K. (1998). *Anatomy & physiology: The unity of form and function*. New York: McGraw-Hill.

Scott, A., Fong, E., & Beebe, R. (2002). *Functional anatomy for emergency medical services*. Clifton Park, NY: Thomson Delmar Learning.

Van Wynseberghe, D., Noback, C., & Carola, R. (1995). *Human anatomy & physiology* (3rd ed.). New York: McGraw-Hill.

APPENDIX D

Anatomy of the Heart and Blood Vessels

THE HEART

The heart is located in the mediastinum, which is the region of the body located in the middle of the chest behind the sternum. The heart is approximately the size of an adult's fist and is positioned slightly to the anatomical left of the sternum, with the point of the heart tilted slightly toward the stomach. The study of the heart is known as *cardiology*.

Pericardium

The heart is surrounded by the pericardial sac. The pericardium can be divided into three portions: the visceral pericardium, the parietal pericardium, and the fibrous pericardium. The visceral pericardium, or epicardium, covers the surface of the heart, while the parietal pericardium is a membrane that lines the inner surface of the pericardial sac. The outer surface of the pericardial sac is made of collagen fibers and is called the fibrous pericardium. The space between the parietal pericardium and the visceral pericardium is the pericardial cavity, which is filled with pericardial fluid. The pericardial fluid is secreted by the pericardial membranes and serves as a lubricant, reducing friction between the surface of the heart and the pericardial sac.

Layers of the Heart

The heart wall consists of three layers: the epicardium, the myocardium, and the endocardium (Figure D-1). The layers of the heart are also referred to as tunics. The epicardium, which is the visceral pericardium, is the outermost layer of the heart. It is covered with adipose tissue, which

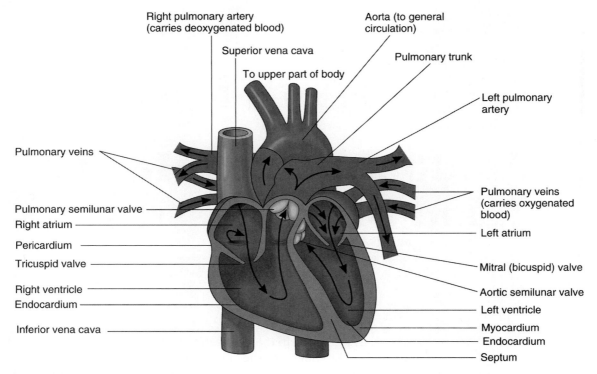

Figure D-1 Pulmonary circulation.

is another name for fat, and contains the coronary blood vessels that supply and drain blood from the heart muscle. The middle layer of the heart wall is the myocardium, which contains cardiac muscle, connective tissue, blood vessels, and nerves. The innermost layer of the heart wall is the endocardium, which consists of endothelium, continuous with the endothelium of the attached blood vessels.

Coronary Arteries and Veins

The heart is too thick to allow for the diffusion of blood from its chambers into the myocardium; therefore, the coronary arteries supply the myocardium with blood, and the coronary veins drain the blood from the myocardium. The left and right coronary arteries are the first branches of the ascending aorta, and they deliver nutrient-rich blood to the myocardium. The blood returns from the myocardium through the middle and great cardiac veins, which drain blood from the cardiac capillaries to a vein known as the coronary sinus. The coronary blood vessels are contained in an indentation known as the coronary sulcus that circumscribes the heart (Figure D-2).

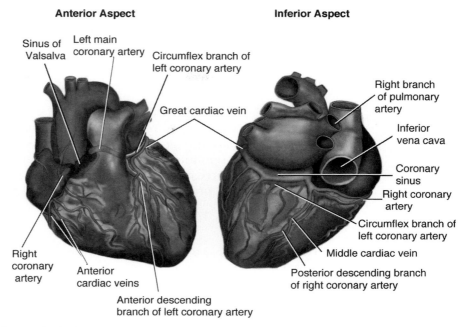

Figure D-2 Coronary arteries and major veins of the heart.

Cardiac Septum

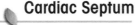

The heart is bilateral and symmetrical in form, and the septum is the wall that divides the left and right sides of the heart. The interatrial septum divides the left atrium from the right atrium. The interventricular septum divides the left ventricle from the right ventricle.

Right Atrium

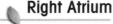

On the interatrial septum of the right atrium is the fossa ovalis, which is a remnant of fetal circulation known as the foramen ovale. In the uterus, the fetus does not need to pump blood through its lungs to receive oxygen because the fetus receives its oxygen supply from the mother through the umbilical cord. The foramen ovale is a hole between the right atrium and the left atrium that allows most of the fetal blood to bypass the right ventricle. The foreamen ovale closes over at birth, due to the increased blood pressure within the left atrium, and becomes the fossa ovalis in the adult heart. The right atrium is the center of drainage during embalming.

Right Ventricle

After leaving the right atrium, the blood enters the right ventricle. The passageway between the right atrium and the right ventricle is the right atrioventricular orifice, which contains the right atrioventricular valve, also known as the tricuspid valve. The right atrioventricular valve prevents the backflow of blood into the right atrium.

For the blood to leave the right ventricle, it must go through the pulmonary trunk orifice, which leads to the pulmonary arteries. To prevent the blood from flowing back into the right ventricle after it enters the pulmonary trunk artery, the pulmonary semilunar valve closes. The pulmonary semilunar valve gets its name from its three crescent-shaped cusps, and it opens and closes according to the changes in pressure exerted by the flow of blood.

Left Atrium

The blood returns to the left atrium from the four pulmonary veins. The holes through which the blood passes are the pulmonary venous orifices. The blood then passes into the left ventricle, which is the largest and the strongest chamber of the heart.

Left Ventricle

The left ventricle allows blood to enter from the left atrium through the left atrioventricular orifice. The left atrioventricular valve prevents the backflow of blood into the left atrium. It is also known by the names mitral valve and bicuspid valve. The left atrioventricular valve differs from the right atrioventricular valve in that the left atrioventricular valve has two cusps instead of three. The blood leaves the left ventricle through the aortic orifice and enters the ascending aorta. The aortic semilunar valve prevents the blood from reentering the left ventricle.

Physiology of the Atrioventricular Valves

The atrioventricular valves prevent the backflow of blood into the atria from the ventricles, as illustrated in Figure D-3. The valves are stabilized by the presence of the chordae tendineae and the papillary muscles. Each of the cusps of the atrioventricular valves attaches to small papillary muscles through "strings" called chordae tendineae. The atrioventricular valves open into the ventricles when the positive pressure of the blood is exerted during atrial contraction. The valves close when the ventricles begin to contract, preventing the backflow of blood into the atria. To prevent the valves from opening backwards into the atria, the papillary muscles contract, holding the valves in place by putting tension on the chordae tendineae.

Blood Pressure

Contraction of the myocardium is referred to as *systole*. *Diastole* refers to the dilation and lengthening of the cardiac wall of the heart after beating, which is

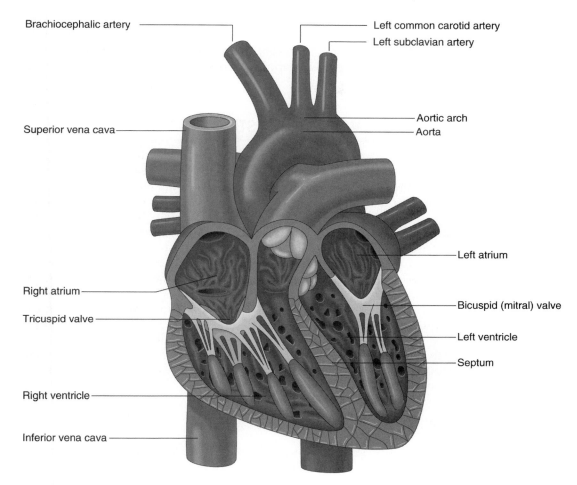

Brachiocephalic artery

Left common carotid artery

Left subclavian artery

Aortic arch

Aorta

Superior vena cava

Left atrium

Right atrium

Bicuspid (mitral) valve

Tricuspid valve

Left ventricle

Septum

Right ventricle

Inferior vena cava

Figure D-3 Blood flow into, around, and out of the heart.

relaxation of the myocardium. Blood pressure is a numeric representation between the systolic pressure, which is the first number, and the diastolic pressure, which is the second number. A typical blood pressure of 120 over 80 indicates that the heart muscle is exerting 120 millimeters of mercury of pressure during contraction and exerting 80 millimeters of mercury of pressure during its relaxing period.

Nervous Stimulation

For the heart to beat in its prescribed order, its beating is synchronized by nervous stimulation. The characteristic "lub-dub" sound of the heart is created by the contraction of the atria and the subsequent contraction of the ventricles. The nervous impulse is sent across the heart beginning at the superior right atrium at a point known as the sinoatrial node, which sends the nervous impulse across the atria causing the heart to make the "lub" sound. The "dub" sound results from the contraction of the ventricles, which occurs when the atrioventricular node conducts a nervous impulse across them. The typical resting heart beat is about 72 beats per minute.

THE BLOOD VASCULAR SYSTEM

The blood vascular system is a closed system, and the study of the blood vessels is known as *angiology*. There are no openings in the circulatory system through which the blood is lost. Instead, the blood circulates over and over again, being replaced only when there is a break in the system or when the cells die.

From the heart, the blood enters the aorta, which directs the blood to the arterial system, depicted in Figure D-4. The larger arteries move the blood along to smaller arterioles, which transport the blood to the tissues through capillary beds. Internal respiration, which is the exchange of oxygen for carbon dioxide, takes place between the connective tissues of the cells and the endothelium of the capillaries.

The deoxygenated blood drains from the capillary beds into the small venules of the body, which lead to the larger veins. The venous blood vascular system is illustrated in Figure D-5. The veins all lead back to the venae cavae, which drain into the right atrium of the heart. After pulmonary circulation through the lungs, the blood enters the left ventricle of the heart. The blood repeats this journey about every 30 seconds.

Arteries and Veins

Both the arteries and the veins contain three layers in their walls: the tunica interna, the tunica media, and the tunica externa. The tunica interna, which is also known as the tunica intima, is the innermost layer of arteries and veins, containing an endothelial lining and elastic connective tissue fibers. The arteries contain a thick layer of elastic fiber that veins do not contain, known as the internal elastic membrane.

The tunica media contains concentric layers of smooth muscle within a structural framework of connective tissue. The connective tissue anchors the layers of the blood vessels together. An external elastic membrane lies between the tunica media and the tunica externa. Vasoconstriction is a process whereby the smooth muscle of the tunica media constricts, narrowing the diameter of the blood vessel's lumen, which is the opening through which the blood flows. The diameter of the lumen increases as a result of vasodilation, which is the relaxation of the muscles of the tunica media.

The outermost layer of blood vessels is the tunica externa, or tunica adventitia, which forms a connective tissue sheath around the vessels. The connective tissue of the tunica externa combines with the surrounding structures and anchors the blood vessel in place.

The study of veins is known as *phlebology*. About two-thirds of the body's blood can be found in the veins at any given moment. Superficial veins are more

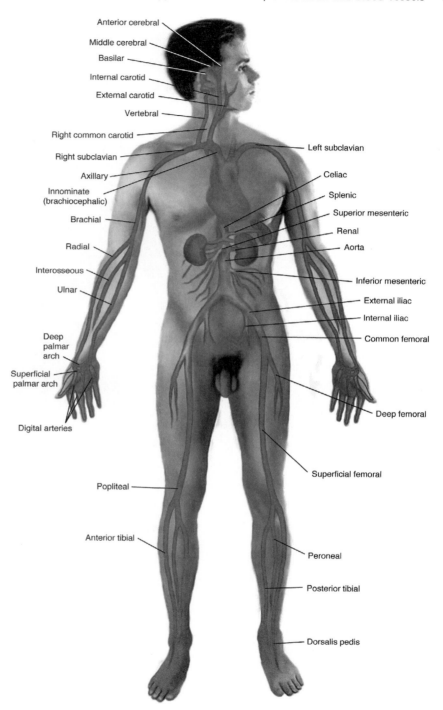

Anterior cerebral
Middle cerebral
Basilar
Internal carotid
External carotid
Vertebral
Right common carotid
Right subclavian
Axillary
Innominate
(brachiocephalic)
Brachial
Radial
Interosseous
Ulnar
Deep
palmar
arch
Superficial
palmar arch
Digital arteries
Popliteal
Anterior tibial

Left subclavian
Celiac
Splenic
Superior mesenteric
Renal
Aorta
Inferior mesenteric
External iliac
Internal iliac
Common femoral
Deep femoral
Superficial femoral
Peroneal
Posterior tibial
Dorsalis pedis

Figure D-4 Major arteries of the body.

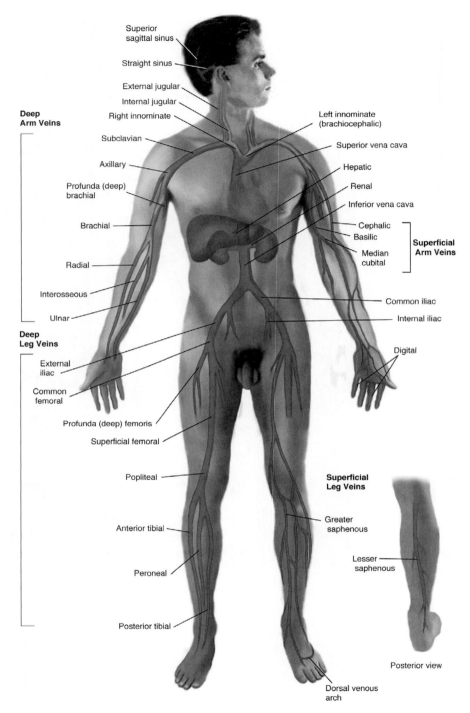

Figure D-5 Major veins of the body.

abundant in the extremities, where they gather blood from the venules. Veins contain paired semilunar bicuspid valves that prevent the backflow of blood into the venules. The valves are most predominant in the legs, where gravity pulls the blood away from the heart. Skeletal muscle surrounding the veins aids in the movement of blood toward the heart.

Bibliography

Saladin, K. (1998). *Anatomy & Physiology: The unity of form and function*. New York: McGraw-Hill.

Scott, A., Fong, E., & Beebe, R. (2002). *Functional anatomy for emergency medical services*. Clifton Park, NY: Thomson Delmar Learning.

Van Wynseberghe, D., Noback, C., & Carola, R. (1995). *Human anatomy & physiology* (3rd ed.). New York: McGraw-Hill.

APPENDIX E

Anatomy of the Digestive System

THE DIGESTIVE SYSTEM

The embalmer should be familiar with the digestive system in order to appreciate the body's internal anatomy, which is illustrated in Figure E-1. In order to properly aspirate the abdominal cavity, embalmers have established topographical landmarks as trocar guides. Also, the biochemical properties of digestion are closely related to the process of decomposition of the dead human remains. Both processes are influenced by the ability of water to break down chemical substances in a process known as hydrolysis.

HISTOLOGY OF THE DIGESTIVE TRACT

The layers of the alimentary canal are the mucosa, the submucosa, the muscularis, and the serosa. The mucosa lines the digestive tract and the serosa covers the wall of the digestive tract. The mucosa is a lubricating, secreting, and absorbing layer of epithelial tissue that protects the lining of the digestive tract from the passing food by reducing friction. The mucosa is also functional in immunity against invading microorganisms. In the stomach, the mucosa's surface area is increased by the presence of folds known as rugae.

The submucosa contains blood vessels and nerves. Certain areas of the submucosa also contain lymphoid nodules. The submucosa contains secretory glands in the esophagus and in the duodenum of the small intestine.

The muscularis moves food along the lumen of the digestive tract via a wave of smooth muscle contractions known as peristalsis. Most regions of the digestive tract contain an inner circular layer of smooth

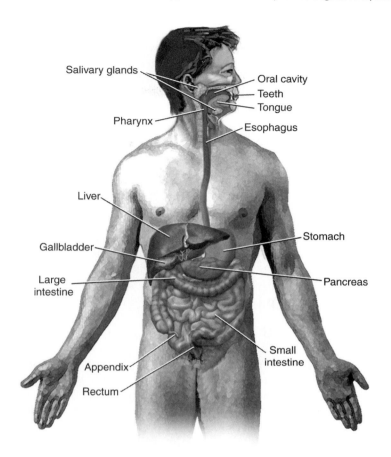

Figure E-1 Digestive system.

muscle, and an outer longitudinal layer of smooth muscle. The stomach contains a third layer of oblique muscle that runs diagonally over the stomach.

The mesentery is a layer of connective tissue serosa that attaches the viscera to the abdominal wall. The serosa can contain blood vessels, nerves, and lymphatics. It may also consist of epithelium that covers the digestive tube and digestive organs. In areas devoid of epithelium, such as the esophagus, the serosa is known as the adventitia. There is a portion of serosa, known as the visceral peritoneum, that covers the organs.

There are two specialized types of mesentery covering the organs of the digestive system. The greater omentum is a folded membrane extending from the greater curvature of the stomach to the dorsal abdominal wall continuing into the pelvic region. The lesser omentum extends from the liver to the lesser curvature of the stomach. The greater omentum contains plasma cells, eosinophils, macrophages, and monocytes. It protects the peritoneum from microbial infections.

Digestive Tract

The digestive system comprises the alimentary canal and the accessory organs of digestion. The alimentary canal consists of the mouth, pharynx, esophagus, stomach, small intestine, large intestine, rectum, and anus. The part of the alimentary canal inferior to the diaphragm is known as the gastrointestinal (GI) tract.

Mouth

The mouth is lined with stratified squamous epithelium. The roof of the mouth is formed by the hard and soft palates. The hard palate is formed by the palatine process of the maxillary bone and the palate bones. The soft palate is located posterior to the hard palate. The dangling tissue supported by the soft palate is the uvula. The uvula helps prevent materials from entering the pharynx prematurely. Food that is ready to be swallowed is called a bolus, and the act of swallowing is known as deglutition.

Pharynx

After the food is broken down through the physical action of the teeth and the chemical action of the saliva, it enters the pharynx. The pharynx is divided into three regions: the nasopharynx, the oropharynx, and the laryngopharynx. The nasopharynx is superior to the soft palate. The oropharynx is located between the soft palate and the epiglottis. The laryngopharynx is posterior to the epiglottis adjoining the esophagus. The nasopharynx conveys only air and is lined with pseudostratified ciliated epithelium. The oropharynx and the laryngopharynx require lubrication for the passage of swallowed food and are lined with stratified squamous epithelium.

Esophagus

The lining of the esophagus secretes lubricating mucus that reduces friction between the bolus and the lining of the esophagus during peristalsis. Each end of the relaxed esophagus is closed by a sphincter muscle. The upper sphincter is known as the superior esophageal sphincter, and the inferior is known as the lower esophageal sphincter or, alternatively, as the cardiac sphincter. If the esophageal sphincter does not remain closed and allows hydrochloric acid to enter the esophagus from the stomach, the resultant disorder is referred to as heartburn.

Stomach

The swallowed bolus of food enters the stomach, which is also known as the gaster, from the esophagus. Figure E-2 depicts the stomach as a sac, shaped like a boxing glove, with the palm facing up. The greater curvature of the stomach is on the inferior side of the stomach, and the lesser curvature is on the superior

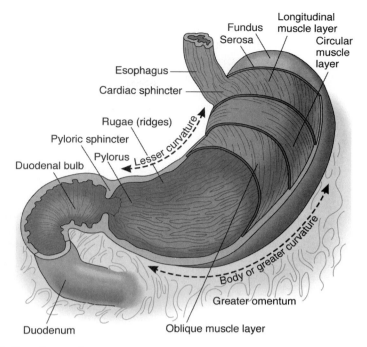

Figure E-2 The stomach.

side of the stomach. The stomach is protected by the left rib cage and is just inferior to the diaphragm. The cardiac orifice of the esophagus opens to allow food to enter the stomach. Food exits the stomach through the pyloric orifice at its opposite end. The four regions of the stomach are the cardiac region, the fundus, the body, and the pyloric region.

The muscularis layer of the stomach contains three directions of smooth muscle fibers: longitudinal, circular, and oblique. The outermost, longitudinal layer is most prominent along the lesser and greater curvatures. The middle, circular layer wraps around the body of the stomach and thickens to become the pyloric sphincter. The innermost, oblique layer covers the fundus and parallels the curvatures of the stomach.

The empty stomach contains a mucous membrane containing many folds known as rugae. As the simple columnar epithelium expands with food, the rugae flatten. The stomach churns, secreting gastric juices that mix with the ingested food, creating a liquid mixture called chyme. The stomach also secretes hydrochloric acid, providing a suitable pH level for digestive enzymes such as gastric lipase, pepsinogen, and intrinsic factor.

Small Intestine

When the chyme leaves the stomach, it enters the small intestine. The small intestine is divided into three segments: the duodenum, the jejunum, and the ileum. The primary function of the small intestine is to further digest the chyme and to begin the absorption of nutrients. Up to 99 percent of the absorption of nutrients occurs in the small intestine, while the remainder occurs in the large intestine.

The mucosa of the small intestine is specialized for absorption and contains pilicae circulares, villi, and glands that secrete intestinal juices. Pilicae circulares are small folds that increase the surface area of the intestinal mucosa allowing for increased absorption of nutrients. Unlike the rugae of the stomach, the pilicae circulares are not removed by enlargement of the small intestine. The villi of the small intestine aid in the absorption of nutrients, and they help move the chyme along the digestive tract. Villi are fingerlike projections that contain blood capillaries and lacteals that aid in the absorption of fats. Chyle is a milk-like, alkaline secretion of the lacteals and lymphatic vessels of the intestine that helps digest fats and protect the body from disease-causing microorganisms.

The duodenum is the first, and shortest, section of the small intestine. The chyme is mixed with pancreatic and liver secretions in the duodenum. The jejunum and the ileum are suspended from the dorsal abdominal wall by the mesentery. The majority of absorption of nutrients takes place in the jejunum and the ileum. The jejunum is located between the duodenum and the ileum. The ileum joins the cecum of the large intestine at the ileocecal juncture, where the ileocecal valve prevents the chyme from flowing backwards into the small intestine from the large intestine.

Large Intestine

The large intestine reabsorbs water and compacts the chyme into feces. The large intestine also absorbs vitamins released by the action of beneficial bacteria that aid in digestion. The large intestine is divided into the cecum, the colon, and the rectum.

The large intestine is covered with three layers of longitudinal smooth muscle known as the taeniae coli. Fat-filled pouches, called epiploic appendages, appear at the juncture of the taeniae coli and the visceral peritoneum. The taenia coli are not as long as the large intestine so small saculations, known as haustra, occur on the surface of the large intestine. These pouches allow the large intestine to distend and elongate.

Cecum.   The ileum of the small intestine joins with the large intestine at the cecum, which is shaped like a sac with a tail known as the appendix. The appendix contains an abundance of lymphoid tissue that aids in the immune response.

It is important during aspiration of the deceased that the cecum be thoroughly aspirated by the embalmer because it often contains a high concentration of microorganisms. Translocation of microbes during the postmortem interval accelerates decomposition of the deceased.

Colon.   The colon is divided into four sections: the ascending colon, the transverse colon, the descending colon, and the sigmoid colon. The ascending colon extends from the cecum superiorly to the liver, where it makes a 90-degree bend called the hepatic flexure. The transverse colon begins at the hepatic flexure and crosses over the abdomen until it reaches the spleen, where it makes a downward 90-degree bend called the left splenic flexure. The descending colon continues from the splenic flexure to the rim of the pelvis, where the colon makes an S-shaped turn and becomes the sigmoid colon. The sigmoid colon follows across the pelvis to the middle of the sacrum, where it joins with the rectum.

Rectum and Anus

The rectum curves along the sacrum and coccyx. At the end of these vertebra, the rectum continues as the anal canal, which makes a sharp inferior and posterior turn. The anal canal opens at the anus, which contains the internal anal sphincter and the external anal sphincter. The internal anal sphincter is an involuntary muscle that remains closed, while the external anal sphincter muscle is under voluntary control.

The loss of muscle tension after death may cause relaxation of the external and internal anal sphincters, resulting in fecal purge from the anus. Packing the anus with cotton soaked in cavity fluid is a standard practice for many embalmers. Care must be taken not to leave any cotton protruding from the anus, as it may act as a wick, drawing fluids from the anus out of the body.

The rectum has no mesentery, no epiploic appendages, no haustra, and no taeniae coli. The complex of venous blood vessels in the rectum is known as the hemorrhoidal plexus. These veins may become enlarged, twisted, and blood-filled. This inflammatory condition is known as hemorrhoids.

ACCESSORY ORGANS OF DIGESTION

The accessory organs of the digestive system produce secretions that aid in the chemical breakdown of the food. These organs include the teeth, tongue, salivary glands, liver, gallbladder, and pancreas.

Teeth

The teeth tear food into smaller, more manageable pieces. The process of chewing is termed mastication. There are 32 teeth in the adult mouth. The most anterior teeth are the incisors, which cut and tear the food. The canine teeth are located on the lateral portion of the mouth, and the bicuspids are located behind the canines. The three teeth behind to the bicuspids are the molars. The most posterior molars are commonly known as the wisdom teeth.

Often, people do not receive proper dental care, resulting in loose, cracked, broken, or missing teeth. It is important for the embalmer to avoid reaching inside the mouth, in favor of the use of embalming instruments whenever possible. Even healthy teeth are sharp, but broken teeth are even more likely to result in injury to the embalmer's fingers. It is also important when using a needle injector to close the mouth, that the embalmer avoid injecting the needle too close to the base of any teeth. It is possible for the force of the needle injector to dislodge loose or fragile teeth.

Salivary Glands

As the teeth macerate the food, tearing it into small, digestible pieces, the salivary glands secrete saliva, beginning the chemical digestion of the food particles. Saliva is a watery substance that contains amylase, which is an enzyme that begins the digestion of complex carbohydrates. There are three salivary glands: the sublingual salivary glands, the parotid salivary glands, and the submandibular salivary glands. They are located under the tongue, near the ear, and along the inner surface of the mandible, respectively.

Tongue

The tongue is comprised primarily of muscle and connective tissue, and is covered in mucosa. The underside of the tongue is smooth and is not involved in tasting food. The superior surface of the tongue has a valvety texture due to the presence of papillae. The tongue is attached to the floor of the mouth by a band of tissue known as the lingual frenum. At the base of the lingual frenum are Warton's ducts, which release saliva from the submaxillary salivary glands. The sublingual salivary glands empty through a series of ducts in the tissues surrounding Warton's ducts. The muscular movement of the tongue aids in chewing and swallowing.

Liver

The liver, which is also known as the hepar, is located just below the diaphragm, and it is the largest of the digestive organs. The liver has a doorway, known as the porta hepatis, through which blood vessels, lymphatic vessels, nerves, and ducts gain passage. The hepatic artery, a branch of the celiac artery, supplies the liver with oxygenated blood, while the hepatic portal vein drains the entire nutrient-rich venous blood supply from the gastrointestinal tract toward the liver. The hepatic veins transport the liver's venous blood to the inferior vena cava.

The liver produces bile, which drains into the right and left hepatic ducts (Figure E-3). The hepatic ducts join with the gallbladder's cystic duct to form the common bile duct, which joins the main pancreatic duct becoming the hepatopancreatic duct. The hepatopancreatic duct becomes the hepatopancreatic ampulla, which travels through the wall of the intestinal duodenum. In the duodenum of the small intestine, the ampulla becomes the duodenal papilla or papilla of Vater, which is commonly, but inaccurately, referred to as the ampulla of Vater. This system of ducts allows both bile and pancreatic juices to enter the duodenum of the small intestine.

Physiology of the Liver. The liver has over 200 known functions, which can be classified into four groups: metabolic functions, hematological functions, storage functions, and bile-related functions. The functional unit of the liver is the lobule, which contains a central vein. The blood is filtered by Kupffer cells neighboring the central veins. Kupffer cells destroy worn-out red blood cells, white

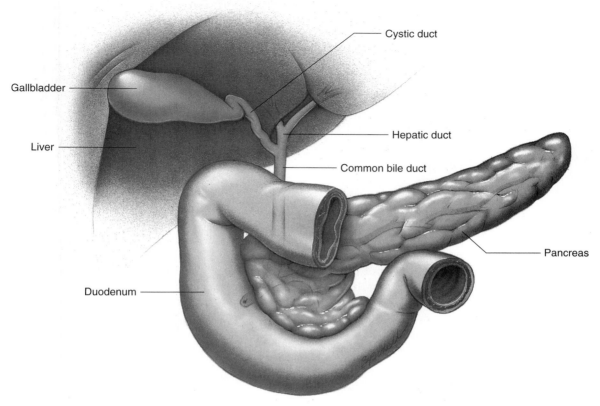

Figure E-3 The liver, gallbladder, and pancreas.

blood cells, microorganisms, and toxins. The liver then recycles materials of value and eliminates waste products.

The liver regulates the amount of blood sugar, which is glucose. Glycogenesis occurs when the blood glucose level is too high, and the liver stores glucose in the form of glycogen. Glycogenolysis is the conversion of glycogen back to glucose, when the blood glucose level is too low. The liver also utilizes fats to synthesize lipoproteins, cholesterol, and phospholipids. Both the breakdown of fatty acids into acetyl coenzyme A and the formation of ketone bodies are also accomplished in the liver.

The liver is the largest blood reservoir in the body. The liver's hematological functions include removal of old or damaged red blood cells, removal of pathogens from circulation, and synthesis of plasma proteins, which transport nutrients and establish blood clotting systems in the blood. The liver also synthesizes albumins, which maintain the blood's osmotic pressure and blood volume.

The liver secretes bile salts into the duodenum, aiding in the digestion of fats. These bile salts are reabsorbed in the ileum and are returned to the liver, where they are resecreted into the duodenum. Bile receives its greenish-black pigmentation from the hemoglobin of ruptured red blood cells. Feces receives its color from a product of the breakdown of bile pigments. The presence of the bile pigment bilirubin in extracellular fluids causes jaundice.

Many diseases and pathological conditions have a negative effect on liver function. The liver is easily affected because it is a detoxifying center in the body. Jaundice, dehydration, edema, and blood clots may all be signs of liver damage. Part Two of this book includes a description of hepatitis, which is a viral infection of the liver that can cause serious illness and death if contracted by the embalmer.

Gallbladder

The gallbladder, which is also known as the cholecyst, is a pear-shaped organ located on the visceral wall of the liver. Bile is produced in the liver and stored in the gallbladder by the following process. At the duodenum, the common bile duct is surrounded by the sphincter of the common bile duct. The hepatopancreatic ampulla is surrounded by the sphincter of Oddi. If cholecystokinin, a hormone, is not released from the small intestine, the sphincters will remain closed, causing the bile to fill the common bile duct and enter the gallbladder. The release of cholecystokinin from the small intestine's wall is regulated by the presence of high amounts of lipids and partially digested proteins in the chyme. When appropriate, the gallbladder contracts, forcing the bile into this system of ducts that lead to the duodenum.

Pancreas

The pancreas is located behind the stomach. When the chyme is emptied from the stomach into the duodenum, it is mixed with secretions from the liver and the pancreas. The pancreas is behind the peritoneum and is connected to the posterior abdominal wall.

The glandular tissues of the pancreas are divided into two categories: endocrine and exocrine. The most significant endocrine secretion of the pancreas is insulin, which is integral to the metabolism of sugar in the body. Insulin is produced in the islets of Langerhans within the pancreas. The pancreas also secretes pancreatic juice consisting of water, ions, digestive enzymes, and buffers, which are salts. The water helps break down the chyme through the process of hydrolysis, and buffers regulate the acid pH of the chyme as it leaves the stomach.

Bibliography

Saladin, K. (1998). *Anatomy & physiology: The unity of form and function*. New York: McGraw-Hill.

Scott, A., Fong, E., & Beebe, R. (2002). *Functional anatomy for emergency medical services*. Clifton Park, NY: Thomson Delmar Learning.

Van Wynseberghe, D., Noback, C., & Carola, R. (1995). *Human anatomy & physiology* (3rd ed.). New York: McGraw-Hill.

APPENDIX F

Anatomy of the Respiratory System

THE RESPIRATORY SYSTEM

The human body cannot survive without oxygen. People have been known to survive without food and water for relatively long periods of time, but humans cannot survive for more than about five minutes without breathing.

Figure F-1 depicts the location of the organs of the respiratory system. The mechanical process in which air is inhaled and exhaled is called ventilation. The process of exchanging inspired oxygen for carbon dioxide is known as respiration, and it is classified into external respiration and internal respiration (Figure F-2). External respiration occurs in the lungs as carbon dioxide and oxygen are exchanged between the blood and the tissues of the lungs, while internal respiration takes place between the blood and the body's tissues, when carbon dioxide is exchanged for oxygen.

Trachea

The trachea is located in front of the esophagus, and it is formed of 16 to 20 C-shaped cartilaginous rings that maintain its shape. The rings are connected by fibroelastic cartilage and longitudinal smooth muscle, allowing the trachea to extend and flex. They are open on the posterior side of the trachea, allowing the esophagus to extend slightly as food passes through it. The trachea is lined with mucus-secreting, ciliated epithelial cells that direct mucus, trapped particles of dust, and microorganisms to the pharynx to be swallowed or spit out (expectorated).

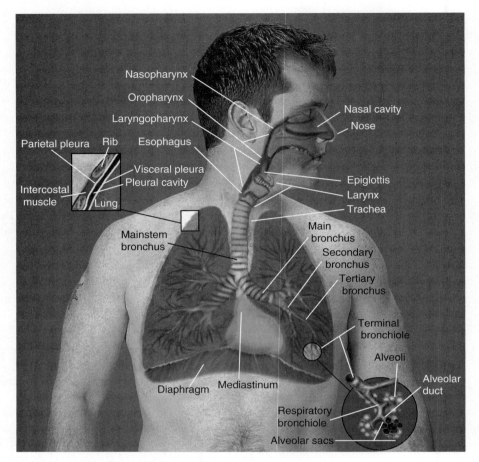

Figure F-1 The respiratory system.

 ## Bronchi and Bronchioles

The trachea divides into the left and right bronchi. The right bronchus is more vertical and larger than the left. The left bronchus branches into two primary bronchioles within the left lung, while the right bronchus branches into three primary bronchioles in the right lung. The bronchioles continue to branch, forming smaller and smaller bronchioles until they become alveolar ducts leading to microscopic sacs called alveoli.

 ## Alveoli

Each lung is filled with microscopic sacs called alveoli, which provide the lungs with 20 times the surface area of the skin. This large surface area provides space for gaseous exchange with the blood capillaries that surround each alveolus.

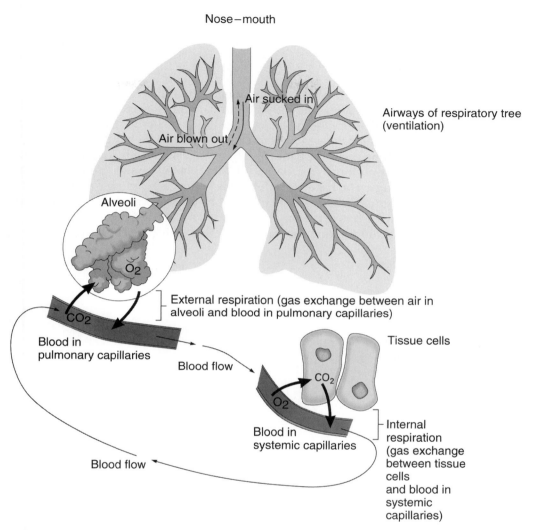

Figure F-2 Respiration.

The capillary lumen has such a small diameter that red blood cells must pass through in single file.

The alveoli are lined with simple squamous epithelium and cuboidal secretory epithelium. The simple squamous layer of epithelium allows gaseous exchange to take place between the alveoli and the capillary beds, while the cuboidal secretory epithelium lubricates the alveoli with a surface active agent. Lung surfactant is a phospholipid-based substance that reduces the surface tension of the alveoli, preventing them from collapsing. The more than 300 million alveolar sacs must maintain their viability because the red blood cell is in a position to exchange nutrients and waste for less than a second within the alveolus.

Dehydration of lung surfactant causes injury that inhibits the effective exchange of gases in the lungs.

 ## Lungs

The left lung is narrower and longer than the right. The left lung also contains only two lobes, while the right lung contains three lobes. The left lung has one fewer lobe because the heart is positioned where the third lobe would otherwise be. The left lung contains a cardiac notch at the point that the heart is located. Each lung contains a hilus on its medial surface through which the bronchiole tubes, pulmonary blood vessels, lymphatic vessels, and nerves enter and exit the lungs. The base of each lung is concave, forming to the curvature of the diaphragm. Each lung is surrounded by the visceral pleura and the parietal pleura. The two layers of pleura are separated by a fluid-filled pleural space. The visceral pleura slides along the parietal pleura with every breath.

Bibliography

Saladin, K. (1998). *Anatomy & physiology: The unity of form and function*. New York: McGraw-Hill.

Scott, A., Fong, E., & Beebe, R. (2002). *Functional anatomy for emergency medical services*. Clifton Park, NY: Thomson Delmar Learning.

Van Wynseberghe, D., Noback, C., & Carola, R. (1995). *Human anatomy & physiology* (3rd ed.). New York: McGraw-Hill.

APPENDIX G

Anatomy of the Urinary System

THE URINARY SYSTEM

The urinary system functions in the removal of naturally occurring toxins from the body. It is also integral in the maintenance of water balance in the body's tissues. The regulation of water affects total blood volume, which, in turn, regulates blood pressure. The urinary system also helps eliminate self-induced poisons from the body, such as narcotics and alcohol. In addition, the urinary system has a crucial role in the homeostatic maintenance of acid-base levels in the tissues. The urinary system includes the kidneys, the ureters, the urinary bladder, and the urethra, which are illustrated in Figure G-1. The study of the urinary system is known as *urology*.

Kidneys

There are two bean-shaped kidneys in the body, which are also known as the renal glands (Figure G-2). They are located just above the waistline, on either side of the vertebral column, approximately between vertebrae T12 and L3. The right kidney is situated slightly inferior to the left kidney due to the presence of the liver. The kidneys are behind the stomach, spleen, and pancreas.

Blood is supplied to the kidney via the renal artery. The renal artery is a branch of the abdominal aorta. The blood drains from the kidney through the renal vein, which returns the blood to the inferior vena cava. These blood vessels are accompanied by lymphatic vessels. Approximately one-fourth of the blood pumped by the heart each minute passes through the kidneys for filtration. Only about 1/1000th of the blood is converted into urine.

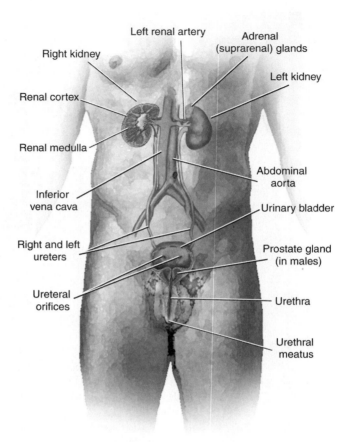

Figure G-1 Structures of the urinary system.

The kidneys are protected by the rib cage, and each is covered by the renal capsule, the perirenal fat, and the renal fascia. The kidneys can be divided into three major areas: the renal pelvis, the renal medulla, and the renal cortex. The renal pelvis contains the major and minor calyces, which form a cavity within the central portion of the kidney for the collection of urine prior to entering the ureters. The renal medulla, which is located between the renal pelvis and the renal cortex, contains the pyramids and the renal columns. The pyramids and columns contain the nephrons that actually filter the blood to form urine. The renal cortex surrounds the medulla and contains blood and lymphatic vessels.

Nephron. The nephron, or renal tubule, is the functional unit of the kidneys. Each kidney contains approximately 1 million nephrons lined with epithelial tissue. Each nephron begins as a renal corpuscle, composed of a double-walled, cuplike structure called the glomerular capsule (Figure G-3).

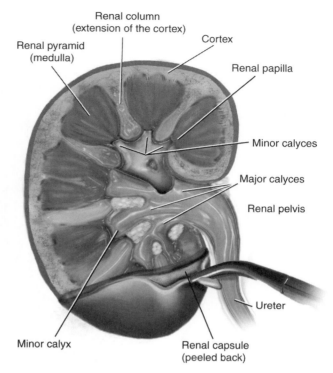

Renal column
(extension of the cortex)

Cortex

Renal pyramid
(medulla)

Renal papilla

Minor calyces

Major calyces

Renal pelvis

Ureter

Minor calyx

Renal capsule
(peeled back)

Figure G-2 Structures of the kidney.

The glomerular capsule surrounds a knot of blood vessels known as the glomerulus. The proximal convoluted tubule extends from the glomerular capsule to the medulla. Within the medulla, an elongation and straightening of the tubule occurs known as the loop of the nephron, which is also referred to as the loop of Henle. The loop of the nephron then returns toward the cortex as the distal convoluted tubule, which is near the proximal convoluted tubule. The tubule then joins with the collecting tubules which descend through the medulla terminating at the renal papillae, thereby conducting formed urine to the renal pelvis.

Filtration and the Production of Urine. Figure G-4 illustrates how the kidneys filter the blood and produce urine. Blood enters the kidney for filtration through the renal artery, which branches into ever smaller arteries. After passing through the glomerulus, the blood is recollected by efferent arterioles. These arterioles have a smaller diameter than the previous blood vessels, resulting in an increased blood pressure within the capillaries of the glomerulus. The high pressure of the blood in the capillaries results in the plasma portion of the blood being forced into the glomerulus through a process known as pressure filtration.

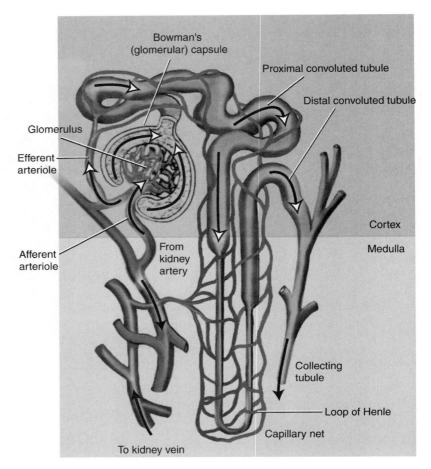

Figure G-3 Structures of the nephrons.

The plasma, filtered out in the glomerulus, is known as glomerular filtrate, and it contains water, electrolytes, sugars, urea, amino acids, polypeptids, and a variety of other dissolved solutes. The glomerular filtrate enters the proximal convoluted tubule from the glomerular capsule. The proximal convoluted tubule is a twisted, coiled tube that contains cuboidal epithelial cells in its lumen. The cells of the lumen contain microvilli that reabsorb water, electrolytes, glucose, and some amino acids and small polypeptides from the glomerular filtrate. The glomerular filtrate, passing through the loop of the nephron, becomes more or less concentrated as influenced by the presence of antidiuretic hormone, which is released by the anterior pituitary gland to regulate the production of urine.

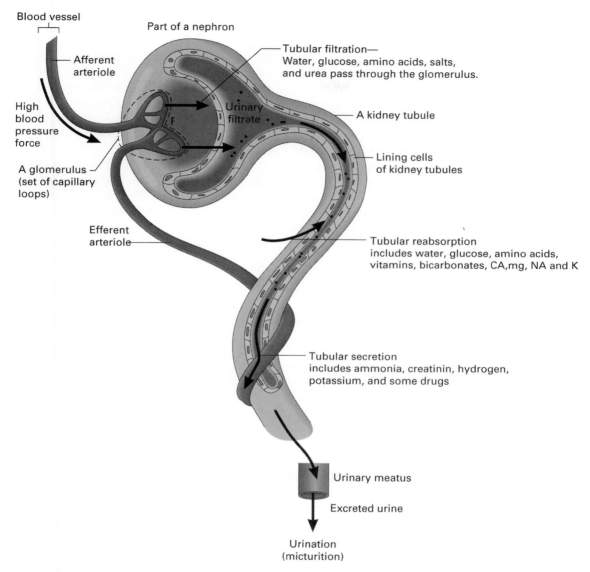

Figure G-4 Processes and structures of the nephron.

Once formed, the urine passes through the collecting duct within the medulla, which opens into a minor calyx. The urine travels from the minor calyx into one of the major calyces, which empty into the renal pelvis. The ureter joins the renal pelvis and transports the urine to the urinary bladder. The urine can then be eliminated from the body through the urethra.

Ureters

The urine moves from the renal pelvis into the ureters, which transport the urine from the kidneys to the base of the urinary bladder. Urine is unable to reenter the ureter from the bladder because the ureters extend obliquely into the bladder wall at their distal end. As the bladder fills with urine, the ureters are compressed. The ureter contains three layers of tissue: the tunica mucosa, the tunica muscularis, and the tunica adventitia.

The innermost layer of the ureter is the tunica mucosa, which consists of transitional epithelium that is able to stretch and change shape. The middle layer is the tunica muscularis, which consists of two layers of smooth muscle tissue that extend longitudinally and circularly. The inferior portion of the ureter contains an additional layer of longitudinal muscle. The tunica adventitia covers the ureters and helps them maintain their position within the abdominopelvic cavity.

Urinary Bladder

After traveling the distance of the ureters, the urine enters the urinary bladder, which is a muscular sac that contains epithelial tissue. The layers of the bladder are the tunica mucosa, the tunica muscularis, and the tunica serosa. The tunica mucosa consists of transitional epithelium that forms folds when the bladder is empty. The tunica muscularis surrounds the bladder with three directions of smooth muscle fibers. The tunica serosa covers the exterior surface of the urinary bladder, secreting lubricants that reduce the friction between the bladder and its adjacent organs as the bladder fills. The process of emptying the bladder is known as micturation, urination, or voiding the bladder.

Urethra

The urine is eliminated from the body through the urethra. In the male, the urethra is part of the reproductive system. The urethra functions not only to remove urine from the body but also to transport ejaculate. During sex, seminal fluid enters the urethra to neutralize any remaining urine. The bulbolurethral gland encompasses the urethra and prevents urine from entering the penis during intercourse. The female urethra is located between the clitoris and the vaginal vestibule. The urethra is about one and a half inches long in the female and about eight inches long in the male. The urethra is lined with mucus-secreting cells along its entire length.

Bibliography

Saladin, K. (1998). *Anatomy & physiology: The unity of form and function*. New York: McGraw-Hill.

Scott, A., Fong, E., & Beebe, R. (2002). *Functional anatomy for emergency medical services*. Clifton Park, NY: Thomson Delmar Learning.

Van Wynseberghe, D., Noback, C., & Carola, R. (1995). *Human anatomy & physiology* (3rd ed.). New York: McGraw-Hill.

APPENDIX H

Anatomy of the Nervous System

THE NERVOUS SYSTEM

The nervous system is divided into the central nervous system (CNS) and the peripheral nervous system (PNS). The CNS consists of the brain and spinal cord, which receive, evaluate, monitor, and transmit nervous impulses that coordinate the multitude of functions of the body. The PNS is subdivided into the sensory, or afferent, nervous system and the motor, or efferent, nervous system. The peripheral nervous system consists of the cranial nerves and the spinal nerves, which transmit nervous impulses to and from the brain and spinal cord.

Neurons

The functional unit of nervous tissue is the neuron, which is a single cell within nervous tissue. Nerves are bundles of neurons, which contain three parts: the soma, the axon, and the dendrites, as illustrated in Figure H-1. Nervous system cells that provide neurons structure and hold them together are known as glial cells.

Soma. The size and shape of the soma, which is also referred to as the cell body, varies from neuron to neuron, but all somas contain the nucleus and organelles such as the endoplasmic reticulum, lysosomes, and mitochondria. The soma also contains neurotubules and neurofilaments. Neurotubules are proteins that aid in the transmission of nervous impulses, while the neurofilaments act as a structural framework within the soma. In cases of Alzheimer's disease, many neuron cell bodies in the cerebral cortex contain tangled neurotubules and neurofilaments.

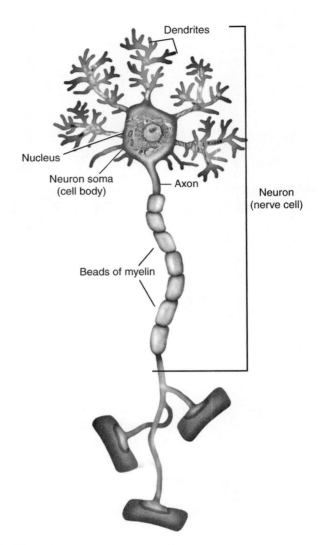

Figure H-1 A neuron.

Dendrites and Axons. The cell body is surrounded by dendrites, which are branchlike structures that help transmit nervous impulses toward the soma. Axons direct nervous impulses toward neighboring cell bodies, glands, or muscle tissue. Neurons contain many dendrites radiating from their cell body, while only one axon is typically present.

Axons come in all manner of sizes. Axons in the cerebrum are less than 1 millimeter in length, while those of the sciatic nerve are long enough to reach from the spinal cord to the foot. Axon branches, which are located at the end of the axon, usually contain small swellings known as end bulbs. These end bulbs are the site of neurotransmitter release, which allows the nervous impulse to cross the synaptic junction chemically. A synapse is the space between neurons.

Myelin. The axon of some neurons is covered in a fatty, phospholipid substance known as myelin, which is often found in a sheath surrounding the axon. The myelin sheath insulates the axon of one neuron from the axon of a neighboring neuron, which inhibits the nervous impulse of one axon from jumping to the axon of an adjacent neuron. Myelin aids in the rapid conduction of nervous impulses, as well as insulating individual axons.

The myelin sheath contains small gaps that allow the nervous impulse to jump from one space to another along the axon. These gaps cause an overall increase in the rate of impulse transmission. Just imagine that a nervous impulse needs to be carried the distance between the foot and the base of the spinal cord. If the impulse traveled the entire distance of the axon, it would take longer than if it could jump from one space to another along the path, skipping parts of the axon. These gaps in the myelin sheath are known as nodes of Ranvier. The cells that surround the myelin, which create the nodes of Ranvier, are called Schwann cells. These Schwann cells only exist in the peripheral nervous system. Myelinated axons in the central nervous system are covered with oligodendrocytes instead of Schwann cells.

Neurotransmitters

A synapse is the space between neurons, as opposed to a neuromuscular junction, which is the space between a neuron and a muscle cell. Neurotransmitters are biochemicals that bind at receptor sites surrounding the soma of neurons, and they are released from the end bulbs of axons. If enough receptor sites are bound with neurotransmitters, a nervous impulse is transmitted to the dendrites of neighboring cells. If conditions are met within the neighboring cell, it transmits a nervous impulse, sending the electrochemical message along its way. This process is repeated until the message has reached its destination. Acetylcholine is a common neurotransmitter.

Meninges

The central nervous system includes the brain and spinal cord, which are both covered with three protective membranes known as meninges (Figure H-2). The outermost meninx is the dura mater, which is formed of two fused layers of thick tissue that line the inside of the skull and the vertebral foramen. The vertebral foramen is the hole in the center of each vertebra that allows the passage of the spinal cord through the bone. The meninges separate in areas of the cranium allowing venous blood to drain from the brain.

The middle meninx, the arachnoid membrane, is located deep in the dura mater. The arachnoid covers both the brain and spinal cord and is similar in structure to a spider's web. The area between the arachnoid and the pia mater is called the subarachnoid space, which is filled with cerebrospinal fluid produced in the ventricles of the brain.

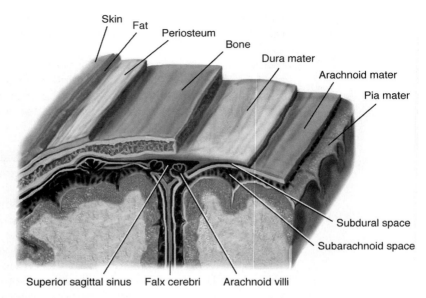

Figure H–2 Cranial meninges.

The deepest meninx is the extremely thin pia mater, which covers the surface of the brain and spinal cord. The pia mater is shiny and transparent and contains most of the blood vessels that supply the brain.

 Brain

The three major divisions of the brain—which is also known as the encephalon—are the cerebrum, the cerebellum, and the brain stem (Figure H-3). These three divisions are associated with cognition, motor control and sensation, and communication between the brain and spinal cord, respectively.

Cerebrum. The cerebrum is covered with an outer layer of gray matter called the cerebral cortex, which is a thin, folded layer of tissue on the surface of the brain. The hills created by the folds are known as gyri, and the valleys are called sulci. These elevations and depressions increase the surface area of gray matter within the cerebrum. The two hemispheres of the cerebrum control opposite sides of the body, and they join together at the corpus callosum, which is a massive bundle of axons.

There are five lobes in the cerebrum, which are illustrated in Figure H-4. The respective functions of the lobes are presented in Figure H-5. The frontal lobe is associated with speech and the ability to determine ethical and moral behavior. The parietal lobe is associated with evaluating the five basic senses. The temporal lobe provides the body with a sense of hearing, balance, and emotion. The occipital lobe is associated with vision. The insula is the only one of the five lobes of the brain that cannot be seen from the exterior surface of the

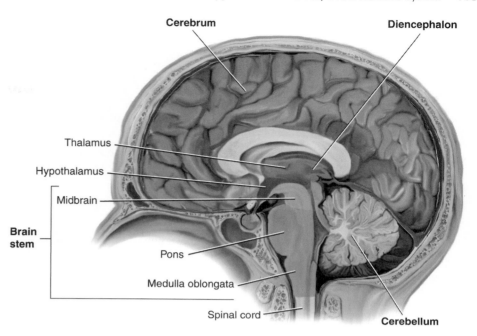

Figure H-3 Cross section of the brain.

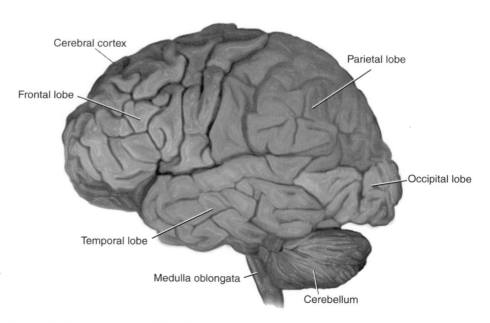

Figure H-4 Lateral view of the brain.

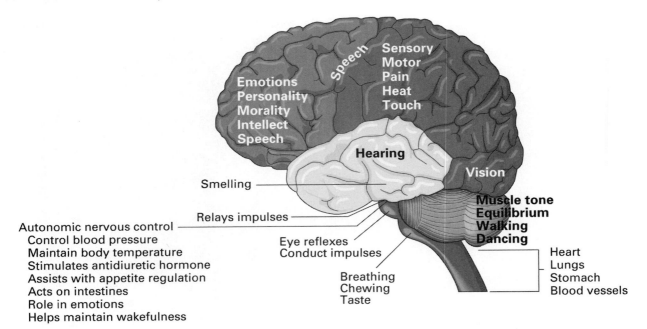

Figure H–5 Cerebral functions.

brain, and its function is assumed to be control of gastrointestinal and visceral activities.

Cerebellum. The cerebellum controls the body's motor functions and sensations, and it is responsible for the coordination of large muscle movement, such as movement of the limbs and torso. The cerebellum itself does not initiate movement; however, it does help control the tension, speed, direction, and tone of the muscles involved in both large and small muscle movement. The cerebellum controls these movements by monitoring the position of the body parts in relation to each other and their surrounding environment. The cerebellum is the second largest part of the brain.

Brain Stem. The brain stem relays messages between the spinal cord and the cerebellum. The base of the brain stem passes through the foramen magnum of the occipital bone to merge with the spinal cord. Ten of the twelve cranial nerves emerge from the brainstem—the olfactory nerve and the optic nerve do not. The brainstem contains the midbrain, the pons, and the medulla oblongata. These three portions of the brainstem allow gross muscle movement and sensory perception.

Medulla Oblongata. The medulla oblongata is the most inferior portion of the brain stem, and it is actually a continuation of the spinal cord. The medulla oblongata registers carbon dioxide levels in the blood, and it regulates the constriction and dilation of the body's blood vessels. Coughing, sneezing, and swallowing are also controlled by the medulla oblongata. In addition, the medulla oblongata is the site at which the nerve pathways cross over between the hemispheres of the brain.

Pons. The pons is superior to the medulla oblongata and helps regulate respiration and the senses of touch, pain, and temperature. The pons contains motor neuron pathways that allow for the movement of muscles, and it contains fibers that allow the two sides of the cerebellum to communicate with each other.

Midbrain. The most superior portion of the brain stem is the midbrain, which controls such functions of the body as movement of the eye, pupil dilation, and relaying of sensations of sound. The midbrain also plays a role in subconscious muscle activity including movement during sleep and twitching.

Thalamus and Hypothalamus. The thalamus and the hypothalamus are located in the diencephalon, which is a region of the cerebrum. The thalamus decodes the five basic senses, and it starts and stops voluntary muscle movement according to the stimuli it decodes (e.g., turning the head towards a sound). The hypothalamus regulates homeostasis in the body.

Homeostasis is the ability of the body to maintain a dynamic equilibrium among its many systems. The hypothalamus determines hunger and satiation. It also senses the body's need for fluids as well as regulating temperature, metabolism, and blood sugar levels. The sleep centers in the brain are located near the hypothalamus, and their proximity to each other and their shared hormone release explains feelings of sleepiness after heavy meals and wakefulness in the presence of cool air and bright light. This area of the brain is related to the experience of sundowning among some persons with Alzheimer's.

Ventricles. The brain contains four ventricles, which are the production centers and pathways through which cerebrospinal fluid (CSF) flows. CSF is found in both the brain and spinal cord, and it functions to cushion the brain and spinal cord as well as filter waste products from the central nervous system. The cerebrospinal fluid drains from the brain into the venous blood drainage found in the layers of the meninges. Figure H-6 illustrates the flow of CSF within the cranium.

Spinal Cord

The spinal cord is the part of the CNS extending from the foramen magnum to about the first lumbar vertebra. At the level of the lumbar vertebra, the roots of the spinal nerves join with the terminal portion of the spinal cord, forming the cauda equina, which is a cluster of nervous tissue resembling a horse's tail. The spinal cord is surrounded by the same three meninges that cover the brain and by cerebrospinal fluid.

There are three myelinated columns of nerve fibers called funiculi in the spinal cord. These columns, which extend the entire length of the spinal cord, are the anterior (ventral) column, the posterior (dorsal) column, and the lateral column. Each funiculus is divided into ascending and descending tracts. The

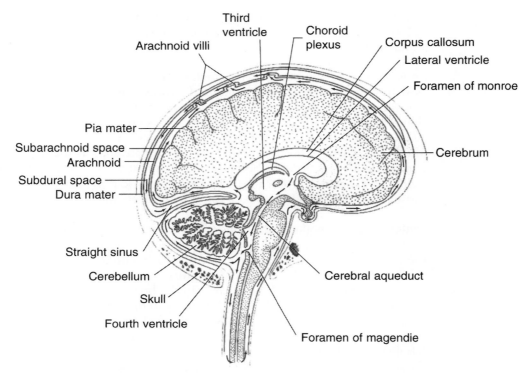

Figure H-6 Circulation of cerebrospinal fluid.

ascending tract is made up of sensory fibers that transmit nervous impulses toward the brain, while the descending tract consists of motor fibers that transmit impulses to the efferent neurons in the peripheral nervous system.

The gray matter of the spinal cord has a characteristic H pattern, and some say its shape resembles that of a butterfly. The gray matter consists of unmyelinated neurons and glial cells. Gray matter is divided into three columns of neurons known as the posterior, anterior, and lateral horns, which extend from the cervical region to the level of the sacrum. The two dorsal horns function in sensory input, while the two ventral horns function in motor output. The lateral horns are only found in the thoracic and upper lumbar levels of the spinal cord, and they contain cell bodies of motor neurons that aid in the regulation of the viscera.

 ## Spinal Nerves

The peripheral nervous system consists of the spinal nerves and the 12 cranial nerves. The spinal nerves are located throughout the body and lead to and from the spinal cord. The cranial nerves are also located throughout the body, however, they are attached directly to the brain stem, with the exception of the olfactory nerve and the optic nerve, which attach to the inferior surface of the brain.

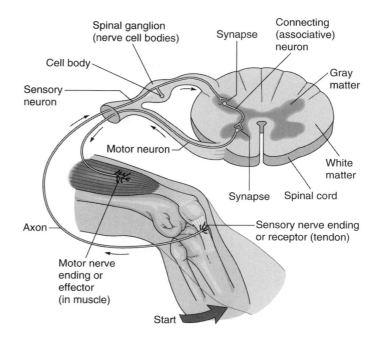

Figure H-7 Structures and functions of the spinal cord.

Spinal nerves, which are part of the PNS, attach to the spinal cord at the dorsal and ventral spinal roots (Figure H-7). The ventral spinal roots emerge from either side of the spinal cord and contain motor nerve fibers. The dorsal spinal roots also emerge from the spinal cord in pairs and contain sensory nerve fibers. The ventral spinal roots contain the axons of motor neurons whose cell bodies are in the gray matter of the spinal cord. In contrast, the cell bodies of sensory neurons, whose axons make up the dorsal roots, are found in the PNS, outside of the spinal cord in the dorsal root ganglia. Sensations are received in the posterior aspect of the spinal cord, while nervous impulses that move muscle originate from the anterior aspect of the spinal cord.

Cranial Nerves

Besides the spinal nerves, the PNS also contains the cranial nerves. The cranial nerves differ from the spinal nerves in that they do not attach to the spinal cord. They arise directly from the brain, bypassing the spinal cord entirely. There are twelve pairs of cranial nerves:

1. Olfactory nerve—sense of smell
2. Optic nerve—sense of vision
3. Oculomotor nerve—motor control of lens and pupil of eyeball
4. Trochlear nerve—inferior and lateral motor control of muscles of the eyeball
5. Trigeminal nerve—sensation from eyeball, cheek, and upper lip, controls chewing

6. Abducens nerve—lateral motor control of muscles of the eyeball
7. Facial nerve—sense of taste and movement of facial muscles
8. Vestibulocochlear nerve—sense of hearing and equilibrium
9. Glossopharyngeal nerve—sensation of the tongue and motor control of swallowing
10. Vagus nerve—sensation of respiratory system and digestive system
11. Accessory nerve—voice production and movement of the head and neck
12. Hypoglossal nerve—movement of tongue during speech and swallowing

Bibliography

Saladin, K. (1998). *Anatomy & physiology: The unity of form and function*. New York: McGraw-Hill.

Scott, A., Fong, E., & Beebe, R. (2002). *Functional anatomy for emergency medical services*. Clifton Park, NY: Thomson Delmar Learning.

Van Wynseberghe, D., Noback, C., & Carola, R. (1995). *Human anatomy & physiology* (3rd ed.). New York: McGraw-Hill.

APPENDIX I

Anatomy of the Female Reproductive System

THE FEMALE REPRODUCTIVE SYSTEM

Figure I-1 provides an overview of the female reproductive system. Although obviously different from the male reproductive system, its general design is quite similar.

Ovaries

Each ovary is covered in a white, fibrous sac known as the tunica albuguinia. Ovaries contain both an inner layer, known as the stroma, and an outer germinal layer. The stroma contains the follicles that hold the immature eggs, which are also known as oocytes. The egg matures and is released in the germinal layer. The corpus luteum is a temporary tissue of the ovary that secretes hormones regulating the development and release of eggs. Figure I-2 illustrates the location of the ovaries.

Female Sex Hormones

The sex hormones are named after the female reproductive system, even in the male. Follicle stimulating hormone (FSH) and leutinizing hormone (LH) cause the ovaries and the testicles to secrete sex hormones. Examples of female sex hormones include estrogen, progesterone, and human chorionic gonadotropin. Estrogen and progesterone cause the development of female sex traits and the regulation of the menstrual cycle. Human chorionic gonadotropin (hCG) prevents the lining of the uterus from sloughing off after fertilization of the egg.

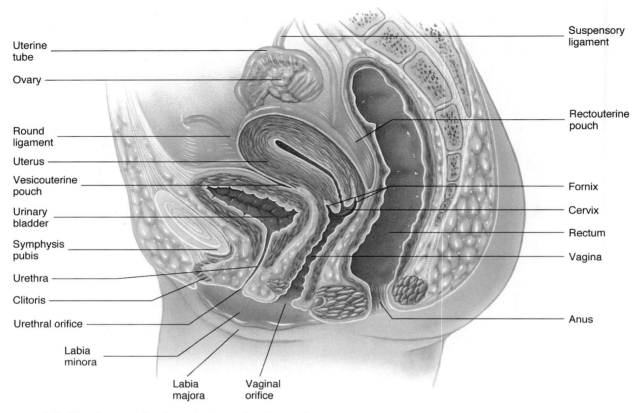

Figure I-1 Structures of the female reproductive system.

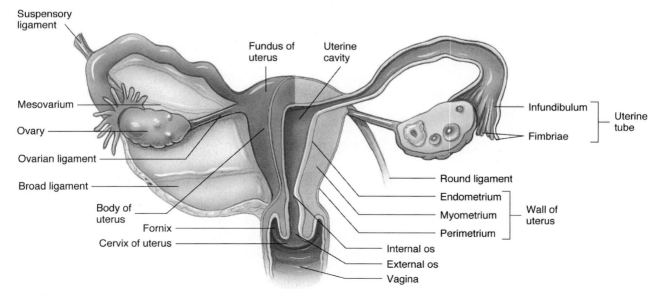

Figure I-2 Position of the ovaries, uterine tubes, uterus, and vagina.

Fallopian Tubes

The ovaries are indirectly connected to the uterus by two tubes, which are known as either uterine tubes or fallopian tubes. The superior end of the uterine tube opens in the abdominal cavity near the ovary, while the inferior end opens into the uterus. Featherlike fimbrae, which contain ciliated cells that direct the released follicle from the ovary into the uterine tube, may overlap the ovary.

The uterine tube consists of three layers, including the serous membrane, the muscularis, and the mucous membrane. The serous membrane is part of the visceral peritoneum that surrounds the outer surface of the uterine tube, while the muscularis contains smooth muscle that, under hormonal control, propels the follicle toward the uterus through peristaltic contractions. The mucous membrane contains ciliated, simple columnar epithelium. The secretions of the mucous membrane provide nutrients to the follicle, while the ciliated cells help fan the follicle toward the uterus.

Uterus

The entire female reproductive system is said to have the shape of a ram's head. The fundus is the most superior region of the uterus and represents the cranial portion of the ram's head. The body is the largest portion of the uterus and is the site where the fertilized egg embeds. The cervix is the opening of the uterus to the vaginal canal.

The perimetrium of the uterus forms the two broad ligaments that connect the uterus to the abdominal wall, stabilizing the uterus. The myometrium contains three layers of smooth muscle tissue. The outer layer of muscle extends in a longitudinal direction throughout the myometirum. The middle muscle layer contains muscle in random directions. The inner layer contains spiral and longitudinal muscle fibers.

The endometrium has a deep, velvety texture that is highly vascular and contains several tubular glands. Each month, the stratum functionalis layer of the endometrium, when not embedded with a fertilized egg, is shed along with blood and glandular secretions through the cervix and vagina. The breakdown of the endothelium adds to the menstrual flow during menstruation. The stratum basalis layer of the endometrium remains intact. If the endometrium does contain an embedded fertilized egg, the endothelium houses the developing embryo.

Vagina

The vagina is located inferior to the cervix of the uterus, posterior to the urinary bladder and the urethra. The vagina is located anterior to the anus and rectum and has the following functions:

- Provides a means for the depositing of sperm during intercourse
- Allows for the removal of menstrual tissues
- Serves as the birth canal during childbirth

The acidic environment of the vagina is due to the fermentation of bacteria that surround the vaginal epithelium. This acidic pH level helps prevent the growth of infectious microbes. During ovulation, more alkaline secretions are produced by the glands of the cervix to accommodate the introduction of sperm.

External Genitalia

The external genitalia are the mons pubis, the clitoris, the labia majora, the labia minor, the vestibular glands, and the vaginal vestibule (Figure I-3). These structures are collectively known as the vulva. The mons pubis is a layer of fat that covers the pubic bone. The clitoris contains many nerve endings and is capable of becoming erect during sexual stimulation. The labia major and labia minor serve as protective covers for the vaginal and urethral orifices. The vestibular glands secrete alkaline solutions during intercourse, which neutralize the acidic pH level of the vagina for the survival of more sperm.

Menstrual Cycle

Men are fertile almost all of their adult lives. Women, however, are only fertile for a few days each month. The delicately balanced course of events leading to female fertility is known as the menstrual cycle. The average menstrual cycle is 28 days in length, although it may be as short as 21 days or as long as 40 days.

During the first five days of the cycle, the stroma functionalis of the endometrium of the uterus sloughs off, causing menstruation. The corpus luteum

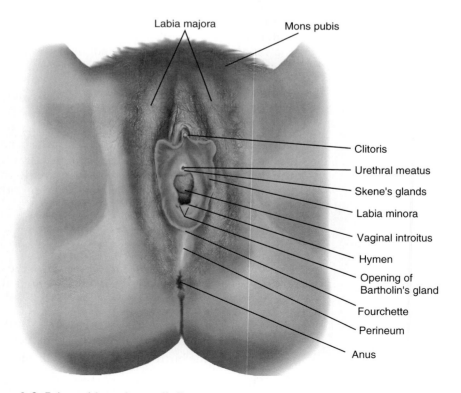

Figure I-3 External female genitalia.

Appendix I Anatomy of the Female Reproductive System **483**

is not producing significant quantities of estrogen or progesterone during this time.

On day 6, the hypothalamus of the brain secretes FSH, promoting the development of the follicle within the ovary. On days 7 through 12, estrogen is produced by the dominant follicle and the production of FSH is inhibited. The presence of estrogen stimulates the thickening of the endometrium.

On day 13, elevated estrogen levels promote the secretion of LH from the anterior pituitary gland. This surge of LH causes the release of the egg on day 14 through the rupturing of the follicle, in a process known as ovulation. The endometrium continues to develop until days 15 through 25, when secretions of estrogen and progesterone maintain the fertile endometrium. This period of fertility lasts between 10 and 16 days.

If the egg is not fertilized, about day 25, in the absence of estrogen and progesterone, the endometrium begins to slough off, and menstruation begins again. The cycle then repeats itself.

Mammary Glands

The breasts are included as part of the female reproductive system because their function is to secrete milk for nourishment of human offspring. They consist of glandular tissue, fat, lactiferous ducts and sinuses, the nipple, and the areola (Figure I-4). The process of milk production is termed lactation. Females

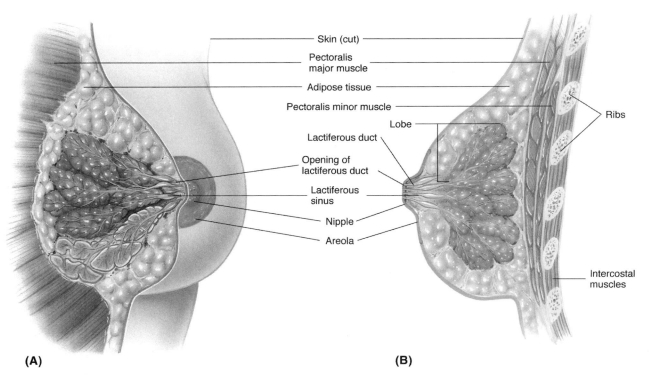

(A) **(B)**

Figure I-4 Mammary glands: (A) Anterior view and (B) sagittal view.

produce milk in response to release of a hormone known as prolactin. The breast itself is located on a layer of deep fascia that separates the breast tissue from the muscles of the chest. The breast's size is determined by the amount of fat it contains, while the amount of lactiferous tissue remains fairly constant among women.

The glandular tissue that secretes milk inside the breast contains lobes of compound areolar glands. The lactiferous ducts lead from the many areolar glands inside of each breast to the lactiferous sinus, which is situated behind the nipple. The lactiferous sinus stores the milk until it is ready to be released.

Bibliography

Saladin, K. (1998). *Anatomy & physiology: The unity of form and function*. New York: McGraw-Hill.

Scott, A., Fong, E., & Beebe, R. (2002). *Functional anatomy for emergency medical services*. Clifton Park, NY: Thomson Delmar Learning.

Van Wynseberghe, D., Noback, C., & Carola, R. (1995). *Human anatomy & physiology* (3rd ed.). New York: McGraw-Hill.

APPENDIX J

Anatomy of the Male Reproductive System

THE MALE REPRODUCTIVE SYSTEM

Figure J-1 provides an overview of the male reproductive system.

Testicles

The testicles are the production site of sperm. During fetal development, the testes are formed below the kidneys. By the time the male is born, they have descended into the scrotum, which is divided into two compartments with each compartment containing one testis. Each testicle is surrounded by a fibrous sac of white membrane known as the tunica albuginea. The tunica albuginea is also found in the female reproductive system surrounding each ovary.

The testicles are located outside the abdominopelvic cavity in the scrotum to encourage the production of sperm. In order for sperm to be produced, the temperature of the testicles must be lower than the normal temperature of the body. The cremaster muscle lines the inside of the scrotum and raises or lowers the testicles to adjust their temperature.

Each testicle contains approximately 800 seminiferous tubules, which serve two distinct, yet synergistic, purposes in the male reproductive system (Figure J-2). First, the seminiferous tubules produce sperm. Second, the seminiferous tubules aid the sperm in their maturing. The spermatogenic portion of the seminiferous tubule is the production site of thousands of sperm each second in a healthy, young male, while the sustenacular portion of the seminiferous tubule provides nutrients to the developing sperm. In addition to sperm, the testicles also produce sex hormones known as androgens. The cells within the testicle that

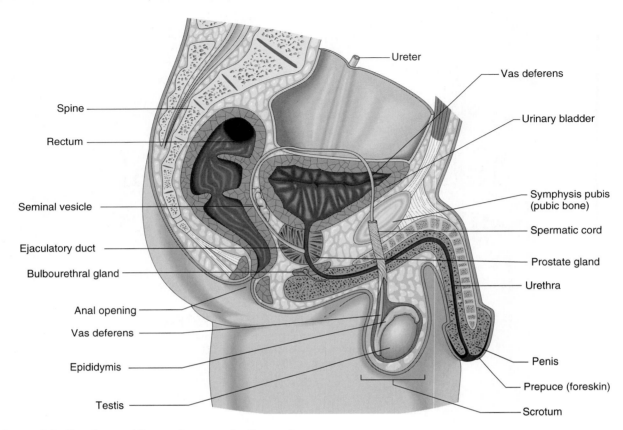

Figure J-1 Structures of the male reproductive system.

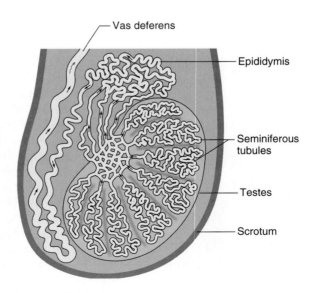

Figure J-2 Structures of the testicle.

produce the androgens are called interstitial cells, and the primary androgen they produce is testosterone.

Epididymis

Atop each testis is a coiled tubule known as the epididymis. It serves three purposes:

1. Storage of the sperm until they are mature
2. Provides a duct system for the sperm to travel from the testes to the vas deferens and, eventually, to the ejaculatory duct
3. Provides peristaltic movement by means of a circular, smooth muscle that contracts to transport the sperm toward the vas deferens and ejaculatory duct

Spermatic Cord. The spermatic cord, which is also known as the ductus deferens or vas deferens, is a storage center for sperm prior to entering the ejaculatory duct. Each spermatic cord is approximately 18 inches long and begins at the superior curvature of each testicle and then travels around the urinary bladder, at which point it passes through the abdominal wall. The spermatic cords then empty their contents into the ejaculatory duct, which becomes the urethra in the penis.

The spermatic cord is an important structure related to both hernias and vasectomies. If the abdominal muscle should prolapse through a weakened area created by the spermatic cord, an inguinal hernia occurs. The spermatic cord can be felt through the scrotum on top of each testicle. The term vasectomy is derived from the removal of part of the vas deferens. A vasectomy prevents the sperm from entering the ejaculatory duct because the spermatic cord has been clamped or severed.

Penis

The penis has two major functions: (1) removal of urine from the urinary bladder and (2) ejaculation of sperm. Both urine and semen are transported through the penis by the urethra, which is a tube extending from the urinary bladder longitudinally through the penis to its tip. The glans, which is the alternate name for the tip of the penis, is covered by the foreskin or prepuce, which may be surgically removed during a circumcision for cultural or religious reasons.

Erections are controlled by the central nervous system. The hypothalamus of the brain and the sacral plexus of the spinal cord cause parasympathetic vasodilation of the arterioles of the penis. During an erection, the arteries of the penis dilate allowing blood to flow into the erectile tissues of the penis, engorging the tissue with blood. The pressure exerted on the engorged tissue compresses the veins of the penis.

Glands of the Male Reproductive System

The seminal vesicles, which produce seminal fluid or semen, are located between the spermatic cord and the ejaculatory ducts. The prostate gland is located at the base of the penis, where it surrounds the urethra. Both the seminal vesicles and the prostate gland secrete fluids, providing nutrients to the sperm and aiding in buffering the acidic vaginal environment. The bulbourethral glands are two small glands located inferior to the prostate gland, which secrete clear, alkaline fluids that neutralize the remaining urine in the male's urethra. The bulbourethral fluids also act as a lubricant in the urethra.

Bibliography

Saladin, K. (1998). *Anatomy & physiology: The unity of form and function*. New York: McGraw-Hill.

Scott, A., Fong, E., & Beebe, R. (2002). *Functional anatomy for emergency medical services*. Clifton Park, NY: Thomson Delmar Learning.

Van Wynseberghe, D., Noback, C., & Carola, R. (1995). *Human anatomy & physiology* (3rd ed.). New York: McGraw-Hill.

APPENDIX K

Anatomy of the Skeletal System

THE SKELETAL SYSTEM

The bones of the body serve many functions besides acting as a framework for the attachment of other structures. Bones function in the production of blood, and they have their own nervous supply and blood vessels. They also act as storage centers for calcium and phosphate. The study of the bones is known as *osteology*, and Figure K-1 identifies many of the bones of the human skeleton.

Histology of Bone

Due to its structure and relatively low water content, bone is dense and durable. Osseous tissue is composed of inorganic salts, such as calcium phosphate and calcium carbonate. When the body needs these reserves, they are extracted from bone. The inorganic salts found in osseus tissue that give bone its hardness are surrounded in fibrous connective material. This matrix of fibers has a leatherlike consistency when the inorganic salts are removed. With age, the bones become less flexible and more brittle, making them susceptible to fracture.

Classifications of Bone

The bones of the body are classified according to their shape and function. Table K-1 lists the six classifications of bones and examples of each.

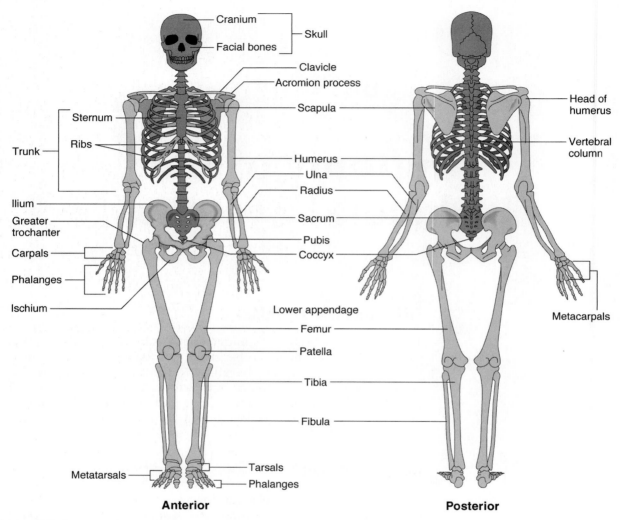

Figure K-1 Bones of the skeleton.

Table K-1 Classification of Human Bones

Classification	Definition	Examples
Long bone	A bone that is longer than it is wide	Arm, forearm, thigh, leg
Short bone	A bone that has equal dimension in all directions	Bones of the wrists and ankles
Flat bone	A bone that is thin or curved	Ribs, sternum (breast bone), scapulae (shoulder blades), cranial bones
Irregular bone	A bone that does not fit easily into any of the other categories	Oddly shaped bones of the spinal column, face, and hips
Seasamoid bone	A bone embedded in a tendon	Patella (knee cap)
Sutural bone (Wormian bone)	A bone that forms between the sutures of the skull	Sutural bones have no names and are unique in each person

PARTS OF LONG BONE

Figure K-2 is an illustration of the parts of a long bone, and it shows how blood vessels are capable of passing through bone. The proximal epiphysis and the distal epiphysis are covered with cartilage, allowing the ends of a long bone to articulate with its point of attachment. Between the two epiphyses is the diaphysis, or shaft. The diaphysis is hollow and contains the medullary cavity, which holds the yellow bone marrow. Red bone marrow is found in the spongy bone. Red bone marrow produces blood cells. The outer surface of a long bone is covered with periosteum containing nerves, lymphatic vessels, and capillaries.

The epiphyseal plate, or growth plate, consists of thick cartilage that provides a framework for the production of bone cells. Long bones grow in length only at the region of the epiphyseal plate; they do not grow in the middle of the bone. Therefore, if the bone is damaged at the epiphyseal plate, the bone may not grow correctly. Fractures of the epiphyseal plate in children may lead to improper growth of their bones—thus the need for proper medical attention whenever bone damage is suspected.

Joints

Figure K-3 depicts the three categories of joints: (1) synarthrotic, those that are immovable, (2) amphiarthrotic, those that are slightly movable, and (3) diarthrotic, those that are freely moving. An immovable joint, like a cranial suture or a sternocostal articulation, would be an example of a synarthrosis. Examples of amphiarthrosis are the pubic symphysis and the sacroiliac articulation. Shoulders, knees, hips, and elbows are all examples of a diarthrosis.

Joints are classified further by their structure. There are three types of structural classifications associated with joints: fibrous, cartilaginous, or synovial. Some joints contain elements from each of these categories. Fibrous

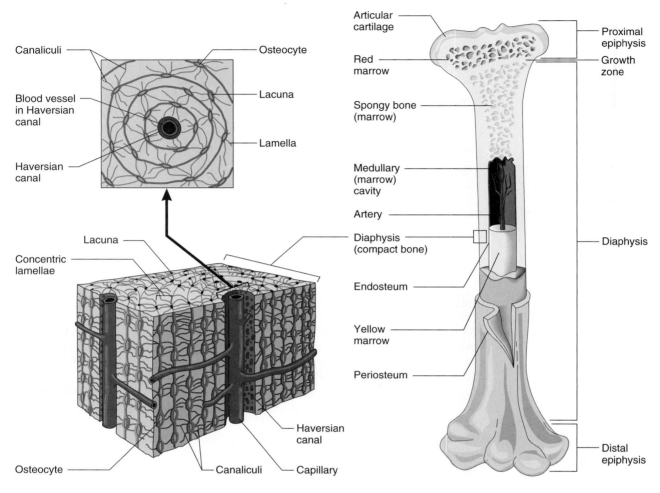

Figure K-2 Structures of a long bone.

joints are those joints held together by connective tissue. There is no cavity created in fibrous joints. Cartilaginous joints are held together by plates of cartilage between the bones, and synovial joints are those joints lubricated by synovial fluid that is held in the joint by a synovial sac. In addition to lubrication, synovial fluid also nourishes the cartilage and absorbs shock. The six types of diarthrotic joints are listed in Table K-2 along with an example of each.

Paranasal Sinuses

There are four groups of paranasal sinuses in the bones of the head, which can be seen in Figure K-4. These air pockets are located in the frontal bone, the

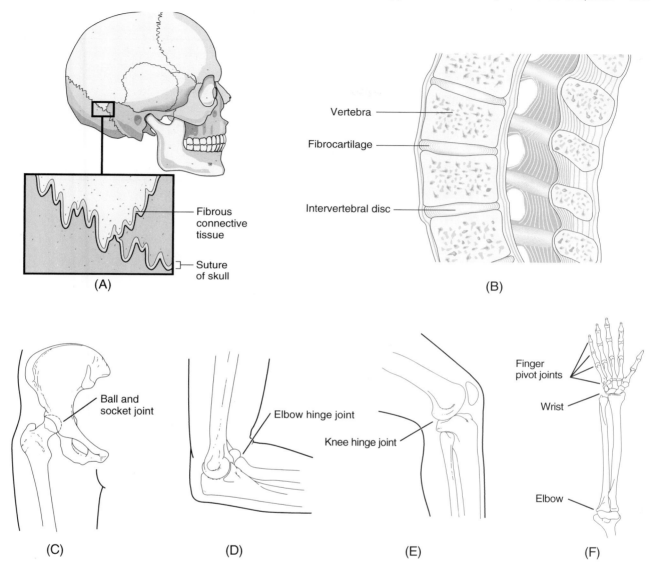

Figure K-3 Types of joints: (A) synarthrosis, (B) amphiarthrosis, (C–F) diarthroses.

ethmoid bone, the sphenoid bone, and the maxillary bones. The purpose of the sinuses is to act as a resonating chamber for the production of sound. These large air pockets also help to lighten the weight of the skull. The sinuses are filled with mucous membranes that drain into the nasal passage through small openings. Infectious microorganisms can travel from the nasal passage into the paranasal sinuses, where they cause inflammation and infection of the tissues.

Table K-2 Diarthrotic Joints

Type	Example
Hinge	Elbow
Ball-and-socket	Hip
Pivot	Base of the skull as it rotates with the axis
Gliding	Articulations of the vertebrae
Saddle	Thumb
Ellipsoidal	Where the fingers meet the palm of the hand

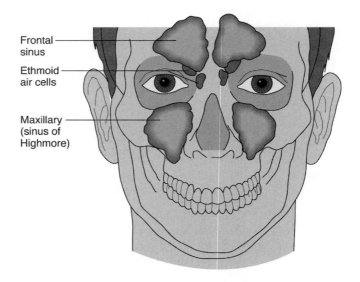

Figure K-4 Paranasal sinuses.

Bibliography

Saladin, K. (1998). *Anatomy & physiology: The unity of form and function.* New York: McGraw-Hill.

Scott, A., Fong, E., & Beebe, R. (2002). *Functional anatomy for emergency medical services.* Clifton Park, NY: Thomson Delmar Learning.

Van Wynseberghe, D., Noback, C., & Carola, R. (1995). *Human anatomy & physiology* (3rd ed.). New York: McGraw-Hill.

APPENDIX L

Anatomy of the Endocrine System

THE ENDOCRINE SYSTEM

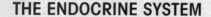

The endocrine system is a regulatory system of the body, communicating through the release of biochemical messengers known as hormones. Endocrine glands are ductless glands containing cells that secrete hormones into extracellular fluid. The hormones enter the bloodstream, where they affect only targeted tissues. Each hormone is not present in the body at all times. Endocrine glands and tissues need not secrete a constant supply of hormones because a small amount of hormone may have a major impact on the tissues that receive that hormone. An individual hormone has an action only on the cells that contain receptor sites for that particular hormone. More specifically, each hormone has an individual chemical composition that reacts only in those targeted cells containing receptor sites in their plasma membranes, nuclei, or cytoplasm for that particular hormone. Figure L-1 indicates the locations of the glands of the endocrine system.

The Pituitary Gland

The pituitary gland is attached to the hypothalamus of the brain by a stalk known as the infundibulum. The gland is nestled in its own bony structure, which is known as the sella turcica. It is divided into two portions: the anterior pituitary and the posterior pituitary.

The posterior pituitary, in conjunction with the hypothalamus, releases two major hormones: oxytocin and antidiretic hormone. The anterior pituitary, in conjunction with the hypothalamus, releases thyroid

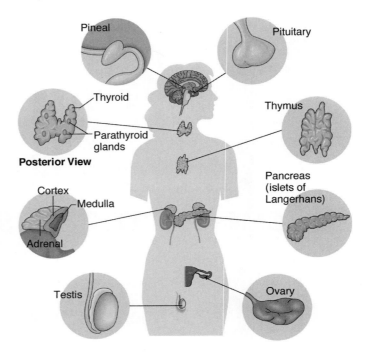

Figure L-1 Glands of the endocrine system.

stimulating hormone; gonadotropins such as leutinizing hormone and follicle stimulating hormone; prolactin; and human growth hormone. Table L-1 lists the hormones secreted by the pituitary gland and their respective functions.

Table L-1 Hormones Secreted by the Pituitary Gland

Hormone	Function
Oxytocin	Stimulates contraction of the uterus during labor and the ejection of milk from the breasts after childbirth
Antidiuretic hormone	Causes the kidneys not to form urine; during bleeding, causes the kidneys to reabsorb water into the bloodstream
Thyroid stimulating hormone	Stimulates the thyroid gland causing it to release thyroid hormones associated with cellular metabolism
Gonadotropins (leutinizing hormone and follicle stimulating hormone)	Cause the gonads to release estrogen and testosterone that give the body its sex-specific traits
Prolactin	Stimulates the production of milk after birth in the female mammary glands
Human growth hormone	Causes the bones and muscles of the body to grow and mature

Pineal Gland

The pineal gland, or pineal body, is located at the posterior end of the third ventricle, deep within the two hemispheres of the cerebrum. This gland is a neuroendocrine transducer, which means that it converts nervous system stimuli into hormones. The pineal gland is believed to function in the sleep-wake cycle of humans. The nervous system senses light through the optic nerve, which passes near the hypothalamus. From the hypothalamus, the nervous system conveys the amount of light registered by the eyes to the pineal gland. The pineal gland secretes a hormone called melatonin, which is derived from serotonin. Melatonin is a sleep-inducing chemical, secreted throughout the darkness of night by the pineal gland. The light of day inhibits the release of melatonin, causing the body to awaken.

Thyroid Gland

The thyroid gland is found in the neck. Its two lobes straddle the left and right sides of the thyroid cartilage, which is more prominent in men and is referred to as the Adam's apple. The thyroid gland secretes two primary hormones: thyroxine and calcitonin. Thryoxine is an iodine-based hormone that increases the rate of cellular metabolism. Calcitonin is a hormone that decreases levels of calcium in the blood. Calcium is an integral component of blood clotting, muscle contraction, and bone development.

The Parathyroid Glands

There are four small parathyroid glands located in the lobes of the thyroid gland. The parathyroid glands secrete parathyroid hormone, which regulates the level of calcium and phosphate in the blood. Parathyroid hormone causes several body processes to be increased, which yields an overall increase in the amount of calcium in the blood. It decreases the concentration of phosphate in the blood by inhibiting its resorption by the kidneys. Phosphate is needed to form ATP, which is an essential source of energy in the cell.

Adrenal Glands

The adrenal glands, or suprarenals, are located at the superior aspect of the kidneys. These glands contain an inner medulla and an outer cortex. The adrenal medulla secretes adrenaline, which is also known as epinephrine, and norepinephrine. The adrenal cortex secretes steroid-based hormones classified as gonadocorticoids, mineralocorticoids, and glucocorticoides.

Epinephrine and norepinephrine are hormones that increase heart rate and blood pressure. They dilate blood vessels and increase the efficiency of muscle contraction. Steroid-based hormones are associated with the production of sex hormones, decreasing the effects of stress, regulating sugar levels in the blood, and reducing inflammation throughout the body. Some of the steroids released by the adrenal cortex are cortisol, cortisone, and aldosterone. Cortisol helps the body respond to stress, maintain blood pressure and cardiovascular function, slow the immune system's inflammatory response, balance the effects of insulin in digesting sugar, and regulate the metabolism of proteins, carbohydrates, and fats.

Bibliography

Saladin, K. (1998). *Anatomy & physiology: The unity of form and function*. New York: McGraw-Hill.

Scott, A., Fong, E., & Beebe, R. (2002). *Functional anatomy for emergency medical services*. Clifton Park, NY: Thomson Delmar Learning.

Van Wynseberghe, D., Noback, C., & Carola, R. (1995). *Human anatomy & physiology* (3rd ed.). New York: McGraw-Hill.

APPENDIX M

Anatomy of the Integumentary System

THE INTEGUMENTARY SYSTEM

The integumentary system provides the embalmer with a first line of defense against the spread of infection. Figure M-1 depicts some of the many characteristic lesions that disease may leave on the surface of the skin and recognition of these signs can alert the embalmer to potential hazards. Because disease transmission through the skin, which is referred to as parenteral transmission, requires blood to blood contact, the intact skin is the best barrier to the spread of microbial diseases.

The skin, hair, and nails make up the integumentary system, which is depicted in Figure M-2. Hair and nails are formed of tough, fibrous material known as keratin. Both hair and nails grow out of specialized skin cells.

Skin and Its Layers

The skin is divided into layers known as strata. Skin has four main layers, or strata. The most superficial stratum of the skin is the stratum corneum. The stratum corneum consists of many dead, flat, interlocking cells. This dry barrier inhibits microbial growth. It is lubricated by lipid (fat) secretions from the integumentary glands. The stratum corneum is water-resistant but not waterproof. The cells in the stratum corneum take approximately 14 days to reach this layer from the deeper layers of the skin. The cells remain in the stratum corneum approximately two weeks, after which time, they slough off and are replaced in a process known as necrobiosis.

The next two layers of the skin are the stratum lucidum and the stratum granulosum. The stratum lucidum is superficial to the stratum

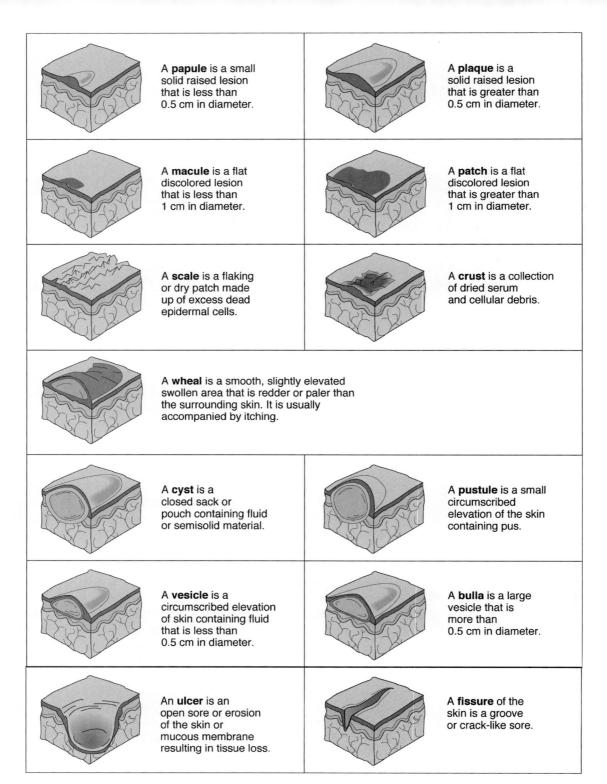

Figure M-1 Skin lesions.

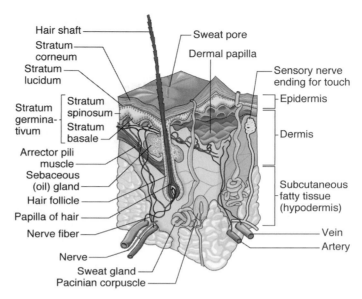

Figure M–2 Cross section of skin.

granulosum. Due to the action of proteins found in these layers of the skin, hair and nails are able to form. These layers also produce the necessary cells to create thick skin on the palms of the hands and soles of the feet. These areas of the body have thicker skin because they are the most likely areas of the body to be in contact with the surrounding environment, resulting in the highest likelihood of cellular erosion.

The deepest stratum of the skin is the stratum germinativum, which is divided into two layers known as the stratum spinosum and the stratum basale. The stratum germinativum is of great importance to the skin because new cells are synthesized in this layer. The new skin cells develop in the stratum germinativum and push their way up through the layers of the skin, until they slough off in the uppermost layers of the epidermis.

Physiology of the Integument

Skin plays a vital role in the synthesis of vitamins and chemicals utilized by the body on a daily basis. Ultraviolet rays from the sun are absorbed by the integument, allowing the digestive system to utilize ingested vitamin D and phosphorus. The absorption of vitamin D also aids in the digestion of calcium, which is integral in muscle contraction, blood clotting, and bone growth.

Skin Color

Skin gets its dark color from a substance known as melanin, which is produced by cells known as melanocytes. The more melanin in the skin, the darker the complexion. Yellow colors in skin are due to the presence of carotene, while pink pigmentation is caused by light reflecting off blood through the skin. The red color of oxygenated blood is from oxyhemoglobin, while the blue color of superficial veins in skin results from deoxyhemoglobin in the blood.

Glands of the Integument

Sebaceous glands produce a substance called sebum, which is an emollient and an antibacterial agent. Sebum is secreted onto the epithelial layer of the skin when small muscles compress the sebaceous gland while elevating the hair follicle. The sebum then flows along the hair follicle to the surface of the skin.

Sweat glands cover the entire body, but are especially concentrated in the soles of the feet and the palms of the hands. These coiled, tubular glands contain ducts that allow them to secrete sweat directly onto the epidermis. Sweat is composed of water and trace amounts of salt and waste products.

Bibliography

Saladin, K. (1998). *Anatomy & physiology: The unity of form and function*. New York: McGraw-Hill.

Scott, A., Fong, E., & Beebe, R. (2002). *Functional anatomy for emergency medical services*. Clifton Park, NY: Thomson Delmar Learning.

Van Wynseberghe, D., Noback, C., & Carola, R. (1995). *Human anatomy & physiology* (3rd ed.). New York: McGraw-Hill.

APPENDIX N

Anatomy of the Lymphatic System

THE LYMPHATIC SYSTEM

The lymphatic system is comprised of vessels in a similar fashion to the blood vasculature, with the exception that the lymphatic system only moves fluid in one direction—from the tissues to the blood vascular system. The lymphatic capillaries lead into ever-larger lymphatic vessels headed toward the trunk of the body, as depicted in Figure N-1. The two major collecting sites for lymph before it enters the venous system are the thoracic duct and the right lymphatic duct.

Thoracic Duct

The thoracic duct collects lymph from the body inferior to the diaphragm and from the left side of the body superior to the diaphragm. The thoracic duct begins in the abdomen, just inferior to the diaphragm, as an expanded area known as the cisterna chili, which collects lymph from the lower abdomen, pelvis, and lower extremities. The thoracic duct continues through the aortic hiatus of the diaphragm and ascends the left side of the vertebral column until it reaches the left clavicle. Lymph from the left side of the head, the left side of the neck, the left side of the thorax, and the left arm is added to the lymph gathered below the diaphragm, and it is all added back to the venous system through the left subclavian vein at a point near the left internal jugular vein. Stated more succinctly, the thoracic duct gathers all the lymph below the diaphragm, and from above the diaphragm on the left side of the body, and returns it to the blood vascular system through the veins.

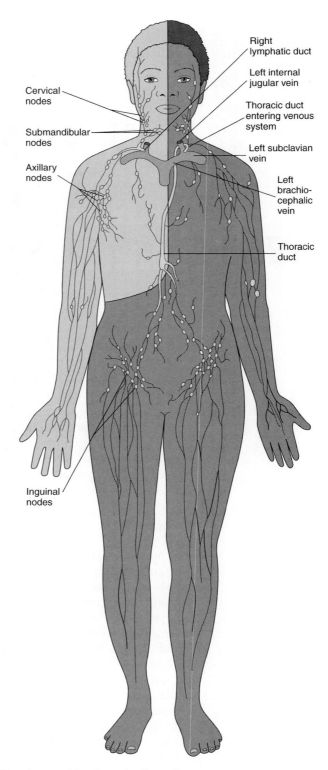

Figure N-1 Structures of the lymphatic system.

Right Lymphatic Duct

The lymph in the upper right quadrant of the body drains into the right lymphatic duct, which is formed by the merger of many smaller lymphatic vessels in the region of the right clavicle. The right lymphatic duct drains into the right subclavian vein near the right internal jugular vein. In other words, the right lymphatic duct drains lymph from the right side of the body above the diaphragm and returns it to the blood vascular system through veins.

Lymphoid Tissues

Lymphoid tissues are divided between aggregations of nodules and actual lymphoid organs. Lymphoid nodules are unencapsulated, connective tissue containing densely packed lymphocytes. They are found deep in the epithelial tissues lining the respiratory, digestive, and urinary tracts.

Peyer's Patches

Aggregated, unencapsulated lymph nodules are also known as Peyer's patches, which are common in the ileum of the small intestine. Peyer's patches are also known as gut-associated lymphoid tissues (GALT) because of their location in the gut of the digestive system. Similar lymphoid tissues are found throughout the mucus-secreting tissues of the body.

The body defends the wall of the small intestine from bacteria and viruses, along with other foreign substances, by reinforcing the mucosal lining of the small intestine with B cells that produce antibodies against specialized antigens. The B cells enter the mucosal lining of the small intestine after a journey from bone marrow.

Inactive B cells are released from the bone marrow and travel to Peyer's patches in the small intestine, where they are activated by antigens in the small intestine. The activated B cells leave Peyer's patches through lymphatic vessels and are transported through the thoracic duct to the venous bloodstream, where they become part of the blood plasma. Eventually, the B cells are carried by the blood to the mucosal lining of the intestine.

Tonsils

The tonsils are two clumps of glandular tissue, on either side of the throat, embedded in a pocket at the side of the palate. The lower edge of each tonsil is beside the tongue in the back of the throat. The tonsils trap bacteria and viruses entering through the throat and produce antibodies to help fight infections. The adenoids are a single clump of tissue in the nasopharynx, located, in the adult, in the throat about an inch above the uvula, which is the piece of tissue that hangs down in the middle of the soft palate.

Lymph Nodes

Lymph nodes are actually small lymphoid organs. Lymphoid organs are covered with a fibrous connective tissue capsule (Figure N-2). Lymph enters the lymph nodes through lymphatic vessels, whereupon the antigens in the lymph trigger the activation of T cells and B cells. The activated lymphocytes in the lymph cross over the walls of blood vessels within the lymph nodes. Lymph nodes are scattered on the lymphatic vessels like beads on a string. The lymph may be filtered several times before it reaches the venous system. Table N-1 lists some of the most prominent locations of lymph nodes in the body.

Spleen

The spleen is located inferior to the diaphragm between the sixth and eleventh ribs, where it is anchored to the stomach by the gastrosplenic ligament. The spleen performs three functions in the body: (1) removal of abnormal blood cells through phagocytosis; (2) storage of the iron it extracts from damaged red blood cells; and (3) initiation of the immune responses by B cells and T cells, when it encounters antigens circulating in the blood.

The spleen also produces red blood cells in the fetus. Later in life, it stores newly formed red blood cells and platelets until they are needed in the bloodstream. The spleen contains so much blood that it serves as a reservoir in times of need. If the body loses blood suddenly through hemorrhaging, the spleen contracts and adds up to 200 ml of blood into the bloodstream in less than one minute.

Thymus

The thymus is located posterior to the sternum in the anterior mediastinum. It is at its largest size in relation to body size during the first year or two after birth. The thymus is at its largest absolute size during puberty, after which it progressively decreases in size and becomes ever-more fibrous, during a process known as involution.

Like all lymphoid organs, the thymus is encapsulated. Fibrous extensions of the capsule divide the thymus into two lobes. Each lobe is further divided

Table N-1 Location of Lymph Nodes in the Body

Cervical lymph nodes	Filter lymph from the head and neck
Axillary lymph nodes	Filter lymph from the upper extremities and breasts
Popliteal and inguinal lymph nodes	Filter lymph from the lower extremities
Thoracic lymph nodes	Filter lymph from the lungs, respiratory passageways, and mediastinal structures
Abdominal lymph nodes	Filter lymph from the urinary and reproductive systems
Intestinal and mesenterial lymph nodes	Filter lymph from the digestive tract

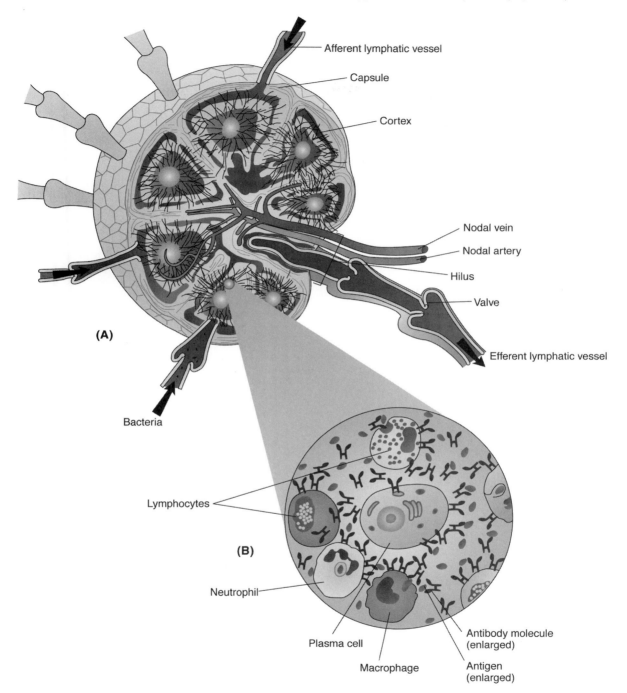

Afferent lymphatic vessel

Capsule

Cortex

Nodal vein

Nodal artery

Hilus

Valve

(A)

Efferent lymphatic vessel

Bacteria

Lymphocytes

(B)

Neutrophil

Plasma cell

Macrophage

Antibody molecule
(enlarged)

Antigen
(enlarged)

Figure N-2 Lymph node: (A) Section through a lymph node showing the flow of lymph. (B) Microscopic detail of bacteria being destroyed within the lymph node.

into smaller lobules. The cortex of the thymus lobules are the production site of T cells, which are not functional against antigens until they enter the bloodstream. Once in the bloodstream, they are transported throughout the body, but especially to the spleen and lymph nodes.

Bibliography

Saladin, K. (1998). *Anatomy & physiology: The unity of form and function*. New York: McGraw-Hill.

Scott, A., Fong, E., & Beebe, R. (2002). *Functional anatomy for emergency medical services*. Clifton Park, NY: Thomson Delmar Learning.

Van Wynseberghe, D., Noback, C., & Carola, R. (1995). *Human anatomy & physiology* (3rd ed.). New York: McGraw-Hill.

APPENDIX O

Answers to Review Questions

CHAPTER 1

Matching

1. d
2. e
3. a
4. c
5. b

Multiple Choice

1. d
2. c
3. a
4. d
5. c

Case Analysis

Lightning

CHAPTER 2

Matching

1. c
2. a
3. e
4. b
5. d

Multiple Choice

1. d
2. c
3. a
4. d
5. b

CHAPTER 3

Matching

1. c
2. e
3. a

4. d
5. b

Multiple Choice

1. a
2. c
3. c
4. d
5. b

CHAPTER 4

Matching

1. d
2. a
3. e
4. c
5. b

Multiple Choice

1. c
2. b
3. d
4. a
5. c

Case Analysis

Cystic fibrosis and diabetes mellitus

CHAPTER 5

Matching

1. d
2. a
3. b
4. c
5. e

Multiple Choice

1. b
2. a
3. c
4. d
5. a

CHAPTER 6

Matching

1. c
2. e
3. a
4. d
5. b

Multiple Choice

1. d
2. a
3. b
4. a
5. c

Case Analysis

Petechia due to vomiting and seizures related to alcohol poisoning.

CHAPTER 7

Matching

1. c
2. b
3. a
4. e
5. d

Multiple Choice

1. a
2. c
3. d
4. b
5. d

Case Analysis

Glioma

CHAPTER 8

Matching

1. e
2. c
3. b
4. a
5. d

Multiple Choice

1. b
2. d
3. a
4. d
5. c

Case Analysis

Polycythemia vera

CHAPTER 9

Matching

1. b
2. a
3. e
4. c
5. d

Multiple Choice

1. b
2. a
3. d
4. c
5. a

Case Analysis

Acute myocardial infarction

CHAPTER 10

Matching

1. e
2. b
3. a
4. c
5. d

Multiple Choice

1. b
2. d
3. c
4. c
5. a

Case Analysis

Appendicitis

CHAPTER 11

Matching

1. d
2. b
3. e
4. c
5. a

Multiple Choice

1. c
2. b
3. a
4. d
5. b

Case Analysis

Hemothorax and atelectasis (collapsed lung)

CHAPTER 12

Matching

1. c
2. d
3. e
4. a
5. b

Multiple Choice

1. d
2. c
3. d
4. a
5. b

Case Analysis

Uremia due to renal failure caused by diabetes mellitus

CHAPTER 13

Matching

1. b
2. e
3. c

4. a
5. d

Multiple Choice

1. b
2. a
3. d
4. a
5. c

Case Analysis

Lou Gehrig's disease (amyotrophic lateral sclerosis)

CHAPTER 14

Matching

1. a
2. c
3. d
4. e
5. b

Multiple Choice

1. c
2. b
3. a
4. d
5. b

Case Analysis

Ovarian cyst

CHAPTER 15

Matching

1. b
2. a
3. d
4. e
5. c

Multiple Choice

1. d
2. a
3. c
4. d
5. b

Case Analysis

Testicular cancer

CHAPTER 16

Matching

1. e
2. c
3. d
4. b
5. a

Multiple Choice

1. b
2. d
3. c
4. b
5. a

Case Analysis

Achondroplasia

CHAPTER 17

Matching

1. d
2. a
3. e
4. c
5. b

Multiple Choice

1. d
2. a
3. c
4. d
5. b

Case Analysis

Diabetes mellitus

CHAPTER 18

Matching

1. d
2. c
3. a
4. e
5. b

Multiple Choice

1. b
2. a
3. c
4. d
5. c

Case Analysis

Psoriasis

CHAPTER 19

Matching

1. c
2. a
3. b
4. e
5. d

Multiple Choice

1. d
2. a
3. d
4. b
5. c

Case Analysis

Hodgkin's lymphoma

CHAPTER 20

Matching

1. d
2. a
3. e
4. c
5. b

Multiple Choice

1. b
2. d
3. a
4. d
5. c

CHAPTER 21

Matching

1. c
2. e
3. a
4. b
5. d

Multiple Choice

1. b
2. a
3. c
4. d
5. c

CHAPTER 22

Matching

1. c
2. e
3. a
4. d
5. b

Multiple Choice

1. c
2. d
3. b
4. d
5. a

CHAPTER 23

Matching

1. c
2. b
3. a

4. d
5. e

Multiple Choice

1. a
2. c
3. b
4. d
5. a

CHAPTER 24

Matching

1. d
2. c
3. e
4. a
5. b

Multiple Choice

1. c
2. a
3. d
4. b
5. a

CHAPTER 25

Matching

1. d
2. a
3. e
4. b
5. c

Multiple Choice

1. a
2. b
3. b
4. d
5. c

Case Analysis

Plague

CHAPTER 26

Matching

1. c
2. b
3. e
4. a
5. d

Multiple Choice

1. b
2. d
3. a
4. b
5. c

Case Analysis

Endemic typhus

CHAPTER 27

Matching

1. e
2. a
3. d
4. b
5. c

Multiple Choice

1. d
2. d
3. c
4. a
5. b

Case Analysis

Secondary fungal respiratory infection due to AIDS

CHAPTER 28

Matching

1. d
2. a
3. e
4. b
5. c

Multiple Choice

1. c
2. a
3. b
4. d
5. a

Case Analysis

Pneumocystosis

Glossary

Abscess—An inflamed area of pus walled off by a membrane.

Acquired—A condition that presents itself after birth.

Acromegaly—Hyperfunction of the anterior lobe of the pituitary gland after ossification has been completed.

Acute—A disease with a more or less rapid onset and short duration.

Addison's disease—A rare endocrine disorder, occurring when the adrenal glands fail to produce enough of the hormones cortisol or aldosterone.

Adhesion—A fibrous band holding parts together that are normally separated, resulting during the healing process after wounds.

Allergies—Having a hypersensitivity to a substance that does not normally cause a reaction.

Amelia—Congenital absence of one or more limbs.

Amyloid—A waxy, translucent, complex protein that resembles starch. Amyloid degeneration is a form of cellular degeneration present in diseases like Alzheimer's disease.

Anasarca—Generalized massive edema in subcutaneous tissue.

Anemia—A decrease in the number of erythrocytes, hemoglobin, or both.

Aneurysm—A localized dilation (abnormal enlargement or bulging) of a blood vessel.

Angina—Chest pain due to lack of oxygenation of the heart muscle resulting from inadequate blood flow.

Antagonism—Mutual opposition or contrary action. The inhibition of one bacterium by another.

Antibodies—Glycoprotein substances developed in response to and interacting specifically with an antigen; also known as immunoglobulins.

Antigen—A foreign substance that stimulates the formation of antibodies that interact specifically with it.

Antisepsis—Preventing or inhibiting the growth of pathogenic microorganisms.

Aplasia—Failure of a tissue or an organ to develop normally due to an absence of cells.

Arrhythmia—Loss of the normal beating rhythm of the heart.

Arteriosclerosis—Disease of the arteries resulting in thickening and the loss of elasticity.

Ascites—Accumulation of free serous fluid in the abdominal cavity.

Asphyxia—The inability to take in necessary amounts of oxygen.

Asthma—A sometimes chronic condition in which the bronchi are hypersensitive to stimuli.

Atelectasis—A collapsed lung or the failure of the lung of a fetus to expand fully at birth. Technically, it is the loss of lung volume due to inadequate expansion of airspaces, which results in inadequate oxygen and carbon dioxide exchange within the lungs.

Atherosclerosis—The most common form of arteriosclerosis, marked by cholesterol, lipid, and calcium deposits in the walls of arteries.

Atrophy—A wasting, decrease in size of an organ or tissue.

Attenuation—Dilution or weakening of the virulence of a microorganism, reducing or abolishing its pathogenicity.

Autolysis—The process by which an organism digests its own cells through enzymes that are naturally present in the cell or in surrounding tissues; this normally occurs after the cell or tissue has died.

Autopsy—A postmortem examination of the organs and tissues of a body to determine cause of death or pathological condition. Also known as a necropsy.

Autotrophic—Self-nourishing, capable of growing in the absence of organic compounds. Organisms that obtain carbon from carbon dioxide.

Bacillus (pl. bacilli)—Any rod shaped microorganism.

Bacteria—A prokaryotic one-celled microorganism of the kingdom Monera, existing as free-living organisms or as parasites, multiplying by binary fission, and having a large range of biochemical properties.

Bacterial colony—A visible group of bacteria growing on a solid medium, presumably arising from a single microorganism.

Bactericides—Agents that destroy bacteria but not necessarily their spores.

Bacteriology—Science that studies bacteria.

Benign—Not recurrent or progressive; nonmalignant.

Binary fission—A method of asexual reproduction in bacteria in which cells split into two parts, each of which develops into a complete individual.

Biological vector—An animal vector in which the disease-causing organism multiplies or develops within the animal prior to becoming infective for a susceptible individual.

Bronchitis—An inflammation of the bronchi, which are the main air passages to the lungs.

Buboes—Infected lymph nodes associated with bubonic plague or other diseases.

Bursitis—Inflammation of the bursae in certain joints of the body.

Cachexia—A state of ill health, malnutrition, and wasting of the body. It may occur in many chronic diseases, malignancies, and infections.

Calcification—The depositing of calcium salts, magnesium, iron, and other minerals within the cells.

Carbuncle—Several communicating boils of the skin and subcutaneous tissues with the production and discharge of pus and dead tissue.

Caseous—Cheeselike. Caseous necrosis is characterized by pink areas of necrotic tissue surrounded by inflammatory granules.

Cause of death—Any injury or disease that produces a physiological derangement in the body that results in the death of the individual. Examples include gunshot wounds, stab wounds, lung cancer, or blood clots.

Cavitation—Formation of cavities in an organ or tissue, frequently seen in some forms of tuberculosis.

Chancre—A hard, primary ulcer due to syphilis infection appearing approximately two to three weeks after infection.

Chemotaxis—The movement of white blood cells to an area of inflammation in response to the release of chemical mediators by neutrophils, monocytes, and injured tissues.

Chlamydia—A large group of nonmotile, gram-negative, intracellular parasites.

Chronic—A disease with a more or less slow onset and long duration.

Cleft palate—Congenitally malformed palate with a fissure along the midline.

Clinical pathology—Study of disease performed in the laboratory by means of body secretions, excretions, and other body fluids.

Coagulase—A bacterial enzyme that causes blood to clot by converting fibrinogen into fibrin.

Coccus (pl. cocci)—A type of bacteria that is spherical or ovoid in form.

Colostomy—A surgical procedure to create an opening of a portion of the colon through the abdominal wall to its skin surface. A colostomy is established in cases of distal obstruction; inflammatory process, including perforation; and when the distal colon or rectum is surgically resected.

Commensalism—The symbiotic relationship of two organisms of different species in which one organism gains some benefit such as protection or nourishment.

Communicable—A disease that may be transmitted directly or indirectly from one individual to another.

Complications—Unfavorable conditions arising during the course of disease.

Concussion—A traumatic head injury of sufficient force to bruise the brain, which often involves the surface of the brain and can cause an extravasation of blood without rupture of the meninges. It can result in temporary loss of consciousness, paralysis, vomiting, and seizures.

Congenital—Condition existing at the time of birth or shortly thereafter.

Congestion—Accumulation of an excess of blood or tissue fluid in a body part.

Contamination—The act of introducing disease germs or infectious material into an area or substance.

Contusion—A bruise, often accompanied by swelling.

Convulsions—Abnormal, violent, and involuntary contraction or series of contractions of the muscles.

Cretinism—A hypothyroid condition of infants and children in which the thyroid gland does not secrete sufficient quantities of thyroid hormones.

Creutzfeldt-Jakob disease—Believed to be caused by a prion, a progressive disease that causes spongiform—porous, like a sponge—degeneration of the brain.

Cryptorchism—Failure of the testis to descend from its intra-abdominal location into the scrotum; also known as cryptorchidism.

Cushing's syndrome—An iatrogenic disorder of the adrenal glands due to chronic glucocorticoid hormone therapy.

Cyanosis—Bluish discoloration of the skin or mucous membrane due to lack of oxygen.

Cyst—A sac within or on the body surface containing air or fluid.

Decubitus ulcer—A pressure sore, a bedsore.

Deficiency—A lack of dietary or metabolic substance that can lead to disease.

Degeneration—The deterioration of tissues with corresponding functional impairment as a result of disease or injury.

Dehydration—Loss of moisture from body tissue that may occur antemortem or postmortem.

Dementia—A progressive, irreversible decline in mental function, marked by memory impairment and, often, deficits in reasoning, judgment, abstract thought, registration, comprehension, learning, task execution, and use of language.

Dermatophytes—A wide variety of fungi that can infect the integumentary system.

Diagnosis—Term denoting the naming of the disease or syndrome; the recognition of the nature of a disease.

Dialysis—A processes of diffusing blood across a semi-permeable membrane to remove toxic materials and to maintain fluid, electrolyte, and acid–base balance in cases of impaired kidney function or absence of the kidneys.

Dilatation—The pathological condition of the heart being enlarged due to a stretching of the muscle fibers, occurring normally, artificially, or as a result of disease.

Diplobacilli—A double bacillus, two being linked end to end to each other.

Diplococci—Any of various spherical bacteria appearing in pairs.

Disinfectant—A chemical or physical agent that kills disease-causing microorganisms; generally used on inanimate objects.

Disinfection—The destruction of pathogenic agents by chemical or physical means directly applied to an inanimate object.

Drug-fast—Resistant, as in bacteria, to the action of a drug or drugs.

Dry gangrene (ischemic necrosis)—Condition that results when the body part that dies had little blood and remains aseptic; occurs when the arteries but not the veins are obstructed.

Dysplasia—Abnormal development of tissue.

Dyspnea—Shortness of breath.

Ecchymosis—Small, nonelevated hemorrhagic patch; extravasation of blood into a tissue. Scientific name for a common bruise.

Eclampsia—The occurrence of seizures during pregnancy, which cannot be attributed to another cause, after the 20th week of gestation.

Ectopic pregnancy—The implantation of the fertilized ovum in a site other than the normal one in the uterine cavity.

Eczema—A general term for a variety of inflammatory skin conditions. It is characterized by dry, red, extremely itchy patches on the skin that may ooze an inflammatory exudate.

Edema—Abnormal accumulation of fluids in tissue or body cavities.

Emaciation—The state of being extremely lean.

Embolism—Sudden obstruction of a blood vessel by debris. Blood clots, cholesterol-containing plaques, masses of bacteria, cancer cells, amniotic fluid, fat from the marrow of broken bones, and injected substances (e.g., air bubbles or particulate matter) all may lodge in blood vessels and obstruct circulation.

Embolus—A mass of undissolved matter present in the bloodstream. Emboli may be solid, liquid, or gaseous. Occlusions of the vessels from emboli usually result in the development of infarcts.

Emphysema—A chronic inflammatory disease of the respiratory system, characterized by the presence of air pockets at the terminal ends of the bronchioles.

Empyema—Pus in the pleural cavity.

Encephalitis—Inflammation of the brain. When used clinically, the term refers to an infection of the brain caused by a virus.

Endemic—A disease that is continuously present in a community.

Endocarditis—Inflammation of the heart valves or the lining of the heart.

Endometriosis—A condition, in which the tissue that normally lines the uterus, which is known as the endometrium, grows in other areas of the body, such as the pelvic area, the surface of the uterus, the ovaries, the intestines, the rectum, or the bladder.

Endometritis—Infection of the endometrium, which is the lining of the uterus.

Endospore—A thick-walled cell produced by a bacterium to enable it to survive unfavorable environmental conditions.

Endotoxin—Bacterial toxin confined within the body of a bacterium freed only when the bacterium is broken down; found only in gram negative bacteria.

Epidemic—Higher than normal appearance of an infectious disease or condition within a given population.

Epidemic typhus (louse-borne typhus)—A disease caused by *Rickettsia prowazekii*, which grows in the intestinal tract of human body lice and flying squirrels in the eastern United States. It is transmitted when the human scratches the wound, rubbing the fecal material into the bite left by the human body louse.

Epilepsy—A chronic neurogenic disease marked by sudden alterations in consciousness and frequently by convulsions. It is a recurrent degenerative disorder of the nervous system marked by repetitive abnormal electrical discharges within the brain known as seizures.

Epistaxis—Bleeding from the nose.

Erythrocytosis—An abnormally high red blood cell count.

Eschar—An anthrax lesion characterized by a central mass of necrotic tissue surrounded by inflammatory vesicles.

Etiology—The study of the cause of disease.

Exacerbate—Increased severity of a disease.

Exogenous infections—Originating outside the body, an organ, or a part of the body.

Exsanguination—Loss of blood to the point where life can no longer be sustained.

Exudate—Any fluid released from the body with a high concentration of protein, cells, or solid debris.

Facultative—Having the capacity to do something that is not compulsory; in particular, having the ability to live or adapt to certain conditions.

Febrile—Term associated with fever.

Fibrillation—A quivering or spontaneous contraction of the individual cardiac cells.

Flagella—Long, whiplike, filament-containing appendages that propel bacteria in liquid.

Focal infection—An infection in which organisms are originally confined to one area but enter the blood or lymph vessel and spread to other parts of the body.

Fomite—Any inanimate object to which infectious material adheres and can be transmitted.

Fulminating—Having rapid and severe onset, usually fatal.

Functional—A condition or disease in which there are changes in physiologic activity, but no recognizable change in anatomy.

Fungi—A group of often filamentous unicellular and multicellular organisms lacking chlorophyll and usually bearing spores.

Fungicides—Agents that destroy fungi and their spores.

Furuncle—An abscess due to pyogenic infection of a sweat gland or hair follicle.

Gangrene—A term used to refer to several types of necrosis.

General infection—An infection that becomes systemic.

General pathology—Deals with the study of the widespread processes of disease such as inflammation, degeneration, necrosis or cellular death, repair, and so on without reference to particular organs or organ systems.

Germicides—Substances that destroy microorganisms but not necessarily their spores.

Goiter—Enlargement of the dysfunctional thyroid gland, often due to iodine deficiency and not associated with inflammation or cancer.

Gout—A form of arthritis due to a metabolic disorder resulting in the depositing of uric acid in the joints.

Grave's disease—A distinct type of hyperthyroidism caused by an autoimmune attack on the thyroid gland.

Gross pathology—Study of changes in structure of the body as a result of disease that are readily seen with the unaided eye.

Gumma—An infectious lesion consisting of a central necrotic mass surrounded by an inflammatory zone and fibrous deterioration of the tissues due to tertiary syphilis.

Hematemesis—Vomiting of blood.

Hematoma—A swelling consisting of a mass of extravascular blood (usually clotted) confined to an organ, tissue, or space and caused by a break in a blood vessel.

Hematuria—Blood in the urine.

Hemophilia—A hereditary bleeding disorder marked by a deficiency of blood clotting proteins.

Hemoptysis—Coughing up blood in the sputum.

Hemorrhage—Escape of blood from the blood vascular system.

Hepatitis—An inflammatory disorder of the liver caused by a virus, commonly hepatitis viruses A, B, and C. Hepatitis B is spread through body fluid contact, and it can lead to either a chronic liver disease or death.

Hereditary—Being genetically transmitted from parent to offspring.

Hernia—Abnormal protrusion of part of an organ through an opening in the wall that normally contains it.

Heterotrophic—Requiring complex organic food from a carbon source in order to grow and develop.

Host—The organism from which a microorganism obtains its nourishment.

Hyaluronidase—A bacterial enzyme that penetrates the body's connective tissues, permitting the easy spread of infection throughout the body.

Hydrocele—Abnormal collection of fluid in any sacculated cavity in the body, especially the scrotum.

Hydrocephalus—Excessive accumulation of cerebrospinal fluid in the ventricles of the brain.

Hydronephrosis—Distention of the pelvis and calyces of one or both kidneys with urine as a result of obstruction.

Hydropericardium—Abnormal accumulation of fluid within the pericardial sac that surrounds the heart.

Hydrothorax—Abnormal accumulation of fluid in the pleural cavity.

Hyperemia—Increase flow of blood in an area of the body. Active hyperemia is due to an excess of arterial blood, while passive hyperemia is due to an excess of venous blood.

Hyperplasia—The increased size of an organ or part due to the excessive but regulated increase in the number of its cells.

Hypertension—High blood pressure based on three readings spread out over several weeks in which blood pressure is higher than 140 millimeters of mercury systolic or 90 millimeters of mercury diastolic.

Hyperthyroidism—Hyperfunction of the thyroid gland.

Hypertrophy—The enlargement of an organ or tissue due to the increase in size of cells composing it.

Hypoplasia—Underdevelopment of a tissue, organ, or the body.

Hypothermia—Body temperature below 80°F (27°C).

Hypoxia—Depletion of oxygen in the cells and tissues.

Iatrogenic—Resulting from the adverse activity of medical treatment.

Icterus—Another name for jaundice.

Idiopathic—Of unknown cause (example: sudden infant death syndrome).

Indigenous flora—Plant life occurring or adapted for living in a specific environment.

Infarction—The formation of an area of necrosis in a tissue caused by obstruction in the artery supplying the area.

Infection—The state or condition in which the body or a part of it is invaded by a pathogenic agent that, under favorable conditions, multiplies and produces injurious effects.

Infestation—The harboring of animal parasites, especially macroscopic forms, such as ticks or mosquitoes.

Infiltration—The process of seepage or diffusion into tissue of substances that are not ordinarily present.

Inflammation—A tissue reaction to irritation, infection, or injury marked by localized heat, swelling, redness, pain, and sometimes loss of function. Inflammation is an immunological defense against injury, infection, or allergy, marked by increases in regional blood flow, immigration of white blood cells, and release of chemical toxins.

Inguinal hernia—A condition in which part of the intestine bulges through a weakened area in the muscles in the inguinal canal, which is located in the groin.

Insecticides—Agents that destroy insects.

Intoxication—State of being intoxicated, especially of being poisoned by a drug or toxic substance.

Intracranial hemorrhage—Extravasation of blood within the skull.

Intussusception—The slipping of one part of the intestine into another part just below it; becoming ensheathed.

Ischemia—Reduction in arterial blood supply.

Ischemic necrosis—*See* dry gangrene.

Jaundice—Condition characterized by excessive concentration of bilirubin in the skin and tissues and deposition of excessive bile pigment in the skin, cornea, body fluids, and mucous membranes with the resulting yellow appearance of the patient.

Larvicides—Agents that destroy insect larvae.

Laryngitis—Inflammation of the larynx (voice box).

Lesion—A circumscribed area of pathologically altered tissue; a single patch in a skin disease.

Leukemia—Cancer of the blood characterized by the appearance of great numbers of immature and abnormal white blood cells, 10 to 100 times that of the normal range.

Leukocytosis—Increase in the number of white blood cells in the blood, but not to be confused with leukemia. It can be caused by infection, inflammation, trauma, or medications (e.g., corticosteroids).

Leukopenia—Abnormal reduction in the number of white blood cells in the blood.

Lipase—A bacterial enzyme that acts with the oils and fats secreted by the sebaceous glands allowing bacteria to colonize in the skin.

Local infection—Infection caused by germs lodging and multiplying at one point in a tissue and remaining there.

Lumpectomy—A procedure during which a surgeon removes a lump and an area of healthy tissue around its edges from the breast.

Lymphadenopathy—Enlargement of lymph nodes.

Lymphangitis—An inflammatory disorder of the lymph vessels, characterized by local and systemic pain.

Lymphoma—Malignancy of lymphoid tissue.

Malaria—A febrile disease of the blood characterized by chills and fever. It is caused by a protozoan and spread by mosquito bite.

Malformation (anomaly)—A defect or deformity.

Malignant—Tending or threatening to produce death; harmful. Concerning cancerous growths: growing worse, resisting treatment.

Manner of death—Explanation of how the cause of death came about. The manner of death is generally classified on death certificates as either natural, homicide, suicide, accident, or undetermined/unclassified.

Mastectomy—The surgical removal of a portion of the breast or the entire breast.

Maximum temperature—Temperature above which bacterial growth will not take place.

Mechanical vector—A living organism or an object that is capable of transmitting infections by carrying the disease agent on its external body part or surface.

Mechanism of death—the physiological derangement produced by the cause of death that results in death.

Examples include bleeding, blood poisoning, or a faulty heart beat.

Medicolegal (forensic) pathology—Study of disease to ascertain cause and manner of death as related to a criminal investigation.

Melena—Black, tarry feces caused by the digestion of blood in the gastrointestinal tract; common in newborns.

Meningitis—An infection of the cerebrospinal fluid, which is the fluid surrounding the spinal cord and brain.

Mesophiles—Bacteria that prefer moderate temperature and develop best at temperatures between 25°C and 40°C.

Metaplasia—Replacement of one type of tissue by a form that is not normally found there.

Metastasis—The spread of cancer from its primary site to a distant location in the body.

Microaerophilic—Requiring little free oxygen.

Microbiology—Scientific study of microorganisms and their effect on other living organisms.

Microscopic pathology (histopathology)—Study of microscopic changes that cells, tissues, and organs undergo as a result of disease.

Minimum temperature—Temperature below which bacterial growth will not take place.

Mixed infection—Infection caused by two or more organisms.

Moist (wet) gangrene—Necrotic tissue that is wet as a result of inadequate venous drainage, accompanied by the invasion of saprophytic bacteria.

Mononucleosis—An infectious inflammatory disease caused by the Epstein-Barr virus.

Morbidity rate—Relative incidence of a disease in the population or number of cases in a given time in a given population.

Morphology—The study of the size, shape, and arrangements of microorganisms.

Mortality rate—Number of deaths in a given time or place or proportion of deaths to a population.

Mumps—An infectious disease of the parotid salivary glands caused by the mumps virus.

Mutualism—A symbiotic relationship in which two different species live in close association to the mutual benefit of each other.

Mycology—The branch of science concerned with the study of fungi.

Mycoplasmas—Bacteria of the Mycoplasma genus that are found in humans, most having no cell wall; the smallest free-living organisms presently known, being intermediate in size between viruses and bacteria.

Myxedema—The clinical manifestations of hypothyroidism that includes an infiltration of the skin by a thick, gelatinous substance formed from the bonding of water and mucopolysaccarides, which gives the skin a waxy or coarsened appearance.

Necrosis—Pathological death of a tissue while still a part of the living organism.

Neoplasms (tumors)—An abnormal mass of tissue exhibiting excessive and uncontrolled multiplication of cells.

Nitrogen—A colorless, odorless inert gas. Nitrogen compounds are found in foods, organic materials, fertilizers, poisons, and explosives. Formaldehyde and nitrogen react to form urotropin, which neutralizes the effectiveness of formaldehyde as an embalming preservative for human remains.

Nosocomial—Infection acquired in a hospital or other healthcare setting.

Occupational disease—A disease with an abnormally high rate of occurrence in members of a particular workforce.

Oophoritis—Inflammation of the ovaries.

Opportunist—An organism that exists as part of the normal flora but that can become pathogenic under certain conditions.

Optimum temperature—Temperature at which organisms grow best.

Orchitis—An acute inflammatory reaction in the testicle.

Organic—A condition or disease in which there is a change in anatomy.

Osmotic pressure—Pressure that develops when two solutions of different concentrations are separated by a semipermeable membrane.

Osteomalacia—A disease marked by softening of the bones due to faulty calcification in adulthood.

Osteomyelitis—Inflammation of bone and bone marrow.

Osteoporosis—Loss of bone mass that occurs throughout the skeleton, resulting in a predisposition to bone fracture.

Pandemic—A disease affecting the majority of the population of a large region or one that is epidemic at the same time in many different parts of the world.

Paralysis—Loss of purposeful muscle movement, usually as a result of neurological disease, drugs, or toxins.

Parasitism—An interactive relationship between two organisms in which one is harmed and other benefits.

Parrot fever—A respiratory disease caused by *Chlamydia psittaci*, which is a gram-negative, obligate intracellular rickettsia.

Pathogen—A microorganism capable of producing disease.

Pathogenesis—The manner in which a disease develops.

Pathogenicity—The state of producing or being able to produce pathological changes and disease.

Pathological anatomy (morbid anatomy)—Study of structural changes in the body caused by disease.

Pathology—Science that deals with the study of disease.

Pericarditis—Inflammation of the membranes that surround the heart.

Petechiae—Antemortem, pinpoint, extravascular blood discolorations visible as small red or purplish hemorrhages of the skin or mucous membranes.

Phagocytosis—A process in which phagocytes (i.e., neutrophils, monocytes, and macrophages) engulf and destroy microorganisms, other foreign antigens, and cell debris.

Phocomelia—Congenital condition in which the proximal portions of the limbs are poorly developed or absent.

Physiological pathology—Study of changes in body functions due to disease.

Pigmentation—Coloration caused by either deposit or lack of coloring material in tissues.

Pleurisy—An inflammatory condition of the pleurae that surround the lungs.

Pneumonia—Infection of the lungs.

Poliomyelitis—A highly contagious infectious disease of the spinal cord caused by the poliovirus.

Polycythemia vera—An increase in total red blood cell mass.

Polydactylism—A birth defect characterized by extra fingers or toes.

Polyp—A growth or mass of tissue that protrudes from a mucous membrane.

Polyuria—Excessive urination.

Prevalence—The number of cases of disease present in a specified population at a given time.

Primary infection—An original infection from which a second one develops

Prion—A small proteinaceous infectious particle that is resistant to most procedures that modify nucleic acids.

Prognosis—Prediction of the outcome of disease.

Prostatitis—Inflammation of the prostate gland.

Protozoa—One-celled organisms of the kingdom Protista; most are unicellular although some are colonial.

Protozoology—Science that deals with the study of protozoa.

Psoriasis—A chronic, inflammatory skin disease, characterized by red, thickened areas with silvery scales, most often on the scalp, elbows, knees, and lower back.

Psychrophiles—Bacteria that prefer cold, thriving at temperatures between 0°C and 25°C.

Purpura—Condition in which spontaneous bleeding occurs in the subcutaneous tissues, causing the appearance of purple patches on the skin.

Purulent—Forming or containing pus.

Pus—Protein-rich fluid containing white blood cells, especially neutrophils, and cell debris produced during inflammation.

Pustule—A small elevation of the skin containing pus.

Rabies—An acute, neurotropic, infectious disease caused by a rhabdovirus known as the rabies virus.

Recurrence—Reappearance of symptoms after a period of remission (abatement)

Regeneration—The replacement of damaged cells with identical cells.

Remission—Temporary cessation of symptoms of disease.

Renal calculi—Kidney stones.

Repair—Physical or mechanical restoration of damages or diseased tissue by the growth of healthy new cells—not necessarily the same type—or by surgery. The replacement of damaged tissue with fibrous connective tissue (scar tissue).

Reservoir—The natural habitat of a disease-causing organism.

Resistance—The ability of an organism to defend itself against infection and disease; the sum total of body mechanisms that interpose barriers to the progress of invasion, multiplication of infectious agents, or damage by their toxic products.

Resolution—The termination of the inflammatory response with the affected part returning to its normal state.

Rickets—A disease of infants and young children caused by deficiency of vitamin D and resulting in defective bone growth.

Rickettsia—A genus of rod-shaped, gram-negative, pathogenic, intracellular parasitic microorganisms.

Rickettsiology—Area of science that studies rickettsia.

Rocky Mountain spotted fever—The most severe rickettsial infection; it is caused by *Rickettsia rickettsii.*

Salpingitis—Inflammation of the fallopian tubes.

Saprophytes—Organisms that only survive on dead or decaying organic matter.

Scoliosis—A developmental disorder of the spine in which the spinal column exhibits a lateral curvature.

Secondary infection—Infection caused by a different organism than the one causing the primary infection.

Seizures—Sudden, uncontrolled discharges of electrical activity in the brain, which may cause convulsions.

Septicemia—Condition characterized by the multiplication of bacteria in blood; commonly known as blood poisoning.

Signs—Objective disturbances produced by disease, observed by a physician, nurse, or other person attending a patient (example: pulse, fever, heart rate)

Special pathology—Deals with the specific features of disease in relation to particular organs or organ systems.

Spina bifida—Congenital defect in which part of the vertebral column is absent or undergoes incomplete closure.

Splenomegaly—An enlargement of the spleen beyond its normal size.

Sporadic—Disease that occurs occasionally in a random or isolated manner

Sporicides—Agents that kill bacterial and mold spores; act as sterilizing agents.

Staphylococci—Gram-positive, nonmotile bacteria that tend to aggregate in irregular, grapelike clusters.

Stenosis—Abnormal constriction of a channel or orifice.

Sterilization—Process of completely removing or destroying all life-forms, endospores, or their products on or in a substance.

Streptobacilli—Bacteria containing gram-negative rods that form a chainlike colony.

Streptococci—Gram-positive spherically shaped bacteria that occur in chains.

Strict (obligate) aerobe—A microbe that can only live in the presence of oxygen.

Strict (obligate) anaerobe—A microbe that can only survive in an environment without oxygen present.

Strict (obligate) parasite—A parasite that is completely dependent on its living host for survival.

Strict (obligate) saprophyte—An organism that can only survive on dead or decaying organic matter.

Sundowning—Confusion or disorientation that increases in the afternoon or evening. It is a common finding in patients with cognitive disorders and tends to improve when the patient is reassured and reoriented.

Surgical pathology—Study of tissue specimens excised surgically in a major or minor operation.

Symbiosis—The living together in close association of different species.

Symptoms—Subjective disturbances caused by disease that are felt or experienced by the patient but are not directly measurable (example: pain, headache).

Syndrome—A set of sign and symptoms associated with a particular disease (e.g., Down syndrome).

Synergism—The harmonious action of two microorganisms producing an effect that neither could produce alone.

Thermophiles—Bacteria that thrive best at high temperatures, between 40°C and 70°C.

Thrombocytopenia—An abnormal decrease in the number of platelets that inhibit blood clotting.

Thrombosis—The formation or presence of an attached blood clot.

Thrombus—A blood clot that obstructs a blood vessel or a cavity of the heart.

Tonsillitis—An inflammation of the tonsils caused by an infection.

Toxemia—Distribution throughout the body of poisonous products of bacteria growing in a focal or local site, thus producing generalized symptoms.

Toxin—A poisonous substance of plant, animal, bacterial, or fungal origin.

Trachoma—A chronic, contagious form of conjunctivitis that is one of the leading causes of blindness in the world.

Trauma—The process or event leading to an injury or wound.

True pathogen—Real or genuine disease-producing organism.

Tsetse fly—A blood-sucking fly found only in Africa that spreads trypanosomes causing African sleeping disease.

Tubal pregnancy—Implantation and development of the fertilized ovum in a uterine tube.

Ulcer—An open sore or lesion of skin or mucous membrane accompanied by sloughing of inflamed necrotic tissue.

Universal precautions—Guidelines designed to protect workers with occupational exposure to bloodborne pathogens.

Uremia—A toxic condition caused by retention in the blood of nitrogenous waste products normally excreted in the urine.

Valvular insufficiency (incompetence)—Failure of a heart valve to close tightly, thus allowing regurgitation of blood.

Vasoconstriction—A decrease in the diameter of a vessel.

Vasodilation—An increase in the diameter of a vessel.

Vesicle—Blisterlike elevation of skin containing serous fluid.

Viricides—Agents that destroy viruses.

Virology—The study of viruses and viral diseases.

Virulence—Relative power and degree of pathogenicity possessed by organisms to produce disease.

Virus—An intracellular, infectious parasite, capable of replicating only in living cells.

Vitiligo—An idiopathic disorder in which the melanocytes stop producing pigment and are destroyed.

Volvulus—A twisting of the bowel on itself due to a prolapsed mesentery, causing obstruction.

Wet gangrene—*See* moist gangrene.

Reference

Venes, D. (Ed.). (2001). *Taber's cyclopedic medical dictionary* (19th ed.). Philadelphia: F. A. Davis.

Index